CONTENTS

Modern Hydrotherapy for the Massage Therapist

Modern Hydrotherapy for the Massage Therapist

Marybetts Sinclair, LMT
Corvallis, Oregon

Wolters Kluwer | Lippincott Williams & Wilkins
Health

Philadelphia · Baltimore · New York · London
Buenos Aires · Hong Kong · Sydney · Tokyo

Acquisitions Editor: John Goucher
Managing Editor: David Payne
Marketing Manager: Nancy Bradshaw
Production Editor: Julie Montalbano
Designer: Risa Clow
Compositor: International Typesetting and Composition

351 West Camden Street   530 Walnut Street
Baltimore, MD 21201   Philadelphia, PA 19106
Printed in China

9

Library of Congress Cataloging-in-Publication Data

Sinclair, Marybetts.
   Modern hydrotherapy for the massage therapist / Marybetts Sinclair.
      p. ; cm.
   Includes bibliographical references and index.
   ISBN-13: 978-0-7817-9209-7
 1. Hydrotherapy. 2. Masseurs. I. Title.
   [DNLM: 1. Hydrotherapy—methods. 2. Massage—methods. WB 520 S616m 2008]
   RM811.S57 2008
   615.8′53—dc22
                                   2007016571

This book is dedicated to those hydrotherapists who have kept an obscure
and out-of-the mainstream tradition alive, who used water healing
not because it was popular, profitable, streamlined patient care or looked trendy,
but because they had faith in the healing powers of the human body

and

to that beautiful and brainy dame, Jeanne Hazleton.
I admire you more than I can say.

PREFACE

PURPOSE

Modern Hydrotherapy for the Massage Therapist has been written to fill in a large gap in the education of today's massage therapist. Today, most licensed therapists have taken only one short course in hydrotherapy, which imparts the most basic information. There are almost no continuing education classes in this subject area and no books that can be used to inspire a therapist to go farther. Without more background in hydrotherapy, today's new massage therapists are in danger of losing a traditionally important adjunct to their hands-on methods.

The purpose of this book, then, is to excite students about hydrotherapy and give them the tools to use hydrotherapy with ease and enjoyment. This will enhance their practices by allowing them to better meet their clients' needs and to create unique treatments that combine their massage and hydrotherapy skills.

THE AUTHOR'S JOURNEY AND APPROACH TO HYDROTHERAPY

When I was licensed as a massage therapist in 1975, the study of hydrotherapy was confined to one short class. The book we used in the course was very old and its language antiquated, making the whole idea of hydrotherapy seem irrelevant and boring. Moreover, hydrotherapy, like massage, was little used in mainstream medicine at the time. What convinced me of the effectiveness of hydrotherapy, therefore, was not what I learned in my formal education but my personal experience.

When I had a serious musculoskeletal injury early in my life, I visited an old-school physical therapist who would treat me with a relaxing soak in a warm whirlpool bath, followed by a rest period, massage, and therapeutic exercises. I found this treatment very healing. Furthermore, I witnessed the effectiveness of hydrotherapy in my professional life. My first job as a massage therapist was giving massages at a health club with a sauna and a swimming pool. My clients used the sauna and pool to extend the relaxing effects of their massages. The physical therapist who worked there frequently used hot moist packs with his patients for their musculoskeletal aches and pains. As I continued to practice and to learn from different teachers and from other massage therapists, it

became more obvious to me that hydrotherapy had a great deal more potential than I had understood. I took further hydrotherapy classes, visited clinics where hydrotherapy was used in a medical context, and began to research this subject. I discovered that there were a great many ways water had been and could be used in medicine and that, furthermore, hydrotherapy had a fascinating history full of patients seeking relief from various maladies, bold experiments with water healing, and colorful personalities.

When I began teaching hydrotherapy for a massage school, however, the available curriculum was just as outdated as what I had encountered in my own education. Students were sometimes terribly confused by antiquated terminology, and treatments that were given a half-century ago by nurses in a hospital setting did not seem relevant to them. It was difficult for them to complete the basic class with a vision of how hydrotherapy could help them with the kind of healing therapy that they wanted to do. They needed a textbook that helped them learn not only about the fascinating past of hydrotherapy but also its potential for massage practice today.

I wrote *Modern Hydrotherapy for the Massage Therapist* to fill that need. It contains information about hydrotherapy's past that places today's massage therapist squarely in the middle of a time-honored tradition. It explains in today's language how hydrotherapy works, and it gives the massage therapist the information he or she needs to use hydrotherapy safely and appropriately. Current research brings the reader up-to-date on the anatomy and physiology of hydrotherapy and scientifically validates many treatments. Furthermore, cautions, contraindications, and notes on proper scope of practice are included throughout to ensure the safety of both client and therapist.

ORGANIZATION AND FEATURES

The first three chapters of the book provide a theoretical foundation for the study of hydrotherapy. Chapter 1, "Introduction to Hydrotherapy," introduces the reader to the field of hydrotherapy and provides a brief history of the therapeutic use of water. Chapter 2, "The Science of Water," discusses the scientific properties of water, and Chapter 3, "Effects of Hydrotherapy," presents the physiological effects of hydrotherapy on the body.

Chapter 4, "Preparing for Hydrotherapy," covers a variety of practical topics that the reader needs to know before practicing hydrotherapy, such as guidelines for buying equipment, cautions and contraindications, and general instructions for performing all hydrotherapy treatments.

Chapters 5 through 11 present an overview and step-by-step instructions for a variety of hydrotherapy treatments, including hot and cold packs and compresses, baths, saunas, steam baths, showers, body wraps, and friction treatments.

The final three chapters demonstrate how hydrotherapy treatments may be applied to specific situations. Chapter 12, "Hydrotherapy Self-Treatments for Health and Wellness," covers how hydrotherapy may be used by the client and the massage therapist as regular self-care treatments for detoxification, tonifying, and prevention of repetitive stress injuries. Chapter 13, "Hydrotherapy and Massage for Musculoskeletal Injuries," and Chapter 14, "Hydrotherapy and Massage for Noninjury Conditions," introduce the reader to how hydrotherapy may be used to address common client injuries and conditions

Finally, the appendices provide hydrotherapy handouts that therapists can give to their clients, information on pool therapy and fever therapy, names and contact information for companies that manufacture hydrotherapy equipment, and answers to all review questions in the book.

The following features are included in the book as learning aids:

- Chapter opening quotations give additional historical perspective on hydrotherapy by experts in a variety of fields from a variety of time periods.

- Chapter objectives clarify the goals of the chapter.
- Boldfaced key terms in the chapter text and the corresponding end-of-book glossary familiarize readers with important terminology.
- Chapter introductions usher in the ideas presented in the chapter.
- Treatment overviews and step-by-step instructions are highlighted in the text for easy referencing.
- Point of Interest boxes highlight interesting facts and concepts related to the content of the chapter and enrich the student's understanding of hydrotherapy.
- Case histories put concepts presented in the text into action, with examples from real massage therapists and actual clients. Chapter summaries give a concise overview of the content of each chapter.
- Review questions at the end of each chapter allow students to review the information they have just read.

FINAL NOTE

Water has profoundly soothing and renewing effects on human beings, and so water treatments have been paired with massage since time out of mind. However, the study of water treatments not only has potential to improve a therapist's skills; it also gives one a deep appreciation for the interconnectedness of humans and their environment. Without contact with the earth through creeks, rivers, oceans, and other natural bodies of water, our emotional and spiritual health is at risk also. Let us all work toward the health not only of our clients but of our natural environment, which nurtures and sustains us all.

ACKNOWLEDGMENTS

First and foremost I owe a debt of gratitude to my sagacious and dashing young editor, David Payne, who so nobly and tactfully waded into an extravagantly large sea (some would say morass) of hydrotherapy material, rife with potentially pretentious scholarly commentary. Although awash in petty details, he managed to keep everything organized and focused, was unbelievably helpful at the photo shoot, and his sharp, experienced, and sometimes pitiless editor's pencil have informed every page of this work. Thanks, David!

This book, labor of love as it has been for me, would also have been impossible without the generosity and expertise of a host of individuals, including long-dead hydrotherapists, professionals in a number of fields, researchers, librarians, friends, and family. I cannot adequately thank all those who took the time out of their busy days to answer obscure and not-so-obscure questions and strange requests for information, put up with long conversations about H_2O, let me experiment on them, and otherwise encouraged, aided, and abetted me.

Some of the professionals who lent a hand include Stephen Noll, PhD; Edward Shorter, PhD; Nancy Dosch, PhD; the reference librarians at the Corvallis Public Library and the National Library of Medicine; Earl Qualls, PT; Woodhall Stopford, MD; Ross Hauser, MD; Agatha Thrash, MD; physical therapists Pam Davidson, Barbara Springer, and Kyla Dunlavey; Helena and Celly of the Uchee Pines Institute; Eric Blake, ND; Letitia Watrous, ND; Keith Miller of the Foundation for the Advancement of Science and Education; Christine Rymal, RN; Jeff Bisbee, recreation therapist; Major Sean Donahue; and my extremely thoughtful and diligent reviewers.

Wonderful helpers at the photo shoot included the staff of the Oregon School of Massage and models Jill Stanard, Kitty Lawrence, Brenda Dick, Jody Altendorf, Smith Sinclair, the lovely Rolfettes, Vanessa, Rainier and Penny Farmer, Bob Heald, Kathy Thielsen, and Ellie Stanard; at the Bethany Athletic Club and La Pointe Spa, Cindy Fellows, Lindsey Poulton, and Jory Fleck-Harding. Special thanks to Susan Soukup and Brenda Dick for helping me organize all the hydro equipment. Thanks to Ray Siderius, owner of Oregon School of Massage, for graciously letting us use the school's hydro room and for his ongoing example of integrity in massage education.

Thanks to Trevor and Bob Heald for a long discussion about water over Cirello's Pizza. Bob also gets a special vote of gratitude for unstinting support in a multitude of ways. Finally, my big-hearted brother Smith, whose support has come in any number of thoughtful and gracious actions and to whom my entire family owes a debt of gratitude—thank you, Smither!

I couldn't have done it without you all.

REVIEWERS

Richard Ceroni, PhD, MeD, MA, LMT
Dean of Education
Ohio Academy of Acupuncture and Oriental Medicine
Suffield, OH

Linda Derick, MA
Director of Education
Connecticut Center for Massage Therapy
Andover, CT

Linda Loney, MD, LCMT
Instructor
Massachusetts Institute of Therapeutic Massage
Newton, MA

Ronald McKendree, BS
Massage Program Coordinator
Keiser College
Melbourne, FL

Roger Olbrot, BA
Director of Education
Myotherapy College of Utah
Salt Lake City, UT

Andrea Robins, MS, LMT
Instructor
Keiser College
New Smyrna Beach, FL

Emily Sibley, BS, LMT
Hydrotherapy Instructor
Downeast School of Massage
Waldoboro, ME

Deborah Taylor, BS, LMT
Instructor
East West College of the Healing Arts
Portland, OR

Agatha Thrash, MD
Uchee Pines Institute
Seale, AL

CONTENTS

Modern Hydrotherapy for the Massage Therapist

INTRODUCTION TO HYDROTHERAPY

If there is magic on this planet, it is contained in water.

—*Loren Eisley, The Immense Journey*

Chapter Objectives

After completing this chapter, the student will be able to:

- Explain several ways in which hydrotherapy can enhance and support the practice of massage.
- Explain the historical development of hydrotherapy in Europe and the United States.
- Describe the appeal of whole-body hydrotherapy, such as baths, saunas, and swimming.
- Give specific examples of both local and whole-body hydrotherapy treatments that have been used in the past.
- Explain how hydrotherapy treatments have changed in different times and cultures.
- Describe how hydrotherapy is used by massage therapists to treat different clienteles.

Although skilled touch and water treatments have been performed differently in different times and cultures, they are among the most ancient of healing modalities and have been used constantly since the dawn of civilization. From the mineral springs of South America to the great baths of Europe (Fig. 1-1) and the Ayurvedic steam treatments of India, and from the Turkish baths of the Muslim world to the **banyas** of Russia and the Native American sweat lodge, peoples the world over have combined hydrotherapy and massage. In private homes, bathhouses, spas, rehabilitation facilities, health clubs, doctors' offices, and hospitals, healers have applied compassionate touch and water to "where it hurts." Ingenious healers have used both whole-body treatments, such as baths, and local treatments, such as foot soaks and herbal compresses, for injury, pain, and nervous tension. Around the world, hydrotherapy and massage have been used not only because they feel good but also because they promote wellness.

In this chapter, you will be introduced to the long and rich history of hydrotherapy and will learn the benefits of incorporating it into your massage practice. In later chapters you will learn exactly how to add treatments to your practice. (Because the range of hydrotherapy treatments is vast, not all of them can be covered in any one book, but you will learn the treatments most suited to the scope of practice of today's massage therapist.)

To see the history of water treatments placed in a chronological context, consult the timeline provided at the end of the chapter (see Fig. 1-16).

The word *hydrotherapy* itself is a combination of two Greek words, *hydor* (water) and *therapeai* (healing). In this book we define *hydrotherapy* as the therapeutic application of water in all its forms, liquid, vapor or solid, to maintain or restore health.

BENEFITS OF USING HYDROTHERAPY IN YOUR MASSAGE PRACTICE

Massage practitioners who are knowledgeable about water treatments can use them during massage sessions in a safe and effective way that genuinely enhances what they can accomplish. Massage therapy students and practitioners may wonder how adding hydrotherapy to massage practice could benefit the clients. Here are some important benefits:

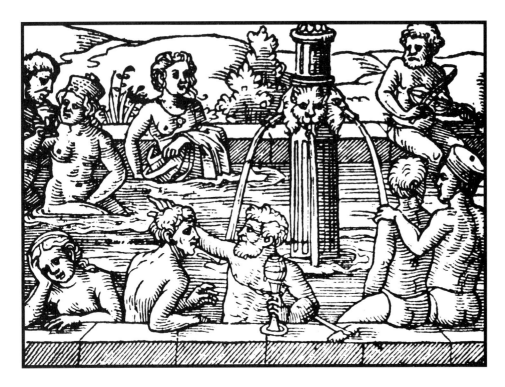

FIGURE 1-1 ■ Outdoor baths, Germany, 1571. Woodcut by Gallus Etschereutter. (Photo courtesy of National Library of Medicine, Bethesda, Maryland.)

- Hydrotherapy can accomplish many of the same therapeutic goals as massage techniques do. Like massage, hydrotherapy can relieve discomfort and pain, stimulate the flow of blood and lymph, make connective tissue easier to stretch, and soothe many aches, pains and injuries.
- Hydrotherapy is relaxing and stress reducing. Robert France, author of *Deep Immersion: The Experience of Water*, has called water "liquid solace."(1) As with massage, the time and personal care given to a person while he or she is receiving a hydrotherapy treatment can be soothing and nurturing and a simple means of escape from a hectic world.
- By cooling a client who is uncomfortably hot or warming a client who is uncomfortably cool, hydrotherapy treatments can make clients more comfortable during a massage session. It is also simpler and more energy efficient to heat or cool the client's body than to heat or cool room air: it is possible to warm a client with a hot water bottle rather than heating the room air or cool a client with an ice pack rather than running an air conditioner.
- Hydrotherapy treatments can provide a variety of types of skin stimulation. Examples include the body-hugging sensation of being surrounded by water; the thermal sensations of warm or cool; the scratchy sensation of a salt glow, dry brush, or cold mitten friction; and the textural sensation of different substances mixed with water. Extra skin sensation can be especially beneficial for those who are receiving less stimulation to their skin than normal, such as elderly, disabled, socially isolated or bedridden clients.

- As a massage therapist, using the information learned in this book, you can move easily into a spa setting. Spas typically have their own signature treatments that new therapists need to learn, but most of what you need to know about hydrotherapy to work in a spa is contained in this book.
- Hydrotherapy can reduce stress on the massage therapist's hands. Many local hydrotherapy treatments can replace the massage strokes needed to warm tissues, relax superficial muscles, and increase local circulation.
- Knowing a variety of treatments allows the massage therapist to be more versatile and more creative. The therapist can fine-tune sessions to individual clients and their specific needs by combining the most appropriate massage techniques with the most suitable water treatments.
- Hydrotherapy treatments can be suggested to clients to help them make progress between sessions, for example using a neutral bath for insomnia, an Epsom salt bath for muscle aches after vigorous exercise, ice applications for low back pain, or a contrast treatment for a sprained ankle.
- Hydrotherapy is an excellent adjunct to any kind of bodywork done for rehabilitation. Cold treatments such as local baths, ice packs, and ice massage stimulate circulation and reduce spasm and pain. Heat treatments soften scar tissue and make muscle tissues easier to stretch.
- Regular hydrotherapy can be part of a health-building regimen. Rather than curing health problems, it can promote health by stimulating circulation and relaxing

skeletal muscles. It can also be a small but significant adjunct to a person's regimen for a particular health problem. For example, a person with chronically cold feet can be given water treatments that increase local circulation, such as cold water treading, hot footbaths with mustard powder, or contrast footbaths.

BRIEF HISTORY OF WESTERN HYDROTHERAPY

Among ancient civilizations, water was sanctified as the source of life, the seminal fluid, the juice of the earth's womb. It formed a common thread in their creation myths. . . . People everywhere feared, revered, or worshipped water deities. Although these gods differed in name and form from culture to culture, all shared the fundamental creative and destructive substance of water.

—Alexis Croutier(5)

The history of medicine is the story of human trial and error, an often hilarious pageant of experimentation, fads and fashions of treatment, and a few time-tested successful remedies. Water treatments have frequently been tried to treat health problems for 3 main reasons: Water has generally been both plentiful and easier to obtain than many other remedies, water treatments are generally very safe, and the effects of water treatments are easy to observe. Often when a new health problem emerges, a variety of remedies are used, and water treatments have almost always been among them. Here we focus only on the history and tradition of European hydrotherapy. However, it is important to note that many other cultures also have well-developed hydrotherapy practices.

HYDROTHERAPY IN ANCIENT GREECE AND OTHER EARLY CULTURES

The origins of using thermal water, mineral waters, and therapeutic mud are too distant to discern, but hydrotherapy has been used since before recorded history for cleansing, relaxation, and as therapy for arthritis pain and injuries. Even before technology was capable of heating and transporting water for bathing, the lure of water treatment was powerful. For example, people have always been drawn to natural hot springs: the attraction of the water's warming and cleansing properties, combined with the chance to float free of gravity, is almost irresistible.

In testament to water's universal appeal, the waters of Baden-Baden in Germany have been used for at least 8000 years, and the waters at Bath, England, were first used by Paleolithic hunters at least 10,000 years ago. Today in Europe there are hundreds of modern spas that were once elaborate establishments located at or near natural hot springs and are still visited because of the curative

properties of the spring waters. Before the technology to build modern saunas existed, primitive sweat baths were also built in numerous locations. In Ireland, for example, sweat houses made of sod and stone, used to treat rheumatism, were constructed as early as the eighth century BCE.(2)

Local hydrotherapy treatments, such as local baths, compresses, fomentations, and applications of cold water, are also found in the most ancient of medical traditions. Water was often used as a solvent for herbal preparations in baths, poultices, plasters, and other preparations.

Spiritual and Religious Function of Water

In the minds of primitive peoples, water was healing because it was associated with supernatural powers and many natural phenomena. Water was sacred not only as the source of life, energy, fertility, and creation, but also as the source of destruction and even death. Although no human, animal, or plant could live without it for long, water might also take life away without warning at any moment, and its power was awesome. (Both the tsunami that struck the coast of Asia in 2004 and Hurricane Katrina, which struck the southern United States in 2005, caused a devastating loss of life, left many thousands injured and/or homeless, and brought about extreme changes in the local ecosystems.) Rainbows, waterfalls, rainstorms, floods, natural springs, the flow of the tides, thunder, lighting, whirlpools, snow, and ice were viewed with awe and respect. So were the animals that inhabited the water. The ocean was a mysterious and often foreboding place.

In cultures the world over, water was associated with powerful deities with incomprehensible cosmic powers. Religious leaders were often physical healers as well, and they used water rituals such as baptism, ritual baths before sacred events, symbolic washing away of disease, and washing of the dead to prepare them for the afterlife. The association of water with birth meant that the physical cleansing of the body often symbolized purification of the soul and was a metaphor for being born again. Even when wounds were bathed, the healing process that began was often thought to be due to the beneficial spirit inherent in the water rather than reducing the likelihood of infection.

All ancient cultures worshipped water gods and goddesses of various kinds, including nymphs and water maidens. Clouds—those cascades of water in the air—were seen as their thrones. In the Old Testament, in Genesis, water was the first element, which existed before the world was created. Elsewhere in the Bible, baths were ordered for skin diseases, for gonorrhea, to cleanse lepers, for menstruating and lying-in women, and to purify those defiled by touching unclean bodies. In Egypt, the temple of Dendera, consecrated to the goddess Hathor, housed an extensive hydrotherapy center approached by a corridor of healing statues. Streams fed stone tanks of different sizes in which the sick bathed in the hope of being cured with the help of the goddess.(3)

In the Greco-Roman tradition, people made pilgrimages to springs to ask for help from their nymphs or gods. These figures or a deity associated with healing (such as the Greek goddess Aphrodite or the Roman goddess Minerva) might intercede on behalf of the suffering mortal. Mineral springs often became shrines dedicated to Aesculapius, the Greek god of medicine.

The Greek Gymnasium

In addition to the religious function of water, bathing for social and medical reasons was an important part of the culture of the ancient Greeks. They were the first to create public baths. In early Greek cities, the Greek gymnasium, which provided inspiration for Roman bathing, incorporated washing and bathing into its regular program. The gymnasium began as a place for Greek men to be trained in athletics but gradually developed into the center of Greek social activity and learning. Total bodily regeneration began with a strenuous workout, followed by bathing and massage. The trio of massage, exercise, and hydrotherapy would occur again and again in European societies.

Beginning with an open-air space with basins and simple showers set aside for athletes to cleanse themselves with cold water after a workout, many early gymnasia were situated near a stream, river, or lake to make bathing after exercising easy. Bathing facilities gradually evolved into various arrangements of individual tubs, a circular pool in the middle, and a hot air baths or saunas. They also used small pools, tubs, primitive showers, and footbaths. As far back as Homer, warm baths were recommended for relieving dejection and low spirits and for reducing fatigue and promoting wound healing. A hot air bath or sauna followed by a cold plunge was the traditional bathing style of the Spartans. Massage—being rubbed or anointed with oils—was an integral part of the Greek bathing experience, usually given both before and after exercise.

Hippocrates and the Medicinal Use of Hydrotherapy

During the time of Hippocrates (460–377 BCE), baths were used not only for cleansing and tonic effects but also for medicinal purposes. A combination of hot and cold baths was used to adjust the bodily humors to bring them into harmony by heating, cooling, moistening, or drying as necessary.(4[p1]) According to Hippocrates, "baths in fresh water moisten and cool; salt baths warm and dry; hot baths taken on an empty stomach reduce and cool; taken after a meal they warm and moisten. Cold baths dry the body and so does total abstinence from bathing." Thermal baths were recommended to cure headaches, promote good respiration, relax joints, and relieve chest and back pains in patients with pneumonia. Neutral baths were prescribed for insomnia. Local treatments were used as well as baths: for example, cold **douches** were used to relieve swelling and painful joints.(5[p119]) Hippocrates also recommended massage to tone and normalize the body.

The Greeks understood the physiological effects of bathing, for example that immersion in a hot bath caused a rise in body temperature, and they understood how hot and cold water applications could manipulate blood flow. Since they had as yet an imperfect understanding of the circulatory system, much careful observation during baths and local treatments must have given them this knowledge. In *Man and Wound in the Ancient World*, pathologist and medical historian Guido Manjo tells us how a Greek physician might have treated an injured carpenter with a deep, profusely bleeding cut on his foot. In this scenario, the injured man would have been laid supine and then the wounded leg raised. The doctor would dip a towel into cold water and wrap it loosely around the ankle to help to check the bleeding. Another towel would be dipped in warm water and wrapped around the patient's head: the idea was evidently to draw blood flow up to the head and away from the injured foot.(6) The cold towel would cause constriction in the blood vessels of the ankle, and the hot towel, dilation of the blood vessels of the head. This treatment is the mirror image of the classic hydrotherapy treatment for a migraine headache—a hot footbath, which limits blood flow to the head and encourages blood flow toward the feet using vasodilating hot water, coupled with vasoconstricting cold compresses to the head and neck (see Chapter 6).

The Greeks also understood the stimulating effect of cold water on the general circulation: according to a Greek physician from the time of Hippocrates, "If a man in good health will cool his body in winter, either by a cold bath or any other means, the greater the degree to which he cools it—provided his body is not altogether frozen—the warmer it becomes again, warmer in fact than he was before, when he has put on his clothes and reached his shelter. Again, if he were to make himself thoroughly warm, either by a hot bath or by a large fire, and afterward to wear the same clothes and stay in the same places as he did when he was chilled, he feels far colder and generally more shivery."(7)

HYDROTHERAPY IN THE ROMAN EMPIRE

The Roman Empire, which had the most elaborate hydrotherapy practices of any ancient culture, existed from 510 BCE to 478 AD. At its height it was the political master of almost the entire Western world. After conquering Greece, Rome adopted much of its culture, art, science, philosophy, and medical practices. Its public water supply schemes and bathing practices were modeled after those of the Greeks as well. The Romans were the direct inheritors of the Greek institution of the gymnasium and the Greek ideal of a balance between mind and body. The views of the Greeks regarding bathing were introduced into the Roman world mainly through the writings of Celsus (b. 25 BCE) and Galen (b. 130 AD). Celsus, who was a medical writer rather than a doctor, passed on the ideas of Greek physicians, so he was a staunch believer in hot bathing therapy, sweating and massage for strengthening those with weak constitutions and curing people with serious health problems. Asclepiades (b. 100 BCE), another Greek physician who practiced in Rome, was also influential. He relied mainly on diet, gentle exercise, massage, and bathing. He invented the shower bath and prescribed cold baths so often that he was given the name the cold bather.

The Romans did not exercise strenuously before their baths as did the Greeks. For them, exercise—and light exercise at that—became only a prelude to bathing. Their emphasis was far more on bathing for relaxation and pleasure. As their technology and wealth grew, the Romans' bathing practices became more elaborate and consumed more resources. For example, the furnaces of one large bath in the city of Rome required 40 lb of firewood per hour to keep bath water and steam rooms heated, as well as many slaves to run them, and both water and firewood had to be brought long distances. In Rome itself, public baths enjoyed the highest priority in official water allocation. Water first came from wells, stored rainwater, and rooftop tanks and later via aqueducts from faraway streams and rivers.

Whole-body immersion and swimming were common treatments for many ailments. Water was also applied locally to various parts of the body and drunk for a wide variety of internal ailments.(4[p2]) During the first and second centuries BCE, cold water was used therapeutically for many diseases and disorders, including skin complaints, gout, wounds, urinary problems, digestive disorders, fevers, eye diseases, paralysis, and convalescence after surgery. Bathing in therapeutic waters was recommended for difficult menstruation and other uterine disorders.(4[p13]) Seawater was believed to have a tonic effect on those suffering from nervousness, arthritis, and consumption: if they were not near the coast, rich Romans such as the emperors Augustus and Nero even had seawater brought inland to them.

As the Romans spread through Europe, they took their knowledge of the benefits of thermal waters with them. Most Roman settlements had not only a public water supply which provided high-quality drinking water but a public bath of some sort. Roman forts and military hospitals

scattered along the borders of the Roman Empire from Scotland to Palestine contained baths as well. Naturally occurring springs were developed wherever they were found. Certain springs were believed to have curative properties for specific ailments. For example, Vitruvius, who was both a famous Roman bath engineer and a historian, recommended sulfur springs for their ability to "abolish muscular weakness by heating and burning poisonous humors from the body." He also recommended alum springs for those with paralysis, alkaline springs for scrofulous tumors, the waters of Albula near Rome for wound healing, and the water from acid springs taken internally to dissolve bladder stones.(5[p119]) Mineral spring baths were prescribed for paralysis, sciatica, psoriasis, rheumatic fever, gout, and other chronic complaints that we now associate with liver and kidney failure, such as jaundice and edema.

For example, the region of Baiae, directly northwest of Mount Vesuvius, contained hundreds of hot mineral springs and was a popular resort for the wealthy pleasure seekers of Roman society. Baiae's hot sulfur springs drew convalescents from across the Roman Empire. Over the centuries natural sweating rooms were created by excavating or carving into the rock chambers, hollows, underground passages, and caves.

The Romans developed and used hot and cold springs in many areas, including England, Spain, Germany, the Czech Republic, France, Switzerland, Rome, and Naples. (Modern spa towns Vichy in France, Baden-Baden in Germany, Spa in Belgium, and Bath in England are just a few of these; all were discovered in the first century AD.) There they also built shrines dedicated to the nymphs and water deities who protected the source and gave it its healing qualities, usually incorporating the local gods and goddesses into their worship as well. Often the healing deity was thought to oversee specific ailments. For example, in one Italian shrine, Ponti di Nona, foot and hand disorders were the special concern of the healing deity, and visitors to its spring hoped to find relief from such problems as fallen arches, torn ligaments, foot wounds and ulcerations, arthritis, clubfoot, and other deformities.(5[p118])

As well as taking advantage of naturally occurring springs, the Romans built artificially heated baths, which evolved from simple small units to complexes that were complete with shops, gymnasia, entertainment, libraries, restaurants, sumptuous gardens, and waterworks displays. For example, the Baths of Diocletian, the largest baths ever built in Rome, covered 32 acres and could accommodate as many as 3000 bathers at a time. Decorated in lavish style, with statues, fountains, decorative columns, mosaic floors, and inner walls covered with Egyptian marble, the ruins of the baths were later turned into a magnificent church by the artist Michelangelo and can be still be seen in Rome today.

Hot rooms and bath water were heated by wood-fired furnaces stoked by slaves from outside the bath itself. These ovens heated air to a high temperature, and this air went directly under the floors of the hot rooms. Steam for the **caldarium** (hot room) was made by filling sunken pools with hot water. Unless floors were especially thick, special shoes had to be worn; otherwise the bathers' feet would be burned by the heated floors. A typical bathing sequence, although this varied somewhat according to place and time, consisted of the following:

Light exercise in the gymnasium.
An hour or so in the **tepidarium** (warm room) while being anointed with oils.
A sweat bath in the caldarium and possibly a plunge in its 104°F hot pool.
Possibly a stay in the **laconium** (dry heat room or sauna).
A trip back to the tepidarium, where the body was cleansed by scraping off oil, dirt, and sweat.
A swim in the cold pool (**frigidarium**).
An application of oils and a massage. Marble slabs called plinths were used for hydrotherapy treatments, cleansing, exfoliation, and massage.

With the fall of the Roman Empire, its highly developed bathing practices came to an end as the great baths and aqueducts that served them fell into disrepair. The last emperor of Rome was deposed in 478 AD, and the final abandonment of most of the baths in Rome came in 537 AD when invading Goths cut off the aqueducts of the city. Invading barbarians destroyed many baths, and weather and time did the rest. However, many of the watering holes that fell into ruins would later be rebuilt as spas.

HYDROTHERAPY IN THE MIDDLE AGES

Europe's water technology now deteriorated to a very primitive level, and only a few monasteries managed to retain the hydrotherapy technology of the past. Because the Roman Catholic church frowned upon bathing in principle, water treatments become less common as well. Although the grand Roman baths fell into disrepair, many continued to be used by local peoples. In a few locations large healing pools were built around thermal springs, and healing arts continued to be practiced at them.(4[p16]) Baiae, the famous Roman resort near Vesuvius, continued as a cure center even in medieval times (although frowned upon by the church), until a major volcanic eruption in 1538 destroyed most of its thermal structures.

Medieval medicine was based almost entirely upon the writings of the Greek physician Galen (130–200 AD), who was a staunch believer in the theory of humoral pathology (the imbalance of humors). He frequently prescribed bathing in the form of cold baths, warm baths, steam, sun, sand, mineral, and herbal baths. A warm bath followed by rubbing with cold water was recommended to lower the temperature in fever. (Agatha Thrash, MD, a modern physician familiar with hydrotherapy, recommends the same treatment to lower fevers.)(8[p25]) Local hydrotherapy treatments included **sitz baths**, **ablutions**, and **fomentations**. In the second century AD, Galen also recommended a sequence of bathing based on the temperature and humidity of bathing rooms. The patient was to move from a room with warm air to an even warmer room with basins of hot water and then to a cold plunge. While his recommendations may have been practical where the ancient Romans had their beloved baths, this was not practical in the Middle Ages. The lack of clean water for drinking and bathing and of resources to heat and transport it must have severely limited the use of bathing for medical treatment. While some large towns had public baths, country people surely bathed less and had fewer changes of clothing than city people. In addition, the church saw public baths, where males and females might bathe together, as scandalous. However, bathing still had its symbolic role in rituals such as those performed on certain saint's days or for those being inducted into knighthood, and in many places hot and mineral springs continued to attract visitors regardless of church policy.

The late Middle Ages in Europe was a period of active and growing interest in the therapeutic use of waters. A thirteenth century manuscript on the thermal baths near Naples, Italy, describes 35 separate baths, each with different properties, that could cure a wide variety of conditions.(9) In many locations, new baths were rebuilt over the old Roman baths and became centers of healing for those with musculoskeletal problems, nervous exhaustion, cardiac and respiratory illnesses, and other conditions. In lepers' hospitals, baths were used as a treatment, and lepers were both dipped and bathed.

In England, regular bathing became fashionable first with aristocratic ladies, following the lead of Queen Eleanor of Castille; however, it required a terrible catastrophe to bring home the importance of personal hygiene to most Europeans. In 1345 the bubonic plague (Black Death) killed at least one-third of Europe's people within a year, and it returned again in the 1360s and 1370s, killing a grand total of 20 million. However horrific the suffering it caused, the Black Death brought about some very important social and ideological changes. The public health tradition of hygiene and prevention was strengthened, so that there were for the first time major efforts to clean streets, collect garbage, empty sewers, and bathe regularly. The custom of bathing at public sweat houses was revived, and withdrawal of bathing privileges was considered a fearful punishment. However, nudity, promiscuity, and fear of illness being spread in the baths led to them being closed periodically. Well-to-do people, of course, could bathe in the comfort of their own homes; some castles had special rooms next to the kitchen where ladies could bathe in groups, soaking in hot water scented with sweet herbs or flowers, then rinsing with rosewater. Or hot water could be carried directly to a lord's bedchamber for use in his personal wooden tub.

HYDROTHERAPY DURING THE RENAISSANCE AND THE INDUSTRIAL REVOLUTION

As the Renaissance began in Europe, medicine began to be put on a more rational basis. Leonardo da Vinci performed dissections in the late 1400s, and the first complete textbook of human anatomy was published in 1543. Unfortunately, epidemics continued to ravage Europe, although never again in proportions like those of the bubonic plague. As always, because water was cheap and relatively plentiful, it was one of the first methods used to treat new illnesses. A hydrotherapy treatment that appears repeatedly for various illnesses is steam, used as a local application or a whole-body steam bath. For example, steam inhalation was prescribed for tuberculosis, and steam baths were given to treat both gout and syphilis.

During this period, interest in and use of mineral springs continued. A 1553 woodcut of the old Roman Bath in Plombières, France, shows it being used by many people on crutches, who most likely had arthritis, polio, or other crippling musculoskeletal conditions. The 166°F water of Plombières contained high levels of sodium sulfate and silicic acid and was reputed to be effective for rheumatism and infertility. Books were written about the beneficial effects of mineral springs. In 1564 one writer described using the waters by bathing in them, drinking them, and using them in a variety of local applications such as douches, **enemas,** local showers on an affected part, fomentations, and applications of mud.(4[p101]). Local hydrotherapy treatments with non-mineral water were in use as well (Fig. 1-2), and the circulatory effects of whole-body treatments were well understood (Fig. 1-3). When the European aristocracy, such as the court of King Louis XIV, had specific health complaints, they often visited spas. (Ironically, Louis XIV, who was born in 1638, was not a visitor to baths anywhere; the "perfumed king" often boasted of having taken only three baths in his entire life!)

Although the process had only begun in the 1400s and would take centuries to complete, over time Western medical beliefs would change. The new foundation of Western medicine would no longer be a mixture of magic and religion but instead pure rationalism. The body would come to be viewed as a machine which was governed by physical principals rather than by humoral pathology. Thus, the terminology around the healing properties of baths and springs began to change as well, and the explanation for their benefits was now given in the language of science. The curative effects of mineral and thermal springs were attributed to the chemicals in the water (such as magnesium sulfate, sodium sulfate, or chloride of lime) or to chemical reactions set in motion by the heat of the water. In 1697 English physician John Floyer claimed that priests who dedicated healing wells to particular saints had deceived common people into thinking their cures were from the merit of the saint rather than the physical virtue of the cold water.

In 1805 French chemist Joseph Gay-Lussac discovered that water was composed of two parts hydrogen and one part oxygen; the change from a spiritual or miraculous explanation of water's healing properties to a scientific explanation was complete.

Despite the new scientific definition of water, its actual cleanliness continued to be questionable. Until this time, little attempt had been made to pipe or channel water from clean sources into cities, but finally contamination of local water became such a serious problem that large cities in Europe and the United States were forced to bring water from distant sources. Contamination of city water was caused not only by heavy concentrations of people living near the banks of rivers but also by chemical and manufacturing industries. These industries took water out of rivers to make their products and then dumped their wastes straight back in them. Finally, however, new channels or aqueducts were built to bring water from pristine sources. Water towers were installed to store water, using pumps powered by horses or windmills. Pumping plant technology improved gradually, powered first by water wheels in rivers, then by steam, and finally by electricity. Cleaner and more readily available water would make water treatments far easier to administer.

Interest in the curative effects of bathing continued, although it was often overshadowed by health fads. Political and economic forces promoted bathing as well. In England, Queen Elizabeth I, fearful that English Roman Catholics who took the waters abroad were gathering to plot against her, encouraged a new cult of public bathing in England. Businessmen rushed in to make money feeding, housing, and providing recreation for invalids and vacationers in towns such as Bath and Buxton. *The History of Hot and Cold Bathing* by John Floyer, which advocated cold bathing, was published in 1697 and was popular enough to be issued in six subsequent editions. Floyer claimed to have been inspired by the remedial use of mineral springs by nearby peasants.

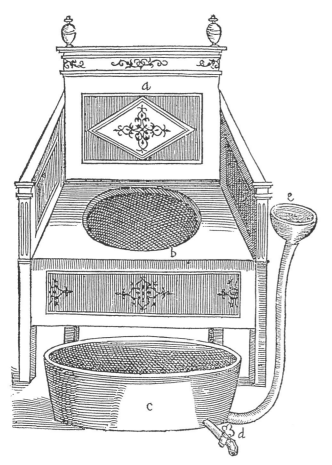

FIGURE 1-2 ■ Steam bath chair, 1564. This chair had an opening in the seat; the user's pelvic area was bathed in steam to alleviate the pain of bladder stones, a common condition of the time. (Photo courtesy of National Library of Medicine, Bethesda, Maryland.)

In 1747 John Wesley published *Primitive Physic*, a book of folk remedies which included many water applications for conditions including asthma, colds, colic, rickets, headaches, whooping cough, rheumatism, swelling, and sciatica. Wesley, a minister and the founder of the Methodist Church, called hydrotherapy "an easy and natural way of curing most disease." Sufferers from minor and major psychiatric illness often patronized spas with a reputation for curing "insane persons." The healing waters of Bath, England, continued to be used year round for a variety of complaints. Sick people continued to drink water from certain mineral springs in the hope that it would heal their ailments (Fig. 1-4). When sea bathing for health was adopted by English royalty, it too gained acceptance, and in 1796 the Royal Sea-Bathing Infirmary was founded in Margate. Many spas which had existed for hundreds of years became more respectable by calling themselves mineral water hospitals. In England, the resort of Bath was renamed the Royal Mineral Water Hospital, and the Bath Charity in the town of Buxton became the Devonshire Royal Water Hospital.

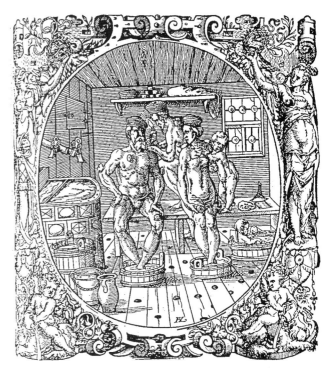

FIGURE 1-3 ■ Sauna and footbath, 1565. A physician in the background supervises while patients not only take a sauna but also have a footbath and undergo cupping. Engraving from *Opus Chyrugicum* by the famous Swiss physician and alchemist Paracelsus, a staunch believer in hydrotherapy and massage. (Photo courtesy of National Library of Medicine, Bethesda, Maryland.)

HYDROTHERAPY IN THE NINETEENTH CENTURY

Despite the continuing advances in medical knowledge and public health leading into the nineteenth century, medical practice itself was still not very effective. The

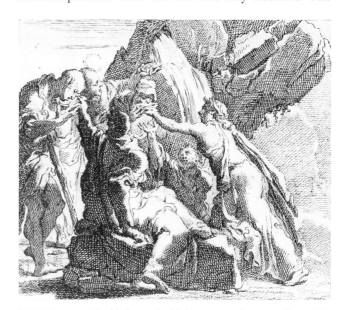

FIGURE 1-4 ■ Disabled people drinking water from a spring which they hope will cure their ailments, by Fernando Bassi, 1768. (Photo courtesy of National Library of Medicine, Bethesda, Maryland.)

mechanistic philosophy that the universe was simply a giant machine continued to guide doctors, and they began to emphasize pathological anatomy, or the study of actual changes in bodily organs by autopsy to learn more about disease.

Priessnitz, Kneipp, and the Hydropathy Movement

Into this environment, just ripe for a new "miracle" method of healing, came water healer Vincent Priessnitz (1799–1851), an uneducated Austrian peasant who developed a collection of water treatments into a natural healing philosophy called **hydropathy**. From direct observation of the effects of cold water treatments on farm animals, himself, and his neighbors, Priessnitz became a believer in the healing effects of water. He noticed that animals' sprains and bruises as well as tumors on horses' hoofs healed faster when they were bathed with cold water. He treated his own fractures and bruises from a serious accident by using cold water and quickly regained his health, contrary to a doctor's prediction. After Priessnitz experimented further with cold water, he also became convinced of the healthy effects of profuse sweating and of his ability to cure gout and rheumatism, common complaints at that time.

Priessnitz believed that all illness was caused by morbid or disease-causing humors that formed inside or outside the human body and were introduced into the blood. These morbid humors came from immoderation (too much food, bad food, use of stimulating liquors, excessive mental excitement, too little exercise), inhalation of noxious air, or lack of cleanliness. Exercise, diet, fresh air, vigorous massage, and above all, water were used to expel the humors and disease from the system. Priessnitz's hydrotherapy treatments included sweat baths, cold baths, wet sheet packs, and many local cold water treatments, such as eye and foot baths. Sweating forced out bad humors and inflammation, wet sheet packs restored healthy circulation and secretions, and cold baths encouraged the natural functions of the skin.

As with so many "miracle" cures of the past, Priessnitz's success was built upon the beliefs of the time (he retained the concept of humors), a germ of truth (the circulatory effects of various types of water applications), and the human taste for novelty. This is not to say that many of Priessnitz's cures were not effective; the effects of many of his hydrotherapy treatments have been validated scientifically. However, the use of water as the primary agent in a medical system was revolutionary. According to this approach, water was employed to cure every type of illness and chronic disability, and no treatment could be successful without water.

Priessnitz became wildly successful. First, he treated his neighbors (Fig. 1-5); then, when his fame spread, the Austrian government was forced to give him a special license to treat patients and to build new roads to help people gain access to his mountain home. In 1840 Priessnitz treated 1600 patients from all over the world using primarily cold water and healthy diet. In 1843 he published *The Cold Water Cure*, which went through many printings and translations into other languages. Physicians from many countries, including the United States, made pilgrimages to his institution and established their own "water cures" back home. In France, Spain, the Czech Republic, the United Kingdom, Austria, Germany, and the United States, these water cures would treat the sick with water as the primary agent. In 1852 there were 24 water cure establishments in England and Ireland alone.(4[p102]) Even physicians who did not specialize in water treatments experimented with various ones. For example, Jean-Marie Charcot, famous French neurologist

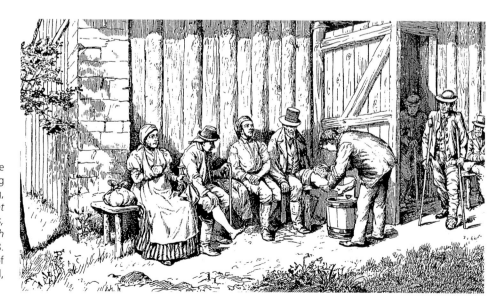

FIGURE 1-5 ■ The beginnings of the water cure: Vincent Priessnitz treating patients with cold water sponging, 1816. (From vom Walde P. *Vincent Priessnitz: His Life and His Works, Published on His One Hundredth Birthday.* Berlin: Wilhelm Moller, 1898. Photo courtesy of National College of Naturopathic Medicine, Portland, Oregon.)

and teacher of Sigmund Freud, experimented with warm circulating water to treat joint inflammation and invented the Charcot shower, a very strong jet of water directed upon the back of a standing patient. Technological progress, such as indoor plumbing which supplied running water, meant that it was possible to use water in large quantities for various hydrotherapy treatments.

Hydropaths could be either folk healers or trained physicians, and they treated a wide variety of medical problems. They generally urged their patients to follow a healthy lifestyle, which included eating unrefined food, drinking lots of water, and exercising regularly. Water treatments included wet packs and dripping sheets, whole-body baths, local baths (sitz baths were a favorite), steam inhalations, **affusions, compresses,** gargles, douches, **sprays,** fomentations, treading in cold water, walking barefoot on snow, and swimming; patients were sponged, wrapped, cooked in saunas, scrubbed, hosed inside and out, sprayed, dunked, bathed and steamed. There seemed no end to the inventive ways that water could be applied to the body. Swedish massage, originally from Swedish masseuses and masseurs who had emigrated to other countries, was frequently offered as part of the regimen. As had occurred so often before, proponents of water treatments found it natural to combine them with diet, exercise, and massage. With hydropathy the health fad of the moment, people on both sides of the Atlantic could satirize the movement (Fig. 1-6).

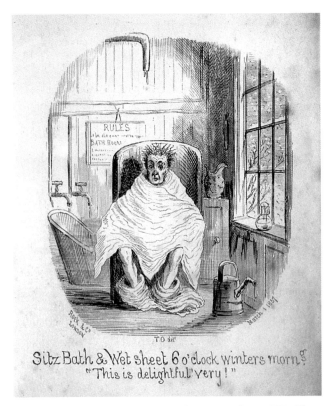

FIGURE 1-6 ■ Satirical drawing by Thomas Onwhyn, 1857. (Photo courtesy of National Library of Medicine, Bethesda, Maryland.)

Twenty years after Priessnitz, Sebastian Kneipp (1821–1897), a Bavarian priest who cured himself of tuberculosis with water treatments and diet, became another internationally prominent lay healer. Kneipp incorporated herbs, exercise, fresh air, nutrition, and emotional treatment into his version of the water cure, which he called nature cure. Body hardening—the strengthening of the body—he considered the best way to preserve health, and as with Priessnitz before him, his treatments were often harsh and rigorous, including ice cold baths and walking barefoot in the snow. Baths of various temperatures and ingredients (from herbs to clays) were common. Gout was treated by using herbal packs, herbal baths, cold washings, and local douches. Warm applications were gradually changed to colder ones until a patient might end up in an ice-cold bath—and not always a local bath, such as a sitz bath, but often the entire body. Patients and doctors who wanted to learn his methods flocked to Bad Wörischofen, the spa town where Kneipp practiced, from many countries in Europe and elsewhere. Kneipp treated royalty and simple peasants alike, including the Archduke Ferdinand of Austria, whose assassination touched off World War I. Kneipp also cured Archduke Ferdinand's father, Archduke Joseph, of Bright's disease, a kidney disorder. (Figure 1-7 shows Kneipp with the two archdukes, whom he has walking barefoot in the snow.) He also treated Pope Leo XIII. Kneipp had a profound influence on the hydropathy movement, and the English edition of his book, *My Water Cure*, went through 50 printings in its first 5 years. Many lay people and numerous orthodox physicians returned from a Kneipp "cure" to establish hydrotherapy practices in their own communities.

Back in the United States, some of the lay people who had healed in European water cures would go on to found alternative colleges, give intense competition to the orthodox (university trained) doctors, and eventually either join conventional medical practice or become naturopathic physicians. Massage, although seen as a secondary therapy, was a popular adjunct to water treatments and used a great deal. In 1892, Kneipp commissioned German-born Benjamin Lust to carry Kneipp's methods to the United States, and in 1902 his American followers changed their work from "Kneipp's water cure" to "naturopathy." Naturopathic medicine has continued as a medical specialty of its own since that time and continues to make far more use of hydrotherapy than does any other branch of medicine.

The Resurgence of Spas

During this period, the upper classes of Europe had both the wealth and the leisure time to retreat to spas for extended periods. This was fortunate, since a typical water cure lasted 24 weeks and required immersion up to the neck for at least 3 hours twice a day, 3 days per

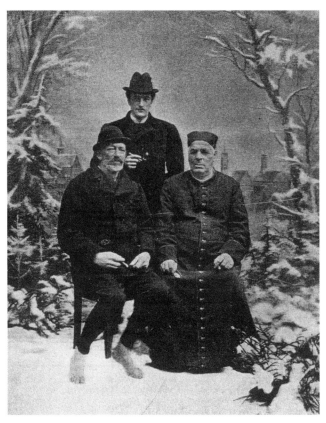

FIGURE 1-7 ■ Sebastian Kneipp with Joseph and Francis Ferdinand, grand dukes of Austria, walking barefoot in the new-fallen snow. Illustration from *Father Kneipp's Teachings* by Paul Wendel, published by Paul Wendel, Brooklyn, New York, 1947. (Photo courtesy of National College of Naturopathic Medicine, Portland, Oregon.)

week.(10[p157]) New technological advances—better plumbing and travel by railroad—made luxury water cures possible at far-flung spas. Rich patients went not only for the healing of physical ailments such as rheumatism and gout and to get fresh air and sunshine but also to see and be seen at fashionable resorts. Well-to-do invalids flocked to try the water treatments, usually receiving massage as well. Amusements such as horse racing, boxing matches, gambling, flirting, and attending the theater softened the rigors of the water cure. Spa therapies also had a strong placebo effect for those with psychosomatic illnesses and "nerves": there are many reports of hysterical paralysis, even blindness, being cured at spas. Upper-class invalids whose emotional pain was being expressed as a physical ailment might become confirmed spa goers, as their doctors referred them to one spa after another.

In Germany the spa resort now called Baden-Baden was discovered by the Romans in 75 AD and named *Aquae Aureliae* (waters of the goddess Aurelia). Used continuously since the time of the Romans, its waters were reputed to be effective for treating obesity, arthritis, rheumatism, heart and circulatory problems, respiratory disorders, and many other maladies. In its mud-pack

rooms, patients were enveloped in mud for half an hour, sprayed with water from hoses, bathed, massaged, and then allowed to rest. By 1830, 15,000 people visited the resort every year, including such luminaries as Queen Victoria, Napoleon III, Kaiser Wilhelm, Chopin, Brahms, Dostoyevsky, Delacroix, and Tolstoy. American author Mark Twain paid a visit to Baden-Baden and wrote, "I fully believe I left my rheumatism there." Bath, England, was another pleasure center as well as a place of healing. Its waters had also been in continuous demand since Roman times, and to bring it up to fashion, the town had a major facelift in the early 1800s, with the renovation of medieval buildings and the construction of magnificent stone buildings in classical style.

These great spas and others, such as Montecatini Terme in Italy and Evian-les-Bains in France (all discovered by the Romans almost 2 millennia ago), adopted the water cure and the hydrotherapy methods of Priessnitz and Kneipp. Many spas had a reputation for healing specific complaints. The fashionable Bad Kreuznach in Germany was known as the ladies' spa, since its waters were supposed to have a rejuvenating effect on inflammatory conditions of the female pelvic organs. Bad Ems was reputed to be healing for throat complaints. In France, Bagnoles de l'Orne had hot radium-impregnated water beneficial for blood vessel problems; the waters of Vittel were said to act on the liver and kidneys to treat arthritis and gout; and the waters of Plombières continued to be used for female infertility.

When John Harvey Kellogg visited Leukerbad, Switzerland, in 1883, the mineral water baths of 95° to 98°F were extremely popular. They were used principally by patients with nervous disorders, rheumatism, psoriasis, and eczema (Fig. 1-8). During their stay at Leukerbad, patients typically entered the baths around 7:00 AM and remained in them until 1:00 PM each day, which explains the need to play chess, write letters, and drink tea to pass the time. A combination water and massage treatment used at a number of famous spas was the Aix douche-massage. During this treatment the patient was massaged by hand and simultaneously sprayed with high-pressure water from a hose; sometimes two masseurs at once performed the treatment, spraying and massaging for up to 15 minutes. This technique was used as part of the treatment for diabetes at Aix-les-Bains in France.(11[p180])

New hydrotherapy techniques were always of interest to Europeans, and when French soldiers stationed in Turkey brought **Turkish baths** and massage techniques back home in the early 1800s, they soon became very popular. Turkish baths were introduced into England in the 1880s and were enthusiastically adopted by the English. (As in the United States, bathrooms with running water would not be available to all citizens until about 1920.) City dwellers patronized public baths, factory owners in large industrial towns provided Turkish

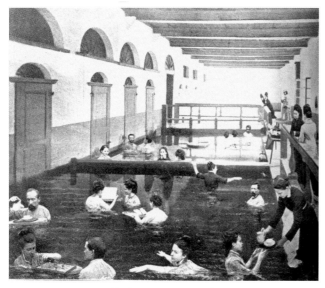

FIGURE 1-8 ■ Neutral bath treatment at Leukerbad Spa, Switzerland, 1883. (From Kellogg JH. *Rational Hydrotherapy*. Battle Creek, MI: Medical Review, 1900, p 565.)

baths for their workers, and mental hospitals tried them for their patients. Soon spas were incorporating a Turkish flavor: in Harrogate, England, which had long been famous for its mineral waters, a new spa with a variety of water treatments opened in 1897. It featured numerous water treatments (including hot pools, intestinal lavage, steam inhalation rooms, and mud baths) and a suite of massage rooms. It was decorated in a grand Moorish design, with Islamic architecture, tile work, and decorations. In the United States too, Turkish baths opened in many large cities around the turn of the century and immediately became very popular. The Turkish baths helped meet the hygiene needs of Americans who had no running water in their homes. The baths often offered massage treatments.

Hydropathy in the United States

I can remember well when the cold water cure was first talked about. I was then about nine years old, and I remember how my mother used to stand me up naked in the backyard every morning and throw buckets of cold water on me, just to see what effect it would have. Personally, I had no curiosity on the subject. And then, when the dousing was over, she would wrap me in a sheet wet with ice water and then wrap blankets around that and put me into bed. I never realized that the treatment was doing me any good physically. But it purified me spiritually. For pretty soon after I was put into bed I would get up a perspiration that was something worth seeing.

—Mark Twain(12)

In the early years of the nineteenth century, the medical climate in the United States was also ripe for health reforms and new techniques. The dismal state of the regular medical profession, combined with the social conditions of the time, was favorable to the development of alternative medical ideas and systems, and so a health reform movement came into existence in the 1820s. It advocated health-promoting practices such as diet and exercise and sought out alternatives to standard medical care, such as homeopathic, water, and herbal remedies.(13) Native American herbal remedies and steam treatments (Box 1-1) were easily incorporated into this growing body of alternative practices. Part of the appeal of the new movement was the lack of toxic and unpleasant remedies. A steam bath with herbal inhalation, a massage, and other gentle cures were much more attractive than

---

BOX 1-1 | *Point of Interest*

NATIVE AMERICAN HYDROTHERAPY

Hydrotherapy was part of the culture of the natives of North America for eons before the arrival of Europeans. Many Native American tribes used **sweat lodges** not only to perform religious rituals and stay clean and warm but also for treating illnesses such rheumatism, colds, and fevers. Herbal remedies were also part of sweat lodge therapy. By adding herbs to the water that was sprinkled upon the hot stones in the lodge, participants inhaled herbal steam and absorbed herbal concoctions through the skin. Over time white settlers adopted a variety of Native American medical practices. Steam therapy became popular among white Americans in the early 1800s, and it is believed that the practice was borrowed directly from Native Americans. For example, Samuel Thompson (1769–1860), a self-taught doctor who advocated gentle herbal remedies and steam treatments, learned about them originally from the Abenaki Indians who lived near his home.

Natural thermal springs were also used for hydrotherapy and jealously guarded by Native Americans. In some places, battles were fought when white settlers wanted to take over a natural spring! The waters of what would later become the resort Saratoga Springs were used by Native Americans for heart disease, asthma, and rheumatism. The Creek Indians of Georgia used the mineral waters of what would later become the Warm Springs resort to heal their warriors' wounds. From the time white people arrived in North America, they adopted the hot springs that had been used by Native Americans, much as the Romans adopted natural springs in areas that they conquered.

References
1. Bruchac J. *The Native American Sweat Lodge: History and Legends*. Freedom, CA: Crossing Press, 1993, p 106.
2. Vogel V. *American Indian Medicine*. Norman: University of Oklahoma, 1970.

orthodox treatments, which resulted in a sick person ingesting toxic substances, being given diarrhea-causing substances, losing large quantities of blood, vomiting, or having burning material applied to the skin to make blisters. However, the health reform movement also attracted individuals looking for more control over their lives and bodies, women who wanted to be physicians, sanitarians interested in public health, freethinkers who challenged the status quo, and many of those caught up in the temperance movement.

Beginning in the early 1800s, information about water cures came to the United States from European immigrants, from books written by doctors practicing hydropathy in Europe, and from American physicians who traveled to Europe to experience and witness hydropathy for themselves.(14[pp9-24]) Hydrotherapy treatments had a long history in medicine, both in Europe and in the United States, but it was not until the height of Priessnitz's success in the 1830s that his methods crossed the Atlantic in earnest. Then, American patients who had been treated at water cures in Europe began to return to the United States, fired with passion to share the benefits they had experienced. Joel Shew, an American who had become an invalid from overexposure to mercury, iodine, and bromine, was one of these. He regained his health at Priessnitz's water cure and then returned to the United States. He established his own water cure in Lebanon Springs, New York, and wrote *The Water-Cure Manual*. Robert and William Wesselhoeft, two German immigrants who had been healed by Priessnitz, studied as physicians and set up a water cure establishment in Vermont. A student of theirs, Mary Gove Nichols, began treating her neighbors with cold water. She and her husband founded the American Hydropathic Institute, a coeducational medical school based upon water cure principles, in 1851. Breaking new ground in the heady atmosphere of change, women were leaders in the movement; they wrote hydrotherapy books, established water cures, and discussed women's health concerns in an atmosphere of unusual openness.

Between 1840 and 1900, 213 hospitals treating patients primarily with hydrotherapy were opened in the United States. They treated common people as well as famous Americans such as Sojourner Truth, Harriet Beecher Stowe, and Henry Wadsworth Longfellow. At costs ranging from $6 to $10 a week, a patient at a water cure could expect to drink plenty of water; have daily hydrotherapy treatments such as wet sheet packs, heating compresses, sitz baths (the most popular bath), and footbaths; swim when possible; and take a cold bath after vigorous exercise. Water would be used as either a stimulant or a sedative, depending on the case. Water treatments were thought to strengthen the nervous and circulatory systems, restore the body's secretions, and fill the patient's system with healthy new blood. Massage was another mainstay of the program, and even weak people who were

unable to exercise in other ways would still be bathed, rubbed, and kneaded.

As Europeans were doing, some Americans made extreme claims about the water cure, promising that it could heal almost all illnesses; this led to criticism, especially by orthodox physicians, that hydropathy was a medical cult. Hydropaths claimed that even in the case of incurable diseases, water treatments would result in the patient's body being stronger and healthier than before. Hydropaths lectured on hygiene, health, diet, and exercise with almost fanatical conviction to anyone who would listen. Patients provided glowing testimonials of miraculous cures and the joys of treatment: in 1851 one guest at a hydropathic rest cure wrote, "It is a happy change from poisonous drugs to pure cold water. Would to heaven I had come here when I was first taken sick; instead of being butchered by pill givers. How many hours of pain and anguish I might have been spared."(15) As the popularity of hydropathy spread, there were not only more than 200 residential water cures, there were also thousands of lay healers and even some short-lived colleges. Between 1840 and 1870, hydropathic publications included the *Water-Cure Monthly*, the *Water-Cure World*, *The American Magazine of Homeopathy and Hydropathy*, and *The Water Cure Journal*, which had over 100,000 subscribers during the 1850s (Fig. 1-9). Home health care manuals explained the use of hydrotherapy treatments, massage and exercise.(11[p114]) Even some conventional doctors jumped on the bandwagon and adopted cold water treatments. Cold baths followed by exercise were used for mania, hysteria, and other nervous disorders; cold baths after sweating treatments treated rheumatism and dropsy; and bathing was used during convalescence to prevent fevers.

Hydropathy's popularity reached its climax in the 1850s, perhaps because no one type of medical practice could possibly live up to the extravagant claims of its proponents for long, but water treatments had become familiar to all and would influence American medicine for years to come. A generation after Priessnitz, the success of the Bavarian Sebastian Kneipp inspired another group of Americans to introduce his version of the water cure to the United States, to use water treatments extensively, and to found naturopathic medicine. Although the hydropathic craze had come and gone by the late 1800s, some conventional doctors sought to transform hydropathy into hydrotherapy, a legitimate medical technology. One conventional doctor, Simon Baruch (1840–1921), was dedicated to putting hydrotherapy on a scientific basis to gain its acceptance by orthodox medicine. Throughout his life he tried to contrast hydropathy, the nonscientific form of treatment with water, with hydrotherapy, which was the entirely rational form. Baruch, who studied hydrotherapy in Europe, was a firm believer in the power of cold baths to strengthen the immune system. Water, he wrote, could be used as an

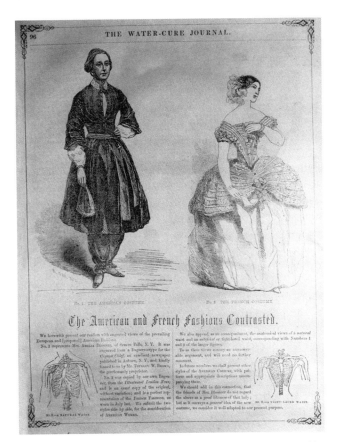

FIGURE 1-9 ■ Page from *Water-Cure Journal*, 1854. A woman with a tightly laced corset and a woman with a natural waist. The "reform dress" (left) was designed in a hydropathic establishment. Wearers of the hydropathic costume cut their hair short for easy drying and felt themselves freed from the bondage of trailing skirts, petticoats, corsets, and corkscrew curls. However, the clothing was considered a badge of radicalism, and its wearers suspected of free love notions and a desire to be free of all feminine graces and restrictions. (Courtesy of Willard Library, Battle Creek, Michigan.)

antipyretic, hypnotic, stimulant, tonic, diaphoretic, purgative, sedative, diuretic, emetic, antiseptic and a local anesthetic.(16) When he returned to the United States from Europe, he became professor of hydrotherapy at Columbia University, taught health care professionals to use water treatments for all disease, and wrote a number of hydrotherapy textbooks, including *An Epitome of Hydrotherapy for Physicians, Architects and Nurses*. Baruch also practiced hydrotherapy on a hospital-wide scale. While he temporarily popularized hydrotherapy by medical doctors in New York State, where he practiced, ultimately Baruch's efforts to win over his orthodox colleagues to hydrotherapy were not successful.

Another of the major players in the American hydropathy movement was the Seventh Day Adventist Church, an American Christian denomination founded in 1844. The Adventists were antislavery, licensed women as ministers, refused to take arms in wartime, and adopted many health reforms that were far ahead of their time, such as abstinence from meat, alcohol, and tobacco. Ellen G. White, a prominent church leader, was a firm believer in natural health remedies, especially in water treatment. She first learned about hydrotherapy through a newspaper article on treatment of diphtheria. White then encouraged Adventists to open institutions using these remedies. "This is our work. Small companies are to go forth to do the work which Christ appointed his disciples. While laboring as evangelists, they can visit the sick, pray with them, and if need be, treat them, not with medication, but with the remedies provided in nature."(17[p22])

The first Adventist health institution, the Western Health Reform Institute of Battle Creek, Michigan, was built in 1866. Ten years later, Adventist physician John Harvey Kellogg became its medical director. The Health Reform Institute burned down in 1902 and was rebuilt

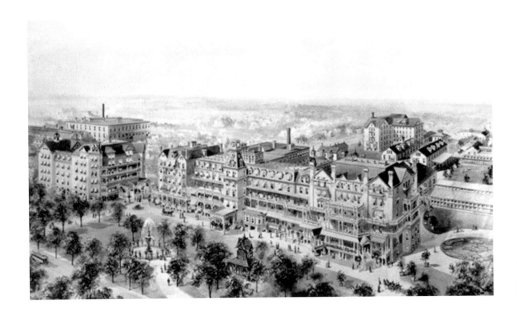

FIGURE 1-10 ■ Battle Creek Sanitarium complex, aerial view, 1900. (Courtesy of Willard Library, Battle Creek, Michigan.)

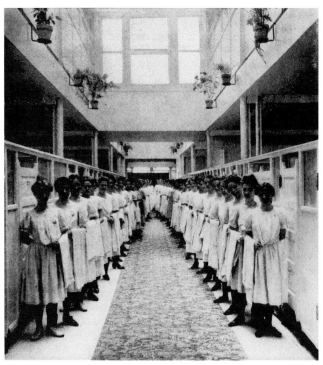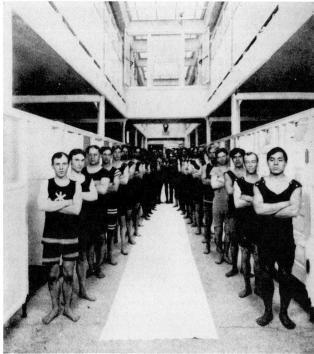

SPECIMEN GROUPS OF BATH ATTENDANTS — EACH AN EXPERT IN HYDRIATIC METHODS

FIGURE 1-11 ■ Female and male bath attendants in the corridors of the Battle Creek Sanitarium bath department. (Photo courtesy of Willard Library, Battle Creek, Michigan.)

and renamed the Battle Creek Sanitarium, a 1200-bed institution built in Italian Renaissance style, that employed many of the most common treatments used in water cures (Fig. 1-10). "The San" drew thousands of chronically ill patients from all over the world and from all walks of life—everyone from President William Howard Taft, Henry Ford, J. C. Penney, Eleanor Roosevelt, and Amelia Earhart to charity cases. It became the leading center for natural healing in North America and Europe, with a thousand patients in treatment there at any given time. Water treatments were given to all patients, who were expected in the Bath Department 40 minutes a day, 6 days a week (Figs. 1-11 and 1-12). Kellogg, sanitarium director who had been trained in both conventional and water cure methods, was committed to transforming water cure methods into legitimate medical practice. He performed many scientific experiments and wrote extensively on health. His book *Rational Hydrotherapy*, published in 1900, has become a classic.(18)

Decline of the Water Cure

In the last quarter of the nineteenth century, hydropathy's popularity in both the United States and Europe began to wane due to a number of factors, including strong opposition from the orthodox medical profession. Although some conventional physicians had adopted water techniques, in general hydropathy was dismissed as useless, its physicians were branded as quacks, and

medical school curricula began to emphasize the use of pharmaceutical drugs. An exception to this was the acceptance of hydrotherapy for treatment of mental illness (Box 1-2). Another factor in the decline of the water cure was the fact that hydropathy was very time consuming. Many water treatments demanded a great deal of time, especially when water had to be carried and heated

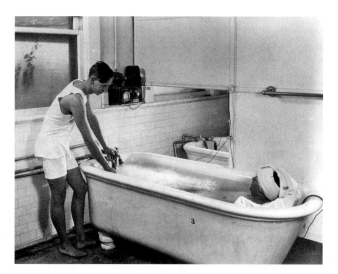

FIGURE 1-12 ■ Patient receiving hydrotherapy treatment, Battle Creek Sanitarium. Note the cold compress on the patient's head. The inlets for hot and cold water, combined with the drain for outflow, allowed the water to be kept at a constant temperature. (Photo courtesy of Willard Library, Battle Creek, Michigan.)

BOX 1-2 | *Point of Interest*

HYDROTHERAPY TREATMENTS FOR PSYCHIATRIC PROBLEMS

One of the most fascinating chapters in the history of Western hydrotherapy is its use for psychiatric problems. In medieval Europe, mentally ill patients were sometimes bowssened (immersed in consecrated waters such as holy wells dedicated to saints or the Virgin Mary) to cure their condition—a kind of primitive shock treatment. Warm baths have always been known to soothe and relax, making them a natural fit for both minor and major psychiatric problems in an era before medication. Europeans had a long tradition of visiting certain spas whose waters were said to be good for minor psychiatric complaints such as anxiety and nervous depression, and so it is not surprising that French doctor Philippe Pinel (1745–1810), the founder of modern psychiatry, recommended warm baths to calm the severely mentally ill patients who lived in asylums.

During the heyday of the hydropathic movement, water treatments were advocated for almost every known ailment, and with their soothing effects, it seemed logical to use them for major mental problems as well as bodily ailments. Management of disruptive or difficult patients presented a dilemma, especially in large institutions. (Stephen Noll, PhD, personal communication with author, November 10, 2004.) However, drugs that were commonly used for calming and sedating the mentally ill and treating insomnia (such as morphine, chloryl hydrate, and barbiturates) were often toxic, addicting, and not curative, making water treatments an attractive alternative.

From the early years of the twentieth century until the 1950s, hydrotherapy was mainstream medicine for mental institutions. Large mental hospitals installed hydrotherapy suites with large-scale hydrotherapeutic equipment such as bathtubs, steam baths, fomentation stations, and sitz baths. Using water for healing in this setting also reflected a change in the conceptualization of mental illness: for the first time, mental problems were conceived as originating in the physical brain, not in the immaterial mind. Therefore a treatment that addressed the body (in the

case of hydrotherapy, through the skin) could be effective, and in the case of hydrotherapy this was done through the skin.

According to Agatha Thrash, MD, water treatments such as neutral baths, wet sheet packs, and warm fomentations made mentally ill patients more comfortable, more compliant, and less likely to be forcibly restrained. Continuous neutral baths, sometimes of many hours' duration, were used to calm restless, agitated, or combative patients, while all stimulation, such as drafts, distractions, and disturbing thoughts, was avoided.(3) For patients who were combative or otherwise unmanageable, the wet sheet pack often not only restrained them but caused a calming sedative effect: after just a few minutes, a patient who was uncooperative became relaxed, often slept for a time, and was quiet and cooperative afterward. Hydrotherapy applications were to be persistently applied over time and not discontinued after a brief trial.

In 1940, psychiatrist and medical hydrologist Rebekah Wright, MD, published *Hydrotherapy in Psychiatric Hospitals*. Wright's work was intended to guide other psychiatrists at mental institutions. It explained the specific hydrotherapy treatments to treat many psychiatric disorders. At the time her book was written, many organic brain diseases and drug addictions, which manifest as problems with thinking, were treated in mental hospitals along with psychiatric disorders. (Today these problems would be treated in nursing or drug treatment facilities.)

References
1. Braslow J. *Mental Ills and Bodily Cures: Psychiatric Treatment in the First Half of the Twentieth Century*. Berkeley: University of California, 1997.
2. Shorter E. *A History of Psychiatry: from the Era of the Asylum to the Age of Prozac*. New York: Wiley, 1997.
3. Thrash A, Thrash C. *Home Remedies: Hydrotherapy, Charcoal, and Other Simple Treatments*. Seale, AL: Thrash, 1981, p 119.
4. Wright R. *Hydrotherapy in Psychiatric Hospitals*. Boston: Tudor, 1940.

by hand, and water cures required people to be gone from home and work for long periods. Modern attitudes do not necessarily endorse time-consuming treatments, even if they are just as effective as the administration of a medication. (According to medical historians Robert and Michele Root-Bernstein, in the last century Western notions of medicine demanded faster cures and less time away from work for patients.(10[p25]) Agatha Thrash, MD, who has written extensively on the use of hydrotherapy for disease, also believes that drug administration may be more popular today primarily because it requires far less time doing hands-on caring for ailing patients.)(8[p1]) And finally, by now patients who were drawn to the water cure because it was the fad of the moment realized that their doctors were serious about lifestyle changes such as diet and exercise and that a fair amount of discipline was required. Long periods of immersion in bathtubs, bland diets, vigorous exercise programs, frequent enemas, and ice cold sitz baths had limited appeal to followers of fashion.

Some of the unorthodox figures who ran hydropathic establishments continued to challenge orthodox medicine by combining hydropathy with chiropractic, massage, and other emerging natural therapies. Benedict Lust (1872–1943) founded the American Naturopathic Association in 1896 and published natural health journals until his death. Naturopath Henry Lindlahr (1852–1925), whose sanitarium in Chicago contained extensive hydrotherapeutic installations, treated hundreds of patients each day by the natural methods he learned from Sebastian Kneipp and at others' European natural healing centers. Naturopath Otis Carroll (1879–1962) practiced for 40 years in Spokane, Washington, where he developed the **constitutional hydrotherapy** treatment. G. K. Abbot believed hydrotherapy saved many lives in the 1918 influenza pandemic, when **derivative** hydrotherapy and cold mitten friction were used to treat pneumonia, a frequent complication of influenza.(8[p3]) The wet sheet pack was also used during the epidemic to treat high fevers accompanied by delirium, restlessness, and insomnia (Table 1-1).

TABLE 1-1 RESULTS OF WET SHEET PACK TREATMENT OF SOLDIERS WITH INFLUENZA ON BOARD THE U.S. HOSPITAL SHIP *SOLACE*, AUGUST 1919

Soldier	Temperature (°F) Before	After	Minutes in Pack	Condition Before Pack Application	Condition After Pack Application
Mc	102.4	101.0	30	Delirious, very restless	Quiet 2 hours
McC	101.8	100.4	45	Delirious	Slept 3 hours
Br	103.4	102.0	75	Restless	Quiet all day
Mil	104.6	99.4	80	Very restless	Slept 3 hours
Mil	99.4	98.6	40	Normal	Normal
Os	104.2	103.2	35	Restless	Normal
O'Q	104.6	102.0	75	Restless	Normal
Cl	105.2	101.0	105	Delirious	Slept in pack
Ru	105.4	100.2	160	Delirious	Quiet
Eu	107.0	102.2	140	Restless	Normal
Gr	104.4	102.4	70	Delirious	Quiet
Go	105.0	103.6	135	Restless	Slept in pack
Go	103.4	103.0	20	Restless	Still restless
Go	103.0	101.2	190	Restless	Slept in pack 3 hours
Sw	104.4	102.6	40	Delirious, very restless	Rested quietly
Sa	105.4	104.6	80	Restless	Quiet
Tr	107.0	102.0	250	Very restless	Slept in pack 4 hours
Ch	105.4	102.4	195	Delirious	Slept in pack 3 hours
Le	104.8	103.4	60	Delirious	Quiet
Ga	102.0	102.0	30	Delirious	Rational
Br	105.4	104.0	190	Delirious	Quiet 4 hours
Gr	102.8	102.4	125	Delirious	Quiet for one hour
Gr	102.6	103.6	90	Moribund	Still delirious
Gu	107.0	105.6	75	Delirious	Rested quietly
Mcf	105.8	103.0	150	Restless	Slept in pack

According to surgeon Edward H. Old, commander of the *Solace*, "During the recent epidemic of influenza a number of the pneumonia cases were delirious and very restless, having to be restrained, these symptoms being beyond control by the use of drugs. Some of the men would remain awake day and night, the whole time in marked delirium. . . the wet sheet pack, as advocated by Dr. Simon Baruch, [using sheets wrung out in 70°F water] was found to be most efficient to quiet the patient in wild delirium or suffering from insomnia. It was our experience that a patient would invariably become normal in the pack and frequently sleep for two to four hours."

Careful reading of the table reveals that only two soldiers did not improve from the application of the pack: the first was a soldier with no fever, whose temperature dropped only 0.4°F, and the second was a feverish soldier whose temperature actually rose 1°F. In all other cases, the core temperature of the soldiers dropped and their condition improved. Even though the wet sheet pack is often given as a sweating treatment, evidently as the heat-dissipating mechanisms of the body were stimulated, core temperatures actually fell.

From Baruch S. *An Epitome of Hydrotherapy for Physicians, Architects and Nurses.* New York: Saunders, 1920, p 63.

HYDROTHERAPY IN THE TWENTIETH CENTURY

Although the rigors of the water cure may have lost their trendiness, that did not reduce the appeal of natural waters, and there was a gradual change toward elegant watering places for the wealthy rather than water cures. Floating in warm water, as always, had great appeal for one and all, especially when running water was not yet standard in all American bathrooms. Figure 1-13 shows a facility built around hot springs; Figure 1-14 shows the type of upscale bathroom still out of reach of many Americans.

Many European water resorts, because they had hydrotherapy facilities already in place, became military hospitals during and after World War I. Both soldiers who needed immediate attention and those recuperating from long-term injuries were cared for. Even American soldiers serving in Europe recuperated at spa towns such as Vittel,

France, and American soldiers with infected wounds were often treated with continuous baths. Whirlpool baths at 100° to 120°F were introduced for treatment of war injuries, including arm and leg stumps, scar tissue, ankyloses following gunshot wounds, recent and chronic sprains, and peripheral nerve injuries. In a 1919 letter to Dr. Simon Baruch, Major William Tindall, director of physiotherapy at the U. S. Army General Hospital in Fort McHenry, Maryland, stated, "We have found that the whirlpool bath is one of the most valuable modalities of this hospital in the treatment of war wounds. . . its soothing warmth changes the cold purple of the swollen and painful hand or foot, leg or arm into a warm red, softening the parts for massage and passive exercise and softening its conductivity for electric treatment. Pain is reduced, and the circulation and nutrition of the part increased." Tindall was convinced of the effectiveness of the whirlpool bath in preparing patients for massage: "One very important feature is the great economy in massage: we have found that

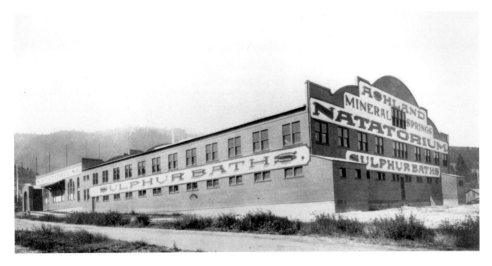

FIGURE 1-13 ■ Ashland, Oregon, mineral springs natatorium. In 1908, local entrepreneurs constructed a large facility over two hot sulfur springs that contained a large covered pool with 58 dressing rooms, balconies around the pool that could seat 500 people, and a ballroom that doubled as an ice skating rink in the winter. (Photo courtesy of the Southern Oregon Historical Society, Medford, Oregon.)

the duration of massage is reduced from thirty to ten minutes. The actual process is easier and less laborious, while the results are in every way superior to those which could be obtained previously."(17[p138])

During the early twentieth century, aquatic or pool therapy was used to treat polio patients, most notably Franklin Delano Roosevelt, thirty-seventh president of the United States. Pool exercise was still relatively new: the first to advocate for it was orthopedic physician Charles Lowman. In 1919 Lowman transformed the lily pond of the Los Angeles Orthopedic Hospital into two therapeutic pools for paralyzed patients to use for

"hydrogymnastics." Roosevelt, paralyzed from the waist down due to polio, first visited Warm Springs, Georgia, in 1924. This town features a natural spring of highly mineralized water containing bicarbonate, silica, calcium, magnesium, sulfate, potassium, sodium, and chloride, which comes out of the ground at a temperature of 88°F. For centuries before the arrival of Europeans, the Creek Indians used the spring to aid in recuperation of their wounded warriors. Later, white people also used the springs, and when pools were built there in the mid-1880s, Warm Springs became a resort and spa called the Merriweather Inn.

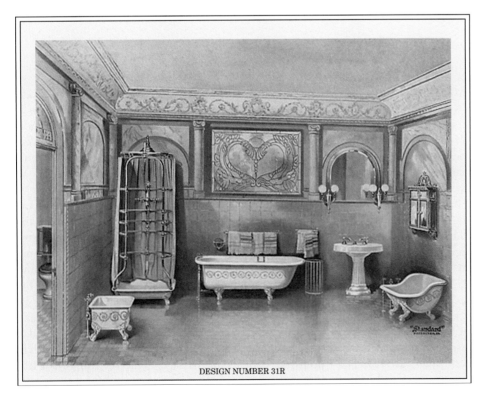

DESIGN NUMBER 31R

FIGURE 1-14 ■ Victorian bathroom, 1903. Note the footbath, which is installed to the left in front of the shower, and the sitz bath to the right. In 1903 not every house contained a bathroom with running water, and certainly only the well-to-do could afford such elaborate appliances. (Photo courtesy of Vintage Plumbing, Los Angeles, California.)

When Roosevelt came to Warm Springs, he spent 2 hours in the warm water every day, both swimming and performing specific exercises (Fig. 1-15); the warmth of the water relieved much of the muscular spasm and discomfort caused by his polio and its mineral-rich composition helped him to float more easily. This meant that exercising in the water was much less tiring, and he could work out for longer periods and greatly increase the strength of his muscles. Roosevelt became an ardent believer in the healing effects of the water, and in 1927 he founded the Warm Springs Institute for Rehabilitation,

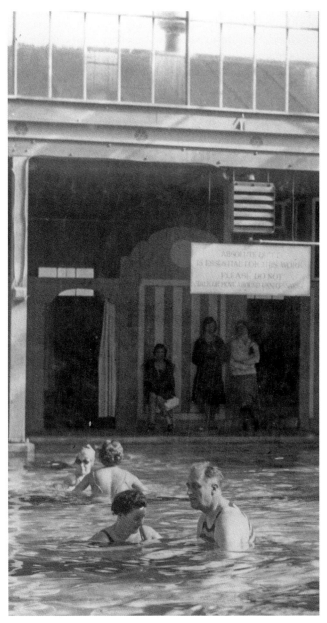

FIGURE 1-15 ■ Franklin Delano Roosevelt and other patients with polio exercising in a warm pool, Warm Springs, Georgia, 1924. FDR is in the center, being assisted by a physical therapist. The sign in the back reads "Absolute quiet is essential for this work. Please do not talk or move around unnecessarily." (Photo courtesy of Franklin Delano Roosevelt National Library, Hyde Park, New York.)

which became a haven for polio survivors. All patients at the institute worked in the pool every morning, then rested in the warm sun. In the water, their exercise consisted of contracting their muscles as much as possible, with therapists guiding and supporting their limbs and providing only a slight extra stretch at the end of each movement. Many patients also received other hydrotherapy treatments, including hot moist packs, percussion douches, and paraffin dips. **Hubbard** tanks, basically small swimming pools in which one person could exercise in warm water, were designed and tested there for use where large pools were not available. (See Box 7-1.)

Although the Battle Creek Sanitarium and similar institutions had shut down during the Great Depression, when their formerly well-to-do patrons were no longer able to afford the cure, water treatments were still used by some in mainstream medicine. Nurses still carried out many of the hydrotherapy treatments prescribed by doctors, nursing schools taught hydrotherapy techniques and massage until the middle of the century (1950), and hydrotherapy continued to be used to treat many medical conditions. For example, the Brand bath, invented by German physician Ernest Brand, was an extreme treatment used to treat the high fever common in typhoid. This bath was given anytime the patient's fever rose over 101°F and during convalescence. The feverish patient was taken directly out of bed into a whole-body bath of 65°F water; there he or she was rubbed vigorously without stopping, while every few minutes, gallons of even colder water were poured over the patient's head. After 15 minutes in the bath, the patient was dried and wrapped in a dry sheet with hot water bottles at the feet. Later, after improved water quality produced a gradual drop in the number of typhoid cases, the Brand bath went out of use. (Although 36 in 100,000 Americans had typhoid in 1900, by 1935 fewer than a tenth of that number did).

After the invention of antibiotics, many hydrotherapy treatments for infectious illnesses were no longer used, but until then water treatments were state of the art in medicine. Both naturopathic and some regular doctors used hydrotherapy treatments to treat infectious diseases and postsurgical infections. The numerous treatments to cool feverish patients included cold affusions, cold baths, wet sheet packs, and cold ablutions combined with friction to the skin. **Contrast treatments** of the chest were routinely given after surgery to prevent pneumonia, and fever treatments—using hot baths or electric light boxes—were used in acute bronchitis, scarlet fever, gonorrhea, influenza, rheumatic fever, syphilis, and other conditions. Such treatments were common until the introduction of penicillin in 1943. A key difference between treatment of these infections with hydrotherapy and treatment with antibiotics is that while both aim to kill the microorganism that causes the disease, hydrotherapy treatments also aim to stimulate the body's defenses.

Chronic illnesses also continued to be treated with hydrotherapy. As late as 1937, the *Journal of the American Medical Association* was publishing articles affirming the value of spa therapy for "chronic disabling conditions, including those affecting the heart and circulation, rheumatic disorders, ailments of the stomach, intestinal tract, gallbladder and liver, nervous conditions, certain disorders of the skin, and some metabolic diseases."(8[p3])

Neutral or tepid baths continued to be used for mental illness—often a chronic illness at this time—and hydrotherapy became a "scientific" treatment in mental hospitals. And finally, nurses who were trained in hydrotherapy techniques were still common in many locations. Retired nurse Barbara Phillips, who grew up in Saskatchewan, Canada, remembers being treated in 1945 by a woman who made house calls when people were ill; Phillips, then 7 years old, was given a contrast treatment of the chest and a mustard plaster, along with massage, to treat a cold. (Phillips, B., personal communication with author, Corvallis, Oregon, November 2005.)

Hydrotherapy and Seventh-Day Adventist and Naturopathic Physicians

In the latter half of the twentieth century, with the advent of antibiotics and other medical advances and a trend toward less labor-intensive treatments, the popularity of hydrotherapy waned even more. Although patients continued to crave personal attention and touch from their health care providers, nurses and physical therapists were no longer trained to perform time-consuming treatments such as hydrotherapy and massage. According to Robert Calvert, author of *The History of Massage*, "Even though massage was an integral part of the initial development of physical therapy, it was quickly replaced by mechanized exercise and manipulation. With the advent of medical technology, the focus of medicine changed from hands-on care to more clinically based medicine, from a small pharmacopoeia to more complex drugs, from simple surgery to more complex surgery. Medicine moved rapidly away from the hands-on, general practice that held out hope for massage becoming more widely accepted as a medical treatment for disease."(11[p114]) The same could be said of hydrotherapy techniques.

Hydrotherapy was still used extensively by a few hardy iconoclasts who were outside of the medical mainstream medicine, including naturopathic physicians and the allopathic physicians of the Seventh Day Adventist Church, whose commitment to follow the teachings of Ellen White led them to prescribe hydrotherapy treatments. These two small groups used hydrotherapy not only for musculoskeletal ailments but also for difficult and challenging diseases. Their commitment to "natural remedies" as opposed to pharmaceuticals and surgery meant that they continued to refine the use of hydrotherapy. For example, both types of physicians might treat patients with hypertension by weaning them from blood pressure medication, using neutral baths and massage to lower the blood pressure temporarily. (In the long term, however, the patient was taught to make lifestyle changes such as losing weight and eating less salt to keep the blood pressure low.) A patient with a diabetic foot ulcer might be treated with contrast leg baths and antimicrobial herbs rather than prescription antibiotics while being counseled on how to prevent ulcers in the future by adopting a healthier lifestyle, including contrast leg baths and regular leg massage to improve local circulation.

After the closing of the Battle Creek Sanitarium, the Seventh Day Adventist Church continued to operate health clinics staffed by allopathic doctors and nurses. In these facilities visitors with every type of serious chronic condition could be treated with natural remedies such as hydrotherapy, massage, exercise, healthy diet, and health education. Wildwood Hospital, near Chattanooga, Tennessee, an Adventist acute care hospital and health education center, was founded in 1942 and still treats inpatients and outpatients with hydrotherapy. Its hydrotherapy department performs about 40 treatments per day, and massage therapy is often combined with them. In 1981, *Home Remedies: Massage, Hydrotherapy, Charcoal and Other Simple Remedies*, by Adventist physicians Agatha and Calvin Thrash, summed up their approach to treating a wide variety of health problems. With 40 years of experience treating patients between them, the Thrashes felt confident that hydrotherapy could be a significant part of a drug-free approach to both acute and chronic illnesses and to a wide variety of musculoskeletal complaints.

Naturopathic physicians also continued to use hydrotherapy and massage in the tradition of the water cure, believing that "heat and water are two of the most powerful therapeutic agents available to any healer."(11[p12]) They continued to experiment with water treatments for new diseases and conditions. Hyperthermia treatments for HIV infection are currently under investigation. In one study by naturopathic physicians, patients with HIV were given a series of very hot baths. Researchers found that after patients' core temperature had been at 102°F for 30 minutes, the virus was 40% inactivated.(19) One important distinction between conventional hydrotherapy and naturopathic hydrotherapy is this: In conventional medicine, the effects of hot and cold water on blood circulation (blood quantity) are well understood and accepted. However, in naturopathic medicine, it is believed that enhanced blood flow through the organs of elimination, such as the skin, liver, kidneys, and bowels, will also improve the quality of the blood itself. Naturopaths believe that water treatments can accomplish this in two ways: First, they can increase desirable elements, such as oxygen, red and white blood cells, and nutrients in the blood. Second, they can decrease undesirable elements such as waste products.(14[p12])

Hydrotherapy and Physical Therapists

Aside from Adventist physicians and naturopathic doctors, however, hydrotherapy became increasingly relegated to the treatment of musculoskeletal conditions, such as arthritis, musculoskeletal injury, chronic pain, and neuromuscular conditions, such as polio. Even in this field, which was founded on the trio of massage, exercise, and water treatments, hydrotherapy became less popular. Physical therapists continued to use local heat treatments and local cold treatments but also continued to decrease the amount of time spent per patient. More elaborate water treatments and massage therapies were increasingly seen as too time consuming and were replaced with therapies that could be applied with equipment, such as diathermy, ultrasound, transcutaneous electrical nerve stimulation (TENS) units, and exercise equipment. Today water treatments are often limited to moist hot packs and applications of ice, and if massage is found in physical therapy, it is generally provided only in small doses and by a physical therapy aide, not by the physical therapist. A small percentage of physical therapists are trained to perform aquatic therapy in a swimming pool.

The autobiography of English physiotherapist Olive Millard, *Under My Thumb*, gives an interesting window on the evolution of physical therapy in Europe. Millard worked as a physiotherapist in Europe from 1913 to 1940. She treated the wounded English soldiers of World War I using hydrotherapy such as whirlpools, paraffin baths, contrast baths, and electric radiant heat, and later she treated patients from many countries and walks of life. Over her years in the profession, Millard saw a decline in the use of both water and massage therapies.(20) However, throughout this period hydrotherapy was always present in at least a small way in the form of hot packs and whirlpools and paraffin baths. The Warm Springs Institute continued to be a place for survivors of polio to benefit from exercising in warm water, but the expense of building swimming pools where there was no naturally occurring warm water made them far less accessible than today.

Two ongoing problems challenged the physical therapy profession: soldiers wounded in various wars (Box 1-3) and the polio epidemics of the twentieth century in developed countries. The first major epidemic in the United States took place in Brooklyn in 1916, and the number of cases increased gradually each year. There were 12,000 cases in 1943, 27,000 in 1948, and 57,000 in 1952. The Salk polio vaccine, first given widely in 1956, finally wiped out polio in the United States. Until a vaccine was available, however, physiotherapists in the United States and abroad continued to look for better ways to treat the effects of the disease. Sister Kenny, a self-taught Australian nurse, popularized the treatment

---

BOX 1-3 | *Point of Interest*

HYDROTHERAPY FOR SOLDIERS

Wars have been fought since prehistory, and injuries occur to soldiers both in combat and in accidents off the battlefield. The list of wartime injuries is extensive. It includes soft-tissue injuries from foreign objects, such as arrows, spears, bullets, and shrapnel; musculoskeletal injuries, such as fractures, dislocations, and amputations; nerve injuries; traumatic brain injuries; and spinal cord injuries. Along with massage, hydrotherapy has been used to treat war injuries from ancient times to the present. Native American warriors used warm springs to promote healing of wounds. Greek warriors took various types of baths to help heal injuries. The ancient Romans not only provided baths for their soldiers in their forts and military hospitals but also used springs in conquered areas as places for their soldiers to recuperate. In this century, the wartime wounded have been treated with a variety of physical therapy modalities, including massage and hydrotherapy. After World War I, American rehabilitation centers for soldiers contained massage rooms, douche rooms, pack rooms, and whirlpool rooms. Contrast baths, contrast douches, paraffin baths, whirlpools, and continuous baths were some of the hydrotherapy treatments used there. Many European and American spa towns, because they had hydrotherapy facilities already in place, became military hospitals. After World War II, treatment of injured soldiers continued to include massage and hydrotherapy; Hubbard tanks and heat lamps were now used as well as whirlpools and other water treatments.

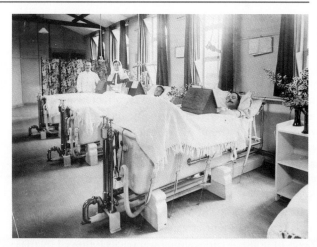

American soldiers being treated for septic wounds with continuous neutral baths. Note the inlet for hot water and outlet to drain cooling water, allowing the water temperature to remain at 98.6°F. Bathtub ward, British Red Cross Society Hospital, Richmond, South Africa, 1919. (Photo courtesy of the National Library of Medicine, Bethesda, Maryland.)

(continued)

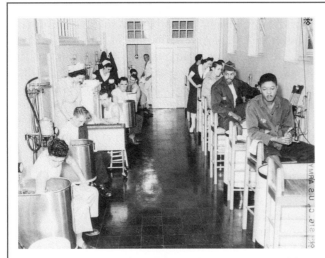

Whirlpool treatments for soldiers with injured arms and legs, U.S. Army Hospital, White Sulphur Springs, West Virginia, 1945. (Photo courtesy of the National Library of Medicine, Bethesda, Maryland.)

Pool exercise did not really catch on until after World War I, because of the expense of building indoor pools. Many soldiers injured in World War II recuperated at spas in Europe and the United States, and pool therapy had developed far more by this time and was increasingly used. Whirlpool baths were part of the physical therapy for soldiers after the both the Korean war and the Vietnam conflict.

Soldiers today continue to receive hydrotherapy for healing and rehabilitation. For example, at Walter Reed National Army Hospital in Washington, DC, the physical therapy department was ready for wounded soldiers returning from Afghanistan and Iraq at the outset of those conflicts and began seeing patients almost immediately. Most of the patients had orthopedic problems stemming from blast injuries (grenades and other explosive devices), trauma (fractures, amputations, disc injuries), gunshot wounds, or motor vehicle accidents. Other problems included traumatic brain injuries and herniated discs. A large percentage

of soldiers use pool therapy to strengthen muscles and maintain range of motion.

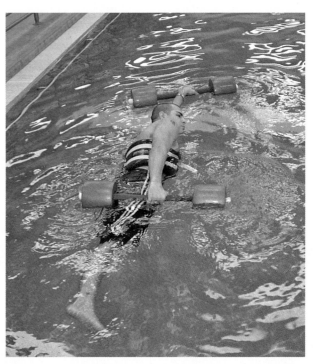

Pool therapy for an American soldier wounded in Afghanistan, physical therapy department, Walter Reed Army Medical Center, Washington DC, 2004. In October 2004, when Private First Class Joey Banegas was 24 years old and serving in Afghanistan, his right femur was amputated 6 inches above the knee in a bomb explosion. (Barbara Springer, PT, and Kyla Dunlavey, PT, telephone interview with author, November 2004.) He is shown working on core stabilization at a therapy pool at Walter Reed Army Hospital 4 months later. (Photo courtesy of the Walter Reed Army Medical Center, Washington, DC.)

of acutely ill polio victims using extremely hot fomentations, one every 30 minutes over affected areas. The intense heat helped relieve pain and loosen muscles, which allowed them to be massaged, stretched, and strengthened. It also helped prevent contractures. This treatment was an advance over the standard treatment, which was to immobilize affected areas with splints.(21) (See Box 6-3.)

In a 1998 radio interview, actor Alan Alda described his Kenny treatment at age 7, when he was in the acute stages of polio. Near-scalding hot packs followed by massage and exercise left him with no residual effects from the disease. According to Alda, the woman who saved his life, aside from his mother, was Sister Kenny. Alda related that before there was a vaccine, most polio sufferers either died or were paralyzed "until Sister Kenny realized that you could get the muscles that had contracted because of this disease—you could get them to open up

again through heat and massage. And just about 2 years before I caught the disease she was invited to come to America and she lectured all over America, and the doctors who treated me learned from her. . . it saved my life."(22) Sister Kenny also favored warm water exercise to reeducate polio-affected muscles, and the large number of postpolio victims who needed therapy spurred the development of this modality.

In both the United States and England, the use of hydrotherapy and massage in both rehabilitation and physical therapy in general has continued to decrease. By contrast, ultrasound, microwaves, exercise regimens, and electrical stimulation, sometimes accompanied with a small amount of massage, are frequently used. Although a few physical therapists are trained to perform aquatic or pool therapy, hydrotherapy treatments are most often limited to local applications of heat and cold for musculoskeletal problems.

Hydrotherapy and Nurses

At the same time that hydrotherapy and massage techniques were steadily decreasing in physical therapy, a parallel movement was also happening in nursing. Although water treatments and massage had been used together throughout history and were cornerstones of the profession of nursing in its early years, their use continued to decline. Modern nursing training in the West began in about the middle of the nineteenth century. At that time, nurses were trained to perform massage along with hydrotherapy treatments such as different types of baths, contrast treatments, and wet sheet wraps, and they used them in clinics, sanitariums, rehabilitation facilities, and hospitals. They performed water treatments prescribed by doctors, and in the hospital the back rub at nighttime was a traditional way for a nurse to help her hospitalized patients sleep without medication. By the middle of the twentieth century, however, nurses spent less time overall with each patient, leaving them little or no time for labor-intensive treatments, and massage was given little or no credibility as an important element in nursing care. By the beginning of the twenty-first century, nursing schools spent no more than a few hours teaching either hydrotherapy treatments (such as hot and cold applications) or massage techniques.

MODERN HYDROTHERAPY AND THE MASSAGE THERAPIST

As has been true throughout human history, whether massage and water treatments were part of mainstream medicine or not, there has continued to be a demand for them by the public. In the heyday of hydropathy, water treatments and massage flourished. Then, as we have seen, both gradually came to be outside of mainstream medicine. Even while massage was being relegated to the lowest rung of the health care ladder, however, it was still being taught and practiced outside medical circles—in public baths, athletic clubs, sanitariums, and spas, often in combination with water treatments. Health clubs, which usually offer steam baths or saunas along with exercise and massage, have a long history in the United States, and the warm water of natural hot springs has continued to be attractive to both sick people and healthy vacationers alike. With the exclusion of massage from mainstream medicine, however, by the middle of the twentieth century the average American came to see massage as either linked to prostitution or as a decadent indulgence for the wealthy, and this view often extended to bathhouses as well. Spas were commonly thought of as fat farms that were primarily for the wealthy middle-aged woman who wanted to dry out or lose weight. Unlike Europe, where serious therapeutic regimens at spas were believed helpful for serious problems and were paid for by health insurance, few people in the United States took them seriously.

Then, in the 1970s, several trends came together to return massage and water treatments to the mainstream. The growth of the human potential movement, a disenchantment with increasingly impersonal mainstream medicine, a renewed interest in wholistic health and "natural" lifestyles, and a far more mobile society with many people living far away from family have all contributed to this revival. While as late as 1975 some states required massage therapists to take annual syphilis tests, by the end of the twentieth century massage therapy had lost its association with prostitution altogether. It emerged as an independent, standalone therapy performed by professional massage therapists, who no longer necessarily have connections to physical therapy, nursing, or exercise therapies. These massage professionals practice in many environments, from spas, athletic clubs, chiropractic offices, and physical therapy clinics to hospitals, hospices, and private offices.

Spas of all kinds have emerged as well, from the day spa to the full-blown spa resort. This growth in spas has been especially marked in the United States, which unlike Europe, did not already have a strong spa tradition. By the year 2000, *spa* was a catchall term that could mean anything from a bathtub with essential oils added to the water to an exclusive health resort in an exotic locale. Spas have become a must-have amenity at resorts and large hotels, where they offer an exotic and ever-changing variety of treatments. Along with massage, true spas generally offer at least one whole-body hydrotherapy treatment, such as a sauna, steam bath, or hot tub. Spas increasingly market themselves as places not only to become more aesthetically pleasing and healthier but also to leave behind stress and tension.

Numerous new spins on spas have appeared, from spas for certain interests (spiritual communication, meditation) to medi-spas, which treat clients who want skin care, minor surgeries, even dental work. In 2004 the prestigious business magazine *Forbes* noted that spas were now big business, especially massage and water treatments. According to *Forbes*, "They're messy, they're wet, and let's face it, some of them sound a little strange, but hydrotherapy services are winning over curious spa clients."(23) Spa products, expanded spa training for massage therapists, and new employment opportunities in spas have helped bring the massage therapist squarely back to the historical association of water treatments and massage.

Today's massage therapist can specialize in many types of therapy and serve many kinds of clientele. A therapist may choose to work in a variety of settings, serving clients with a wide variety of special needs. With almost any group of people, the massage therapist who is knowledgeable about hydrotherapy can use water

| 2000 | 0 | 500 | 1000 | 1500 | 2000 |

BC | AD

2000: Construction of the great palace of Knossus on Crete, complete with bathtubs and a toilet that flushed. Pipes and drains were connected to clay sewers.

460: Birth of Hippocrates

312: Completion of Rome's first city aqueduct and its first great closed sewer, the Cloaca Maxima

33: 170 public and private baths in use in the city of Rome

75: Romans discover springs at Baden-Baden, develop them and name them Aquae Aurelia (waters of Aurelia). The following year, they discover springs at Bath, England, and name them after the Celtic goddess Sulis.

130: Birth of Clarrissimus Galenus (Galen), Greek physician, medical scientist, and medical writer

300: 900 baths operating in the Roman Empire outside of the city of Rome itself

400: Over 1,000 baths operating in the city of Rome, a phenomenal number considering the energy required to transport and heat he water needed for the baths.

537: Invading Goths cut the aqueducts to the city of Rome.

1100's: In Bath, England, the King's Bath is built out of the remains of the old Roman building.

1200's: Hospitals begin to be built in Europe

1242: Warm springs are discovered and immediately developed in Bad Ragaz, Switerland

1353: Karlsbad is discovered by Charles IV

1500: Private bathrooms and showers are introduced in Europe

1697: Publication of *The History of Hot and Cold Bathing* by John Floyer

1799: Birth of Vincent Priessnitz

1810: Construction of the first bathroom in the United States to have a bathtub, a sink, and a toilet, in a private house in Philadelphia

1804: Completion of the first water facility since Roman times to deliver water to an entire town (in Paisley, Scotland)

1821: Birth of Sebastian Kneipp

1829-1842: Vincent Priessnitz treats 7000 people in his Austrian mountain "water-cure"

1840: Birth of Simon Baruch, MD

1847: Ignazso Semmelweiss, MD, introduces the practice of handwashing between patients

1851: First bathtub installed in the White House in Washington, DC, and founding of the American Hydropathic Institute: a co-educational medical school in New York which was based on water-cure principals

1884: Publication of *My Water Cure* by Sebastian Kneipp

1898: Water mains are established in the large cities of Europe and North America, making running water available in the homes of many city-dwellers.

1901: First public baths in the United States opened in New York City, and the publication of *Rational Hydrotherapy* by John Harvey Kellogg

1903: Opening of Battle Creek Sanitarium

1919: First pool specifically for therapeutic exercise at Los Angeles Orthopedic Hospital

1920: Chlorinated drinking water available in cities across the United States

1923: Invention of constitutional hydrotherapy treatment by O.G. Carroll, Spokane, Washington

1927: Franklin Delano Roosevelt founds Warm Springs Institute for Rehabilitation

1928: Invention of Hubbard tank

1940: Publication of *Hydrotherapy in Psychiatric Hospitals* by Rebekah Wright, MD

1942: Public Health Service adopts first set of drinking water standards

1968: Jacuzzi tub patented by inventor Ron Jacuzzi

1980: Invention of Watsu aquatic bodywork by Harold Dull

1981: Publication of *Home Remedies: Hydrotherapy, Massage, Charcoal and Other Simple Remedies* by Adventist physicians Agatha and Calvin Thrash

1991: Founding of International Spa Association

FIGURE 1-16 ■ Timeline of European and American hydrotherapy.

treatments to enhance and complement the massage experience. For example, those working in spas can combine relaxing massage with salt glows, body wraps, and hydrotherapy treatments that require expensive equipment, such as Vichy showers. Those practicing sports massage can use local hot packs, ice massage, contrast baths, and whirlpools. Those working with physically disabled individuals may choose to move into a pool setting and practice Watsu. Those working with geriatric clients will find that hot soaks and paraffin baths ease the pain of osteoarthritis. Those working with children will find them receptive to warm applications, salt glows, and paraffin baths. Those working in a neighborhood health club will find that saunas and steam baths relax clients before massage. Those working with the terminally ill will find that warm baths and local applications of heat help ease pain. Those working in a chiropractic clinic will find hot moist applications and ice massage helpful to loosen muscles and make both the massage therapist and the chiropractor's work easier. Those practicing massage with a psychological slant may choose to incorporate flotation tanks or Watsu in their practice.

New technologies are also making many water treatments easier to do. For example, a steam canopy which fits over a massage table means that steam treatments may now be performed without the massage therapist having to find the money and floor space for a steam cabinet or steam room. New and innovative water treatments are sure to be developed in the twenty-first century, and more ways to make hydrotherapy even easier are soon to come.

CHAPTER SUMMARY

In this chapter you have learned about hydrotherapy's place in the history of medicine and how using water treatments can enhance the practice of massage. Because water is readily available, water treatments have been employed for thousands of years for a wide variety of health needs. (Figure 1-16 places the history of water treatments in a chronological context.) In the past, humans have tried whole-body and local water treatments. They have tried pilgrimages to springs, bathhouses, and spas. They have tried breathing steam, drinking water of various types, swimming, and using water as a solvent for herbs, salts, and minerals. The practice of hydrotherapy changes as a culture, its belief system, and the technology of the times change. However, over the centuries, through much trial and error, humans have discovered which water treatments are most effective. Although not all hydrotherapy treatments have been successful, use of water as a healing agent has recurred many times, particularly in combination with massage and exercise. Hydrotherapy, as we have seen throughout

our tour through history, will continue to be used—although its form may change with the time and place—as long as water is available. The many uses of water include controlling the body temperature, cleansing the body, stimulating the circulation, administering chemical solutions through the skin, providing an excellent medium for therapeutic exercise, encouraging relaxation, and even releasing emotional trauma—and surely more ways to heal with water will be discovered in the future. Massage practitioners who are knowledgeable about the effects and benefits of these treatments have a powerful, versatile tool to complement and enhance their expertise in touch.

REVIEW QUESTIONS

Short Answer

1. List 5 ways in which using hydrotherapy can enhance a massage practice.

   _____

   _____

   _____

   _____

   _____

2. Describe several ways that the healing power of water has been explained in different cultures.

   _____

   _____

3. Explain, step by step, how a typical bather would make his or her way through the different rooms of a Roman bath.

   _____

   _____

Multiple Choice

4. The Romans derived much of their medicine and bathing practices from
   a. Egyptians
   b. Ancient Greeks
   c. Invading Goths
   d. Celtic peoples

5. The water cure methods of Vincent Priessnitz had popular appeal due to all of the following *except*
   a. Actively promoted healthy lifestyle
   b. Novel and different from standard medical practice
   c. Retained concept of humors
   d. Advocated toxic remedies

6. Whole-body baths have been prescribed for all of the following *except*
   a. Thermal effects
   b. Internal cleansing
   c. Tonic effects
   d. Soothing effects

7. Massage has been paired with water treatments in all *except*
   a. Modern nursing training
   b. Roman baths
   c. Priessnitz water cure
   d. Turkish baths

True/False

____ 8. Water is a compound of two parts by weight of oxygen and one part of hydrogen.

____ 9. The wet sheet pack was used in the 1918 flu epidemic to treat high fevers.

____ 10. Historically, insomnia has been treated with continuous cold baths.

____ 11. Historically, local cold applications have been used for local swelling.

Matching

12.

____ 1. Herbal baths   a. Used for mental disorders
____ 2. Cold applications   b. Used for typhoid
____ 3. Continuous baths   c. Used for swelling
____ 4. Brand bath   d. Used for chemical application

13.

____ 1. John Harvey Kellogg   a. Greek physician whose ideas were the basis of medieval medicine
____ 2. Hippocrates   b. American physician and hydrotherapy professor
____ 3. Ignazso Semmelweiss   c. Viennese physician and proponent of handwashing
____ 4. Simon Baruch   d. Greek physician, father of modern medicine
____ 5. Galen   e. American physician, hydrotherapist, and sanitarium director

14.

____ 1. Alkaline springs   a. Bladder stones
____ 2. Sulfur springs   b. Scrofulous tumors
____ 3. Alum springs   c. Muscular weakness
____ 4. Alkaline springs   d. Paralysis

15.

____ 1. Control body temperature   a. Used to relax superficial muscles
____ 2. Adjunct to rehabilitation   b. Soothing effects
____ 3. Reduce stress on therapist's hands c. Mechanical and thermal sensations
____ 4. Stimulate skin   d. Make soft tissues more stretchable
____ 5. Relaxation and stress reduction e. Warm or cool client

16.

____ 1. Fomentations   a. Amputations
____ 2. Body heating treatment b. Deep relaxation
____ 3. Whirlpool   c. War wounds
____ 4. Swimming pool therapy d. Syphilis
____ 5. Watsu   e. Polio

REFERENCES

1. France RL. *Deep Immersion: The Experience of Water*. Sheffield, VT: Green Frigate, 2003, p 35.
2. Bruchac J. *The Native American Sweat Lodge: History and Legends*. Freedom, CA: Crossing Press, 1993, p 15.
3. Halioua B, Ziskind B. *Medicine in the Days of the Pharaohs*. Cambridge, MA: Harvard University, 2005, p 31.
4. Porter R, ed. *The Medical History of Waters and Spa*. London: Wellcome Institute for the History of Medicine, 1990.
5. Phillips E. *Aspects of Greek Medicine*. New York: St. Martin's, 1973, p 119.
6. Manjo G. *Man and Wound in the Ancient World*. Cambridge, MA: Harvard University, 1975, p 150.
7. Jones W. *Philosophy and Medicine in Ancient Greece*. New York: Arno, 1979.
8. Thrash A, Thrash C. *Home Remedies: Hydrotherapy, Charcoal, and Other Simple Treatments*. Seale, AL: Thrash, 1981.
9. Bettman, O., *A Pictorial History of Medicine*. 3rd ed. Springfield, IL: Charles Thomas, 1962, p 100.
10. Root-Bernstein R, Root-Bernstein M. *Honey, Mud, Maggots and Other Medical Marvels: The Science Behind Folk Remedies and Old Wives' Tales*. Boston: Houghton Mifflin, 1997.
11. Calvert R. *The History of Massage: An Illustrated Survey From Around the World*. Rochester, VT: Healing Arts, 2002.
12. Fatout P, ed. *Mark Twain Speaking*. Iowa City: University of Iowa, p 106.
13. Legan M. Hydropathy in America: A Nineteenth Century Panacea. *Bull Hist Med* 1971;45:267.

14. Boyle W, Saine A. *Lectures in Naturopathic Hydrotherapy*. Sandy, OR: Eclectic Medical, 1988.
15. Cayleff S. *Wash and Be Healed: the Water-Cure Movement and Women's Health*. Philadelphia: Temple University, 1987, p 87.
16. Baruch S. *An Epitome of Hydrotherapy for Physicians, Architects and Nurses*. New York: Saunders, 1920, p 14.
17. Numbers R. *Prophetess of Health: A Study of Ellen G. White*. New York: Harper & Row, 1976.
18. Kellogg JH. *Rational Hydrotherapy*. Battle Creek, MI: Modern Medicine, 1923, p 381.
19. Standish L et al. *AIDS and Complementary Medicine*. London: Churchill Livingstone, 2002.
20. Millard O. *Under My Thumb*. London: Christopher Johnson, 1952, p 20.
21. www.cdc.gov/nip/events/polio-vacc-50thtimeline.htm.
22. Alda A. Fresh Air Program. Philadelphia: WHYY National Public Radio, February 3, 1998.
23. Cademartori L. Water, water everywhere. *Forbes Magazine*, November 15, 2004, p 79.

7. Ferrell V. *The Water Therapy Manual*. Altamont, TN: Pilgrims, 1986.
8. Hembry P. *The English Spa, 1560–1815: A Social History*. London: Athone, 1990.
9. Moor FB, Peterson S, Manwell E, et al. *Manual of Hydrotherapy and Massage*. Hagerstown, MD: Review and Herald, 1964.
10. Odent M. *We Are All Water Babies*. Berkeley, CA: Celestial Arts, 1994.
11. Reisner M. *Cadillac Desert: The American West and its Disappearing Water*. New York: Viking Penguin, 1986.
12. Shorter E. *From Paralysis to Fatigue: A History of Psychosomatic Illness in the Modern Era*. New York: Free Press, 1992.
13. Smith N. *Man and Water: A History of Hydro-Technology*. New York: Scribners, 1975.
14. Watson L, Derbyshire J. *The Water Planet: A Celebration of the Wonder of Water*. New York: Crown, 1988.
15. Yegul F. *Baths and Bathing in Classical Antiquity*. Cambridge, MA: MIT, 1992.

RECOMMENDED RESOURCES

1. www.awwa.org (American Water Works Association).
2. Barclay J. *In Good Hands: The History of the Chartered Society of Physiotherapists, 1894-1994*. Oxford, UK: Butterworth-Heinmann, 1994.
3. Bruchac J. *The Native American Sweat Lodge: History and Legends*. Freedom, CA: Crossing, 1993.
4. Coleman P. *Toilets, Bathtubs, Sinks and Sewers: A History of the Bathroom*. New York: Atheneum, 1994.
5. Croutier A. *Taking the Waters: Spirit, Art, Sensuality*. New York: Abbeville, 1992, p 14.
6. Dosch NC. *Exploring Alternatives: The Use of Exercise as a Medical Therapeutic in Mid-nineteenth Century America*. Doctoral dissertation, University of Maryland, 1993.

RECOMMENDED MOVIES

1. *The Cure*. In: *The Chaplin Mutuals*, vol 1: 1917. www.image-entertainment.com. A short film starring Charlie Chaplin, who goes to a sanitarium to dry out and gets in hot water in a hilarious way. A classic massage scene is followed by his being tossed into the healing waters.
2. *Roosevelt at Warm Springs*. HBO-TV movie about Franklin Delano Roosevelt and his involvement with Warm Springs, Georgia, made at Warm Springs.
3. *Sebastian Kneipp*. A 1958 movie directed by Wolfgang Liebenerner, on location in Bad Wörischofen, about the life of Sebastian Kneipp.

THE SCIENCE OF WATER

When color photographs of the earth as it appears from space were first published, it was a revelation: they showed our planet to be astonishingly beautiful. We were taken by surprise. What makes the earth so beautiful is its abundant water. The great expanses of vivid blue ocean with swirling sunlit clouds above them should not have caused surprise, but the reality exceeded everyone's expectations.

—*E. C. Pielou, Fresh Water*

Chapter Objectives

After completing this chapter, the student will be able to:

- State the scientific definition of water.
- Describe several characteristics of water.
- Explain how various characteristics of water make it useful in hydrotherapy treatments.
- Explain how water stores energy and can turn from liquid to vapor or liquid to solid and back again.
- Explain conduction, convection, condensation, evaporation, and radiation and give an example of each.
- Explain why water is important to the maintenance of health.

The purpose of this chapter is to lay a foundation of knowledge about water as a substance, which will help you understand how its unique properties can make it a healing agent and an excellent adjunct to your massage techniques. (Figure 2-1 shows a few of those properties: the water in the bowl takes the shape of the container in which it is placed, its temperature can be readily changed, objects can float in it, and it comes in solid and liquid forms.) You will also learn about the scientific definition of water, its remarkable characteristics, and its essential role in maintaining human life.

WATER DEFINED

We begin our discussion by defining water: it is a colorless, odorless, transparent liquid, each molecule of which is a compound of two atoms of hydrogen and one atom of oxygen (Fig. 2-2). Water can take three forms—liquid, solid, or vapor—and it can readily be changed from one form to another. Water expands slightly when it is heated and contracts slightly when it is cooled, until just before it freezes it expands markedly. Many hydrotherapy treatments use water in its liquid form, which occurs at temperatures between 32° and 212°F (Table 2-1).

The natural beauty of water in streams, waterfalls, raindrops, and other forms is appreciated by everyone. However, because it is the most common substance on our planet, covering more than 70% of its surface, water often seems ordinary, and it is easy to take its remarkable qualities for granted. Water is something of an everyday miracle, though, and without it life on earth would not be possible. Although it may become clouds, rain, snow, or runoff, water in different forms flows continuously between ocean, sky, and land. In this process, known as **the water cycle**, surface water evaporates because of the sun's heat and becomes water vapor in the atmosphere (Fig. 2-3). After condensation, it falls back to earth as

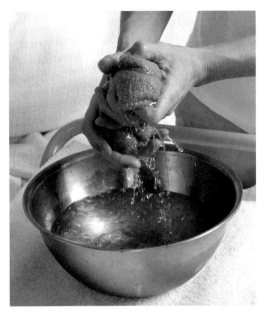

FIGURE 2-1 ■ Water has unique properties that make it an excellent adjunct to massage.

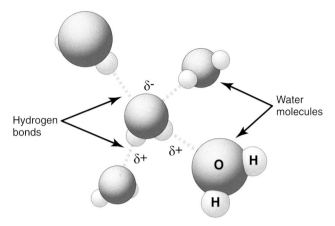

FIGURE 2-2 ■ Water molecules. Each molecule of water is composed of two atoms of hydrogen and one of oxygen. (Reprinted with permission from Prekumar K. *Massage Connection: Anatomy and Physiology.* 2nd ed. Baltimore: Lippincott Williams & Wilkins, 2004, p 20, Fig. 1-14.)

rain or snow and begins the cycle again. The total amount of water on earth remains constant.

Some examples of the major roles that water plays:

1. Water nourishes our bodies, feeds our livestock, and irrigates our crops: all plants and animals, including humans, must have water to grow and to maintain their tissues.
2. Water cleanses our bodies, our clothing, and our towns. The quality of our health and our lives would be vastly different without the hygiene provided by running water.
3. Water is a versatile healing agent: used in thermal, chemical, and mechanical hydrotherapy treatments, it can relieve stress and pain, help heal a variety of musculoskeletal conditions, and provide a wonderful medium for therapeutic exercise.
4. Water not only generates 25% of the world's electricity as it flows over dams, it is also needed to mine coal, drill for oil, and provide nuclear power. In some places, it still runs primitive waterwheels.

5. Almost nothing can be manufactured without the use of water: it takes 100,000 gallons to make one car, 1400 gallons to make a meal of one hamburger, fries, and soda, and 1500 gallons to make a barrel of beer. Furthermore, 69% of fresh water used in the world goes to agriculture (food crops, clothing, animal fodder). The United States uses almost 400 billion gallons every day.
6. Rivers, lakes, and oceans provide a means of transportation for goods and people. All of the great cities of the modern world grew up on waterfronts.
7. Water sports such as swimming, sailing, canoeing, fishing, water skiing, and sailing are an important form of recreation that is deeply important to many people.

CHARACTERISTICS OF WATER

The characteristics of water that make it uniquely useful for healing treatments are discussed next.

TABLE 2-1 FORMS OF WATER			
Temperature Range	Ice <32°F (0°C)	Water 32–212°F (0–100°C)	Steam >212°F (100°C)
Effects of cooling or heating	Molecules move farther apart when cooled, making it less dense than liquid; volume increases by 11% over liquid (100 tsp of liquid makes 111 tsp of ice)	Expands slightly when heated; contracts slightly when cooled	When heated, changes from a liquid to a vapor
Action when applied to the body	Absorbs body heat	Below 98°F, absorbs body heat; at neutral temperature, neither absorbs body heat nor transfers heat to the body; above 98°F transfers heat to the body	Transfers heat to the body

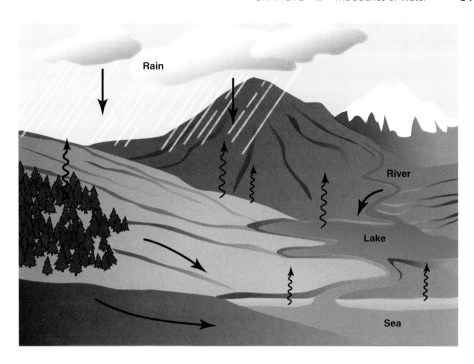

FIGURE 2-3 ■ The water cycle.

ABUNDANT

Although water is a natural resource that must be carefully conserved, it remains one of the most abundant resources for healing. Running water is available in virtually every office and home in the United States, and almost every household has a bathtub or shower which can be used for basic hydrotherapy treatments such as warm baths or contrast showers.

AFFORDABLE

Water is one of the least expensive resources for healing purposes. In the United States, the average price of water is about 0.2¢ per gallon, or $2 for every 1000 gallons. A typical bathtub holds 30 gallons, making a warm bath an inexpensive treatment compared to other types of products used for relaxation, such as prescription medications, nutritional supplements, or products containing herbs or essential oils.

WEIGHS 8 POUNDS/GALLONS

One way to feel the weight of water is to venture into the water of a hot tub, swimming pool, or lake: the deeper you go, the greater the weight and pressure of the water above you. (Dams are much thicker at the base than at the top because the base has to withstand much greater pressure from the accumulated weight of the water pressing down on it.) For this reason, we feel increasing pressure in our ears as we swim deeper. The force water exerts on a submerged body is called **hydrostatic pressure**. A person of

average height who is standing immersed in water up to the neck will be under a water pressure of 1.74 pounds per square inch.(1) At that depth, on average, 700 millileters of blood moves from the limbs to the thorax: with the weight of more water pressing upon the lower part of the body, fluid in the legs is squeezed upward like toothpaste out of a tube. For more information on how this effect of underwater immersion has been used to treat medical problems, see Box 2-1.

VERSATILE

One reason that water can be used for many different healing treatments is its great versatility. Because it can be take many shapes and forms, it is suitable for a wide variety of treatments, from ice to liquid water to steam.

All fluids conform to the size or shape of the container they are put in, and liquid water is no exception. Water can be used in everything from cups for ice massage to sponges full of holes, and from a metal tank in which moist packs are stored to a hose that can apply water at high pressure. This property makes it easy to apply water in a way that conforms to body shapes and contours. For example, for local treatments such as compresses, hot packs, and ice packs, water can be "bent" to conform to body shape, or the whole body or parts of it can be immersed directly in water.

Water can be used in any of three forms by the hydrotherapist. Ice is useful for ice packs and ice massage, liquid water for direct immersion, and steam for treatments such as whole-body steam baths and local steam inhalation.

BOX 2-1 *Point of Interest*

UNDERWATER IMMERSION: USING WATER'S WEIGHT FOR MEDICAL PURPOSES

As discussed previously, a person who is standing in water up to the neck will experience greater hydrostatic pressure on the lower parts of the body than on the upper body, and blood will be squeezed from the limbs to the thorax. The body's blood pressure receptors sense that blood volume is too high, and urination is stimulated to bring it down Then, as water is excreted through urination, water must be pulled from the body's other cells to replenish it. As shown by a decrease in total hemoglobin, packed cell volume, and red blood cell count, the blood becomes diluted during the first hour a person is immersed, as extracellular fluid pulled from cells enters the bloodstream.

These effects mean that deep-water immersion may be an effective treatment for some medical conditions, including certain types of edema, lead-induced gout, lead poisoning, liver disease with **ascites,** kidney disease, and other conditions. For example, in **preeclampsia** a pregnant woman experiences salt retention, a rapid rise in arterial blood pressure, and a buildup of body fluids at the expense of blood volume. This is a dangerous condition which can endanger the health and even lives of both mother and baby. Various diuretic drugs can be used to combat this fluid retention, but their effects on the fetus are not well established, and so a drugless treatment may be preferred. Bathing up to the neck in a pool for a few hours has been found to effectively shift fluids from the limbs into the central body cavity, markedly increasing urination and excretion of salt.(1) Scuba divers who have chronic **lymphedema** have found that the hydrostatic effect of water has a similar effect to that of compression bandaging.(2) Pregnant women in water exercise programs have found that the hydrostatic effect upon the body reduces varicose veins and swelling in their arms and legs, improving overall body circulation and stabilizing blood pressure.(3) Another medical use of this hydrostatic effect, suggested by a physician who supervises marathons, is for cooling an overheated athlete: by immersing the athlete in a tub of ice water which is deep enough to submerge his or her trunk and limbs, the hydrostatic pressure squeezes blood back into the thorax, which helps to maintain normal blood pressure.(4)

References
1. Root-Bernstein R, Root-Bernstein M. *Honey, Mud, Maggots and Other Medical Marvels: The Science Behind Folk Remedies and Old Wives' Tales.* Boston: Houghton Mifflin, 1997, pp 44–58.
2. Chikley B. *Silent Waves: The Theory and Practice of Lymph Drainage Therapy.* Scottsdale, AZ: IHH Publishing, 2001, p 27.
3. Harper B. *Gentle Birth Choices.* Rochester, VT: Healing Arts, 1994, p 10.
4. Roberts W. Tub cooling for exertional heatstroke. *Physician Sports Med* 1998;26(5):1–3.

EASY TO USE

Water is easy to work with. Because it is a thin, mobile liquid—unlike thick liquids such as honey or lotion—it is easy to pour, easy to transfer to containers of various sizes, and easy to clean up when spilled. Furthermore, water volume is easy to measure; its pressure can be easily controlled when it comes out of a spray, shower, or jet; and its temperature is easy to monitor with a water thermometer.

STIMULATES THE SKIN

Cold, warm, or hot water stimulates the temperature receptors in the skin: the classical hydrotherapists called this stimulation the "thermic impression" and made great use of it. For example, a very short cold shower or bath was used not to chill the person but to give a brief impression of chilliness, which would stimulate the body to conserve heat through vasoconstriction. Pressure receptors can be stimulated by treatments which rub, spray, or strike the skin, and proprioceptors in muscles and joints are stimulated by the weightlessness we feel when floating in water. (Many hydrotherapy treatments combine thermal and mechanical sensations, such as a hot shower or a cold mitten friction). When water is mixed with various substances, additional skin stimulation is provided. Both oatmeal and baking soda baths impart distinctly slippery sensations to the skin; seaweed or clay baths give a grittier feel; and vasodilating substances, such as mustard powder, do not actually heat the skin but give a warming sensation.

OBJECTS FLOAT IN IT

Buoyancy is the ability to float. When something is immersed in water, it displaces as much water as it weighs: an 8-pound object placed in a tub of water will displace 8 pounds of water, which is 1 gallon. An 80-pound person will displace 80 pounds of water (10 gallons worth). This displacement is actually an upthrust equal to the weight of the fluid displaced, and it is this buoyant thrust that accounts for the apparent loss of weight that we feel when we get into a pool. Buoyancy is one of the primary attractions of both whole-body baths and water immersion while swimming or receiving Watsu treatment: when we float in water, it actually holds us up, and the pull of gravity is reduced. For those with musculoskeletal problems such as arthritis, or heavy people such as pregnant or obese clients, the sensation of weightlessness is a great relief. Figure 2-4 shows a group of Watsu practitioners using buoyancy by floating in a pool.

AFFECTS BOTH MIND AND BODY

The longer I lay in the clear hot water the purer I felt, and when I stepped out at last and wrapped myself in one of the big, soft, white, hotel bath-towels I felt pure and sweet as a new baby.

—Sylvia Plath, The Bell Jar

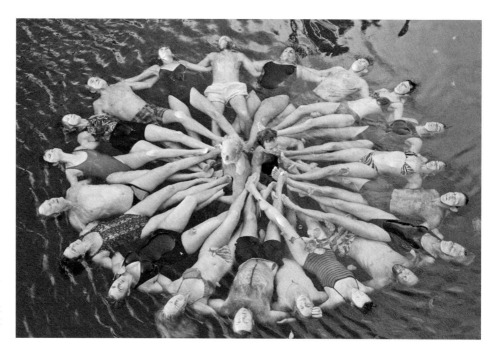

FIGURE 2-4 ■ Buoyancy. Watsu practitioners in a pool, Pahoa, Hawaii, 1994. (Photo courtesy of World Aquatic Bodywork Association, Harbin Hot Springs, California.)

In addition to the objective properties discussed above, sensations of soothing and nurturing are frequently linked with water. As discussed in Chapter 1, people the world over are drawn to thermal springs, to places where they can simply be near running water, or to bodies of water where they can swim and enjoy other water sports. In urban areas, even the water in fountains and bathtubs is relaxing and much sought after, linking city dwellers with rainfall, storms, mist, the shimmer of evaporation on a hot summer day, the tides that are ruled by the moon, snowfall, and rainbows.

Due to its relaxing effect, water immersion has probably always been used to improve mental and emotional states, and as far back as Homer, warm baths were recommended for relieving dejection and low spirits. The early hydrotherapists referred to baths as "hypnotics," and whole-body baths came to be used extensively in psychiatric hospitals during the first half of the twentieth century (see Box 1-2). In modern medicine, water immersion is in use for laboring women: warm baths are so relaxing that in many cases they can ease the pain of contractions and shorten labor, thus reducing the need for pain medication. For the massage therapist, helping clients to relax is of paramount importance, and the mind-body effects of water can help accomplish that goal, using full hot baths, saunas, steam baths, body wraps, moist hot packs, local baths and other water treatments.

Although it cannot be objectively proven, it may be that the soothing effects of water are connected in part to our experience in utero, when we float in amniotic fluid. As much as 1 quart of fluid protects the developing fetus from direct injury, helps maintain its temperature, allows it free movement, and permits hormonal and electrolyte exchange. After birth, many fussy newborns can be immediately soothed by a warm bath, and water continues to have a soothing effect from then on. Watch young children splashing in a pool, and you will see that they are euphoric, without a doubt in their natural element. *Deep Immersion: The Experience of Water*, by Robert France, is devoted entirely to the attraction of water immersion for humans.(2) Healers, scientists, and people who spend much time in or on water, such as swimmers, sailors, and kayakers, discuss its importance to them. Water immersion is a driving force in the lives of a great many people.

ABSORBS AND HOLDS BOTH HEAT AND COLD

Water can absorb and give off heat far more than any other substance. This means that when water is heated to a hot but safe temperature, it is capable of heating a body part or the entire body very efficiently. Cold water also has a great capacity to absorb heat; for example, if an athlete is treated for heatstroke by immersion in an ice water bath, his or her temperature can fall as much as 8°F in 15 minutes.

Because it is readily accessible and can absorb and conduct large quantities of heat, water is used as the standard for measuring **specific heat**, or the number of calories that is required to raise the temperature of 1 gram of water 1°C. (It takes 1 calorie to raise the temperature of 1 gram of water 1°C.) A lot of heat is needed to raise the temperature of liquid water, but water also holds more heat than most substances. Hot water holds twice as much heat as liquid paraffin, for example. When water cools, it gives off a lot of heat. So a hot, moist treatment such as a hot gel pack or **fomentation** gives off a lot of heat as it is in contact with the skin and gradually cools.

When 1 gram of liquid water cools 1°C, 1 calorie of heat is given off. Then should that 1 gram of water reach 0°C, or 32°F, approximately another 80 calories of heat must still be lost to change the water to a solid (ice). These extra calories are known as *latent heat*. Therefore, freezing water gives off large quantities of latent heat, and melting ice absorbs large quantities of latent heat: 1 gram of melting ice absorbs 80 times more heat than 1 gram of water being raised from 0° to 1°C. This makes ice a very powerful treatment.

To change 1 gram of liquid water to 1 gram of water vapor (steam) at 100°C requires approximately 540 calories, which is stored in the water vapor. Only 1 calorie is required to change water at 90°C to water at 91°C, but changing the form of the water requires a great deal of energy to disperse the molecules.

TRANSFERS BOTH HEAT AND COLD

Water is able to not only store heat but to transfer it in the following ways:

- **Conduction** is the transfer of heat by direct contact of one heated or cooled substance with another. For example, when an ice pack is applied to one part of the body, heat is conducted away from the skin onto the ice pack. This is the primary way that temperature exchange is done in hydrotherapy. Water can conduct heat onto the body many times better than air. This is why moist heat penetrates more deeply than dry heat and why hot, moist applications such as cloths wrung out in hot water will heat body tissues far more than even the very hottest dry cloth. **Autoclaves**—closed boilers that produce steam to kill fungus, bacteria, viruses, and other microorganisms—can sterilize surgical instruments, glassware, and other objects with steam in only 15 minutes, whereas it takes at least 2 hours to sterilize them in an oven with dry heat. Water is also many times more effective at inducing cold than air. If you were to go out into 55°F weather for 5 minutes with bare skin, you would feel cold but would quickly rewarm when you went back inside. If you jumped into a 55°F pool for 5 minutes instead, it would take far longer for you to rewarm when you went back inside, because the water would have conducted so much more heat away from your skin and underlying tissues than the air did. (When the *Titanic* sank, the only survivors were the passengers who went directly into the rowboats and remained dry. Even though the water was actually warmer than the air, not a single passenger who went into the water survived, even if he or she was wearing a lifejacket.)
- **Convection** is the process of transferring heat onto or off of a body by moving air or gas. Take, for example, a cold wind blowing warm air from the surface of a hot tub. The wind transfers the heat of the water to the air molecules, cooling the water in the tub much faster than if the air were still. Wind chill is another example of how body heat is lost to the environment through convection. To determine how cold it actually is outside, it is necessary to calculate not only the air temperature but also the speed of the wind, which will strip warm air directly off of a person's body. Moving currents of warm liquid or gas in convection ovens use the same strategy, but for heating: cold air is stripped off the food that is being baked, causing the heat of the warm air to be transferred to the food much faster, thus reducing cooking time.
- **Condensation** is the process which changes water vapor (a gas) into water (a liquid). This can be seen when you drink from a glass or can that is very cold. At first the glass is dry, but then it gets wet on the outside, and water sometimes runs down the side.
- **Radiation** is the transfer of heat through space without two objects touching, through the emission of heat. When a person who is overheated steps out of a warm bath and stands in the cool air with no wind, heat is transferred into the air through radiation. (If a wind comes along, heat will be lost even faster through convection, as discussed earlier.) Radiation is one of the main ways that body heat is lost.
- **Evaporation**, the reverse of condensation, is the process of changing water, a liquid, into water vapor, a gas. This happens when molecules escape from the surface of a liquid and become vapor. The molecules carry their kinetic energy with them, which lowers the temperature of the liquid, so the liquid and its surroundings are cooled. This evaporation is enhanced by air flow (draft) passing over the surface of the liquid, which prevents accumulation of vapor at the surface. Sweating in hot weather cools the body in this manner.

EFFECTIVE SOLVENT

By mixing them with water, a great many substances can be converted from a solid to a liquid state. Half of the known elements on earth are dissolved in our lakes and seas. More substances dissolve in water than in any other liquid, and so it is known as "the universal solvent." Due to its molecular structure, according to biologist Lyle Watson, water is "always grasping at other substances, gathering these around it, never content to be just H_2O."(3) Both seawater and freshwater contain dissolved air. Even a wind ruffling a lake's surface causes the water to absorb oxygen directly from the air, and fish breathe by extracting with their gills the oxygen that is dissolved in water. Because thoroughly saturating many substances with water dissolves them and makes them easier to clean or remove, water is used to clean up all kinds of messes. Many wastes are gotten rid of by simply diluting them with water and then pouring them down a drain.

BOX 2-2 *Point of Interest*

WATER IS EASILY POLLUTED

Pollution is a serious threat to freshwater and eventually to seawater. Industrial effluents and sewage are the two worst offenders. Some polluted water goes directly into streams and rivers, but much of it leaches into the soil and ultimately contaminates the groundwater. The illustration shows how easily water can carry pollutants because of its solvent properties.

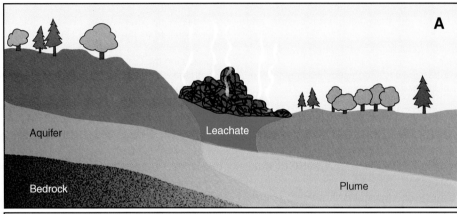

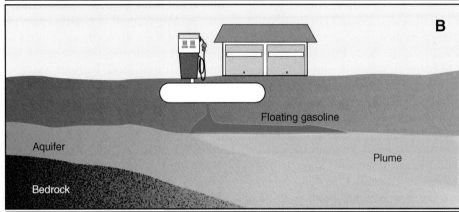

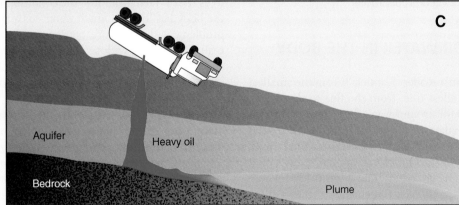

Water is easily polluted due to its properties as a solvent.

These are some common ways that water is polluted:

- Pesticides can be washed from lawns and farms into bodies of water.
- Grease or motor oil on streets can be washed into streams and rivers with rain or down a drain when someone hoses off a driveway, and 1 gallon of gasoline can contaminate approximately 750,000 gallons of water.
- Animal waste can be dropped directly into creeks from animals that are too close to them, or waste from feedlots can be hosed down and enter large waterways.

(continued)

- Dirt from timber harvesting on unstable slopes can run into creeks.
- Violent downpours on paved city streets can carry trash into sewers and rivers.
- Humans who camp near bodies of water can foul them with excrement, soapsuds, or dumped trash.
- Factories that use water to clean up their wastes can dump the used water into waterways, or if the water remains on top of the ground, it can leach into the groundwater.
- Fertilizers, which contain high amounts of nitrogen and phosphorus, can run off from fields into streams and rivers.
- Water can seep into landfills, mix with garbage, and leach into groundwater.
- Debris such as grass clippings, if dumped into stream channels, rob water of life-giving oxygen.

- Along waterways where there is little plant cover, dirt from construction can be washed into streams.
- Dirt at large construction sites can be washed down sewers.
- Rain that is falling through a sky contaminated with vehicle exhausts and industrial smokestack emissions will mix with them, become acid, and pollute the surface water it ultimately drains into.
- Water contaminated with nuclear wastes will eventually end up in the ocean. For example, fallout from the nuclear reactor meltdown in Chernobyl, Ukraine, eventually washed into the Techa River, which flows to the Arctic Sea. Nuclear wastes from the Hanford Nuclear Reservation in Hanford, Washington, have drained into the Columbia River, not only earning the Columbia the title of "the most radioactive river in the world," but resulting in those wastes ending up in the Pacific Ocean.

Unfortunately, due to its excellent solvent properties, water can become polluted with a wide variety of noxious substances (Box 2-2).

Most relevant to massage therapists, however, is how water's solvent abilities can enhance the healing nature of their work. In the health realm, water has traditionally been used as a carrier of medicinal substances which are meant to be absorbed into the body through the skin. Various salts, ground oatmeal, minerals, vinegar, Epsom salt, seaweed, clays, baking soda, essential oils, and a huge variety of herbs are among the substances that are added either to whole-body baths or to smaller amounts of water for soaks, compresses, body wraps, bandages, and poultices. The numerous minerals in seawater can be incorporated in hydrotherapy treatments such as baths and body wraps. Water is also mixed with substances which are applied to the skin as pastes, such as ground herbs, mud, and seaweed preparations.

THE NEED FOR WATER IN THE BODY

According to scientist Robert Kandel, "From the smallest bacterium to the tallest tree, from the flea to the whale, all creatures are built around water."(4) Humans are no exception: water makes up at least two-thirds of our total body weight. Our brain floats in cerebrospinal fluid, which is almost all water. Our blood, our tears, our sweat, and our saliva are largely water. The brain is 75% water, the bones are 22%, and even the enamel of our teeth is 2% water. Someone who weighs 150 pounds is composed of about 100 pounds—more than 10 gallons of water. About 2 gallons of this water is found in the alimentary canal, synovial fluid, saliva, and tears, and most of the rest flows through blood and muscle. Part of our self-awareness is constructed from sensing our own body water, and our language is full of phrases that describe it, such as "It brought tears to my eyes," "I broke out in a cold sweat," or "That made my mouth water."

The cells that make up our vital organs need water to carry out basic chemical reactions. Our bodies require 1 milliliter of water per calorie that we ingest in order to maintain our body temperature at 98.6°F, digest our food, process its nutrients, and eliminate its wastes. We can eat a healthy diet yet still be poorly nourished if we do not have enough water to absorb or digest the nutrients in it. Although we can live about a month without food, without water we die after about 10 days.

An average adult needs to take in 8 to 10 cups of water every day, although this amount varies with the person's body size and lifestyle and with the weather. People living in hot climates sweat more than those living in a cold climate and need to drink more water, and a highly active person exercising in that hot climate will need even more water than a sedentary person who lives there. Dehydration—the condition that occurs when the body has lost too much water—is a far more common problem, with far more consequences, than most of us realize. Every day we lose 3 or 4 pints of water in our urine, another pint disappears as we exhale thousands of times, and another pint or so is lost in sweat, and all of this water absolutely must be replaced.

Because water is critical to life, the human body has many sensitive mechanisms to detect and correct dehydration. Our kidneys continually monitor the amount of water and other chemicals in the blood, making constant adjustments to maintain just the right amount. Water is reused from saliva, enzymes, and intestinal secretions. If the body has more water than it requires, extra urine is made and excreted. When the body has lost too much water, the opposite happens: water is shifted out of the organs and into the bloodstream through osmosis, and less urine is made and excreted. Less saliva is made, too, and the mouth has a dry feeling. (Unfortunately, many people do not feel thirsty until they are very dehydrated, and by that time it is necessary to make a conscious effort to get enough fluids.)

Signs of mild to moderate dehydration include cracked lips, headache, irritability, lethargy, poor appetite, and malaise. If a person is prone to constipation or to urinary tract infections, being dehydrated will make these problems much worse. Because the brain is largely water, even mild dehydration affects its function. Severe dehydration can occur from a high fever, vomiting, diarrhea, or exercising in hot weather. Signs include weakness, dizziness, nausea, irritability, malaise, loss of appetite, dry mouth, sunken eyes, and dark yellow urine. More severe dehydration can be life threatening. Its signs include high body temperature, dangerously low blood pressure, disorientation, apathy, depression, aggression, and permanent damage to the central nervous system, liver, and kidneys. Babies and small children are particularly likely to become dehydrated quickly because of their fast metabolism, small size, and relatively large surface area. Elderly people are also more likely than most to become dehydrated.

Tips on preventing dehydration:

1. Make half of your fluid intake pure water. Try to drink small amounts often rather than huge amounts all at once.
2. Begin each day with 1 glass of water.
3. Serve a glass of water with every meal. Keep a spill-resistant water bottle in the bedroom and fill it every day.
4. Try different drinks that make water taste more interesting, including sparkling water, water flavored with a slice of lemon or a small amount fruit juice, herb teas, broth, hot lemonade, commercial or homemade rehydration drinks, and smoothies made with juice, fresh fruit, crushed ice, and/or yogurt.
5. Because caffeine is a diuretic, any food that contains caffeine, including soda pop, caffeinated tea, and coffee causes the body to lose water. Therefore, drink one glass of pure water for every glass of coffee, black tea, or soda pop.
6. Alcohol also causes the body to lose water. (Salty foods such as potato chips will cause the blood to lose water, as water is retained in the tissues along with the salt.)
7. Eat foods with a high water content, such as milk, lettuce, and watermelon.
8. When exercising on a hot day, drink water before exercising, every 20 minutes during exercise, and after exercise. A half cup each time is a good amount. Have water on the playing field at all times.

The quality of the water you drink is also important. Drinking water which flows through old household plumbing fixtures may have a high lead and copper content. For this reason, in 1987 the U.S. Congress banned the use of lead solder, pipes, and fittings. If you live in an old house with copper pipes, you may want to have your water analyzed to make sure it does not contain lead from the solder used to join the pipes. Home water filter systems can eliminate chlorine, chemical contaminants, parasites, bacteria, and pesticides from your water. Information on the water in your area can be obtained from your county health department. Fluoride, a chemical which discourages tooth decay, is likely to be in your drinking water, as it is added to municipal water systems in many parts of the United States and Europe. The chemical phthalate, a constituent of plastic, has recently been found to be present in some waters sold in plastic bottles; it may leach out of the plastic bottle and into the water.(5)

Hard water—water with an appreciable amount of dissolved minerals in it—may actually be a nutrient. Hard water contains more iron, calcium, magnesium, copper, zinc, nitrate and other minerals, depending upon where the water originates. A number of studies have found that living where the water supply is higher in minerals actually decreases the risk of heart attack, compared to living in an area with soft water.(6)

CHAPTER SUMMARY

This chapter explains how water affects not only our planet but our everyday lives in many ways, and the remarkable properties of water and how they relate to hydrotherapy. These characteristics include water's availability, versatility, ability to float objects, ability to store and conduct different temperatures, solvent ability, tactile qualities, and soothing and nurturing effects. Furthermore, you have learned about water's critical importance to maintain health. After reading this chapter and gaining an appreciation of the uniqueness and primacy of water in our lives, you are ready to look more deeply at the specific ways that water treatments can affect the human body and help heal clients.

REVIEW QUESTIONS

Short Answer

1. Describe three characteristics of water and how they are useful in hydrotherapy treatments.

_____

_____

_____

2. Explain conduction, convection, condensation, evaporation, and radiation, and give an example of each.

_____

_____

3. Explain how water stores energy

_____

_____

4. Explain why water is important to the maintenance of health.

_____

_____

Multiple Choice

5. All but one of the following uses water in a chemical application:
   a. Epsom salt bath
   b. Mud bath
   c. Whirlpool bath
   d. Aromatherapy compress

6. Water is necessary for the body to perform all but one of these functions:
   a. Carry out chemical reactions
   b. Digest food
   c. Absorb nutrients
   d. Control body temperature

7. Buoyancy relieves discomfort in all but one of these conditions:
   a. Obesity
   b. Arthritis
   c. Gallstone
   d. Pregnancy

True/False

___ 8. When an object is submerged in water, the amount of water it displaces weighs the same as the object itself does.

___ 9. Freezing and condensation absorb heat, and melting and condensation give off heat.

___ 10. Local treatments such as compresses, hot packs, and ice packs can "bend" water to conform to body contours.

___ 11. Because of water's ready accessibility and its ability to absorb and conduct large quantities of heat, it is used as the standard for measuring specific heat.

___ 12. The effect produced by the impact of water on the skin is a chemical effect.

Matching

13.
___ 1. Copper pipes   a. Death
___ 2. No water for 10 days   b. Irritability, lethargy
___ 3. 8 to 10 cups   c. Average daily adult requirement
___ 4. Mild dehydration   d. Lead in water

14.
___ 1. Solvent   a. Treats heatstroke
___ 2. Hypnotic   b. Warms body parts
___ 3. Heat absorbing   c. Dissolves other substances
___ 4. Heat conducting d. Whole body bath

15.
___ 1. Convection   a. The process which changes water vapor (a gas) into water (a liquid)
___ 2. Conduction   b. The transfer of heat through space, without two objects touching, through the emission of heat
___ 3. Radiation   c. The transfer of heat by direct contact of one heated or cooled substance with another
___ 4. Condensation d. The giving off of heat by the actual movement of heated liquid or gas

16.
___ 1. 60% to 70% of body weight a. Number of days survival without water is possible
___ 2. Composed of 22% water   b. 10 gallons
___ 3. 80 pounds   c. Water
___ 4. 10   d. Bone

REFERENCES

1. Davis B, Harrison R. *Hydrotherapy in Practice*. London: Churchill Livingston, 1988, p 61.
2. France RL. *Deep Immersion: The Experience of Water*. Sheffield, VT: Green Frigate Books, 2003, p ix.
3. Watson L, Derbyshire J. *The Water Planet: A Celebration of the Wonder of Water*. New York: Crown, 1988, p 23.
4. Kandel R. *Water from Heaven: The Story of Water from the Big Bang to the Rise of Civilization and Beyond*. New York: Columbia University, 2003, p 40.
5. www.nrdc.org/water/drinking/bw. Accessed winter 2005.
6. Kousa A, Moltchanova E, Viik-Kajander M, et al. Geochemistry of ground water and the incidence of acute myocardial infarction in Finland. *J Epidemiol Commun Health* 2004; 58:136.

RECOMMENDED RESOURCES

1. Kandel R. *Water from Heaven: The Story of Water from the Big Bang to the Rise of Civilization and Beyond*. New York: Columbia University, 2003.
2. Kamler K. *Surviving the Extremes: A Doctor's Visit to the Limits of Human Endurance*. New York: Penguin, 2004.
3. Pielou EC. *Fresh Water*. Chicago: University of Chicago, 1998.
4. Prager E. *The Oceans*. New York: McGraw-Hill, 2000.
5. Rothfeder J. *Every Drop for Sale: Our Desperate Battle Over Water in a World About to Run Out*. New York: Jeremy Tarcher/Putman, 2001.
6. Sinclair M, Von Weller A. Don't let the well run dry: The importance of water to your child's health. *Exceptional Parent Magazine*, May 2001, p 45–48.
7. Smith N. *Man and Water: A History of Hydro-Technology*: New York: Scribners, 1975.
8. Water Pollution Control Federation Public Education Program. *Water: The Lost Treasure*. Alexandria, VA: Water Pollution Control Federation, 1989.
9. www.awwa.org: Web site of the American Water Works Association. Contains information on a variety of topics related to water.
10. www.epa.gov/watrhome. Web site of the American Environmental Protection Association. Contains information on a variety of topics related to water.

EFFECTS OF HYDROTHERAPY

Humans must fiercely protect their internal temperature, for it holds the key to all their life functions. The human body is a mass of millions of exquisitely sequenced chemical reactions, which speed up as temperature rises. . . The timing, and thus the temperature of these reactions is so critical that if body temperature varies by more than 4°F from 98.6°F. . . the body's formidable defenses begin to crumble.

—*K. Kamler, Surviving the Extremes: A Doctor's Journey to the Limits of Human Endurance*

Chapter Objectives

After completing this chapter, the student will be able to:

- Describe the basic structures and functions of the circulatory system, the skin, and the nervous system.
- Explain the importance of keeping body core temperature at 98.6°F.
- Explain the physiological effects of local and whole-body heating treatments.
- Discuss the reflex effects of local heat applications.
- Describe the physiological effects of local and whole-body cooling treatments.
- Explain the reflex effects of local cold applications.
- Describe the effects of mechanical hydrotherapy treatments.
- Describe the effects of chemical hydrotherapy treatments.

The human body is an exceptionally fine-tuned organism that is capable of detecting and responding defensively to a huge variety of changes in the outside environment. A vast network of feedback mechanisms informs the body of threats to its homeostasis such as bodily injuries, dangerously high or low core temperatures, and dehydration. Many delicately paced and closely intertwined processes form the body's response to such threats. In this chapter you will learn how hydrotherapy treatments can affect the body in a positive way by taking advantage of its own homeostatic responses.

Depending on which treatments you choose and how you perform them, a wide range of physiological effects can be created. Treatments can stimulate, deeply relax, relieve pain, increase or decrease muscle tone, detoxify, relieve inflammation, soften connective tissue, alter body temperature, and even cause numbness. However, if you are to choose the hydrotherapy treatment that

best suits each client, you must understand how it affects the body and when it can or cannot be properly used. For example, a client with a migraine headache who comes in for massage treatment could also be treated with a hot foot soak and an ice pack to the back of the neck during a session, but not if that person is diabetic. A client who has a severely strained calf muscle could benefit from local ice massage before hands-on treatment, but not if that person has **Raynaud's syndrome.** If you have a sauna or steam bath at your facility, understanding the effects of a whole-body heating treatment can help you understand when it can be beneficial for your clients and when it could be dangerous. Box 3-1 lists some of the principles of hydrotherapy to keep in mind as you choose treatments for your clients. These principles are covered in greater detail later in the chapter.

This chapter also explains how three of the body systems most affected in hydrotherapy, namely the

BOX 3-1 *Point of Interest*

PRINCIPLES OF HYDROTHERAPY

1. *Hydrotherapy treatments use the body's own defensive mechanisms to promote healing.* For example, when a person steps into a short cold shower, the body reacts defensively against the threat of reduced core temperature by increasing many of its metabolic functions. When the cold shower is over, the person experiences an increased flow in surface blood vessels, increased muscle and tissue tone, increased function in the endocrine system, and a prolonged feeling of warmth.
2. *Water plays a different role in different kinds of hydrotherapy treatments.* For example, hot or cold treatments (such as hot or cold packs) affect the body primarily through temperature, and water's role in them is simply to transmit heat or cold. Mechanical treatments, such as frictions, sprays, or whirlpool jets, however, affect the body primarily by using water to apply pressure to the skin in various ways. Finally, chemical treatments which mix substances such as herbs, salts, and essential oils with water affect the body primarily through the chemicals absorbed into the skin. Here water is simply the medium which carries the chemical solution onto the skin. Use of water to heat the skin leads to an increase in local blood flow, which speeds absorption of the chemicals in the water.
3. *Many hydrotherapy treatments have multiple effects.* For example, an application of moist heat may be appreciated mainly to give the client a sensation of warmth, but it can also be used for its fluid-shifting (derivative) effect or for its ability to reduce local muscle spasm.
4. *Hydrotherapy treatments affect more than one body system at the same time.* Any treatment that is applied to the skin also affects the nervous system through the sensory receptors of the skin, and any hot or cold treatment that touches the skin immediately affects not only the nervous system but also the circulatory system. Clever use of reflex relationships can affect other parts of the body with one application.
5. *Hot and cold treatments may be performed specifically to change tissue temperature.* For example, when an overheated client takes a cold shower before receiving a massage on a very hot day, the direct cooling of tissues is the desired effect.
6. *Hot or cold treatments and mechanical treatments can redistribute blood or lymph within the circulatory system.*

For example, a contrast leg bath given to a person with a subacute ankle sprain before massage can reduce edema. Repeatedly dilating and constricting the blood vessels of the foot and lower leg pulls blood flow into and out of the tissues around the ankle, creating a pumping action that ultimately shifts edema out of the area.

7. *Mechanical hydrotherapy treatments stimulate not only the skin but the nerve endings, blood vessels, lymph vessels and muscles it contains.* Treatments such as salt glows, showers, whirlpool jets, percussion douches, brushing, and friction have an intensely stimulating effect that is similar to such massage strokes as tapotement and vibration.
8. *Hydrotherapy treatments can promote the absorption of chemicals into the body through the skin.* Herbs, salts, oils, minerals, and other substances containing beneficial chemicals can be dissolved in water and then applied to the skin through compresses, poultices, packs, steam inhalation, local baths or whole-body baths. For example, Epsom salts contain magnesium sulfate, which has a muscle-relaxing and detoxifying effect due to the presence of magnesium, a moisture-drawing effect due to its salt content, and a detoxifying effect due to the action of the sulfate.
9. *Some hydrotherapy treatments produce their results mainly through their effect upon the nervous system.* For example, ice stroking can deactivate trigger points and release muscle tension long enough for individual muscles to be gently but thoroughly stretched. Application of intense cold is not intended to cause tissue chilling or the fluid-shifting effect of vasoconstriction; instead, the desired effect, numbing the area, is a nervous system effect.

References
1. Buchman D. *The Complete Book of Water Healing*. New York: Instant Improvement, 1994, p 206.
2. Charkoudian N. Skin blood flow in adult human thermoregulation: How it works, when it does not, and why. *Mayo Clin Proc* 2003; 78:603.
3. Guyton A. *Textbook of Medical Physiology*. 8th ed. Philadelphia: Saunders, 1991.
4. Hayes B. *Five Quarts: A Personal and Natural History of Blood*. New York: Ballantine, 2005.
5. Kamler K. *Surviving the Extremes: A Doctor's Journey to the Limits of Human Endurance*. New York: St. Martin's, 2002.
6. Michlovitz S. *Thermal Agents in Rehabilitation*. Philadelphia: FA Davis, 1996.

circulatory, integumentary, and nervous systems, can be manipulated to enhance the practice of massage. (Because the body works as a whole, other systems play a part as well, but here we emphasize the systems most relevant to the practice of massage therapy.) Hydrotherapy treatments are applied to the skin and sensed by the nerves, and that information is communicated to the brain. Then, taking orders from the nervous system, the circulatory system reacts to those treatments. If massage therapists are going to use hydrotherapy treatments, whether they are local or whole body, they need to understand its effects upon these three systems. After a brief review of these body systems, we will consider the thermal (heat and cold),

mechanical, and chemical effects of hydrotherapy on the body.

ANATOMY AND PHYSIOLOGY REVIEW: THE CIRCULATORY SYSTEM, SKIN, AND NERVOUS SYSTEM

Before exploring the physiological effects of hydrotherapy treatments, we will briefly review the anatomy and physiology of three body systems that are particularly affected by them. These are the circulatory system, the skin, and the nervous system.

CIRCULATORY SYSTEM

The human circulatory system consists of blood and lymph, blood and lymphatic vessels, and the heart. It is responsible not only for supplying our cells with nutrients but also for cleansing them of metabolic wastes and foreign matter. Because most hydrotherapy treatments have a strong effect on blood vessels and can shift blood flow from one part of the body to another, it is especially important for anyone using them to understand the circulatory system.

In hydrotherapy terms, it is most useful to conceive of the circulatory system as what physiologist Stephen Vogel has called "a serial arrangement of pipes and pumps."(1) The pipes of the circulatory system are all of the branching tubes that either carry blood away from the heart and to the tissues (major arteries down to tiny arterioles) or carry blood and lymphatic fluid away from the tissues and back towards the heart (large veins down to tiny venules and lymphatic vessels of varying sizes). Arteries lead to all major organs and areas in the body, including the large arteries that supply 3 pints of blood per minute to the brain. Veins and lymphatic vessels drain blood and tissue fluid away from all these organs and areas (Fig. 3-1). Together, arterial, venous and lymphatic vessels form a container for all of the body's blood and lymph. (Fig. 3-2).

Each type of vessel in the circulatory system is specially constructed for the type and amount of fluid that it carries. Larger arteries are constructed to handle not only more blood than smaller arteries but blood that is moving faster and that is under higher pressure as well. Their walls are quite thick and contain both muscle and elastic fibers. Venous and lymphatic vessels carry the blood and lymphatic fluids that are returning to the heart; they are under less pressure and flow more slowly, and so their walls are much thinner and contain no muscle and little or no elastic tissue (Fig. 3-3). Exchange of oxygen, nutrients, and wastes actually takes place in the smallest vessels, the capillaries. There are some 7 billion capillaries in each of us. Human tissues are so densely laced with them that there is a capillary very close to almost every single one of our cells.

The pumps of the circulatory system force blood to flow from the center of the body through its pipes and out to the extremities and then force blood and lymphatic fluid back to the heart, mostly against gravity. These pumps include the heart, large arteries, skeletal muscles (including respiratory muscles), and smooth muscles found in larger lymphatic vessels. The primary pump is the muscular four-chambered heart, which contracts hard enough to raise the pressure of the blood and force it into either the lungs or the aorta. The heart is extremely responsive to the needs of the body. For example, when a person is resting, the heart pumps out about half of the blood that has come in during **diastole** (the rest period after each heartbeat when the heart fills with blood).

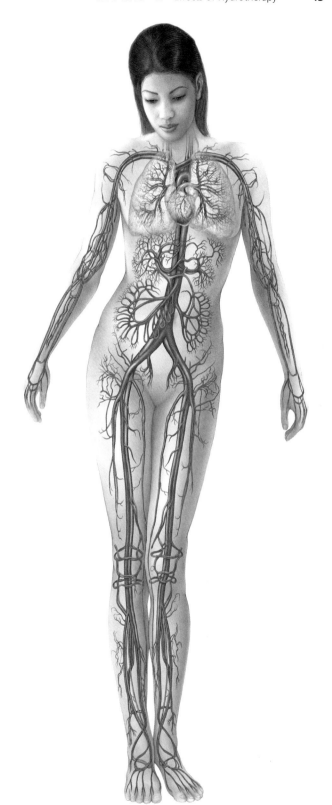

FIGURE 3-1 ■ Arteries and veins of the circulatory system. (Courtesy of Anatomical Chart Co.)

During strenuous exercise, however, it pumps out three-quarters of the blood that flows in during diastole. Incredibly, the delicate and durable human heart pumps about 100,000 times every day.

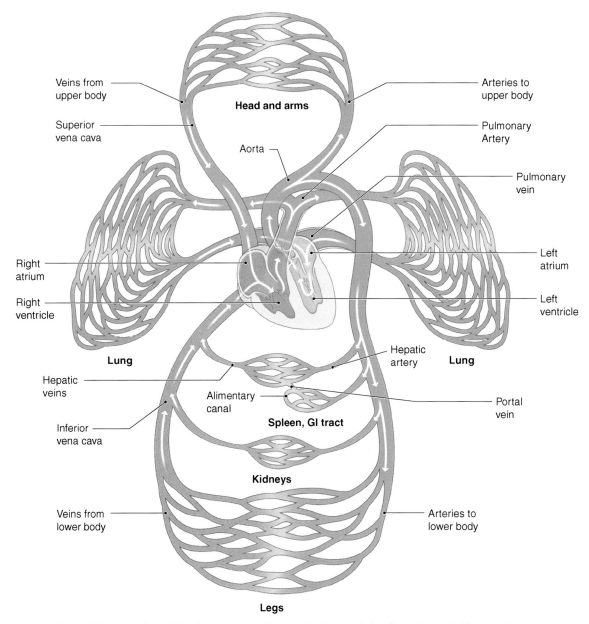

FIGURE 3-2 ■ Schematic plan of circulatory system. (Reprinted with permission from Archer P. *Therapeutic Massage in Athletics*. Baltimore: Lippincott Williams & Wilkins, 2007, p 46.)

In addition to the heart, the largest arteries act as smaller pumps. Because they are made up of both elastic and muscular tissue, the arterial walls stretch with each surge of blood that is pumped into them by the heart and then recoil like a rubber band snapping back. This action channels the intermittent waves of blood into one continuous stream and gives the blood another push onward.

Blood and lymph returning to the heart are pumped by the action of the skeletal muscles. For example, when the calf muscles are contracting and relaxing, the **lumen** (space in the interior) of the vein or lymphatic vessel is squeezed shut, and then when the muscles relax, a suction effect is created. This propels venous blood and lymph forward, speeding up the flow and preventing pooling of blood. Valves in the veins and lymphatic vessels prevent backflow (Fig. 3-4). Without this muscle pump, much of the blood pumped to the legs would not return to the heart. The movements of the respiratory muscles also help propel venous blood and lymph toward the heart. During inhalation, the intrathoracic pressure is less than the intra-abdominal pressure, and this causes suction of the fluids toward the heart.

Finally, smooth muscle in the walls of larger lymphatic vessels plays an important role in fluid transport because when it contracts, it forces lymphatic fluid toward the heart.

Artery

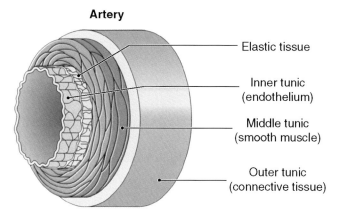

Elastic tissue

Inner tunic
(endothelium)

Middle tunic
(smooth muscle)

Outer tunic
(connective tissue)

FIGURE 3-3 ■ Typical artery showing layers of its wall. (Reprinted with permission from Archer P. *Therapeutic Massage in Athletics*. Baltimore: Lippincott Williams & Wilkins, 2007, p 47.)

Thus far we have discussed the pipes and pumps making up the container that holds blood and lymph. But what is the nature of those fluids? Blood makes up 7% of our body weight. It is composed of water, red blood cells, white blood cells, platelets, proteins, nutrients, antibodies, oxygen, carbon dioxide, and waste products. Urea, lactic acid, and other wastes are transported to the kidneys, liver, lungs, or skin for elimination. Nutrients in blood include water, fats, electrolytes, vitamins, salt, glucose, proteins, and carbohydrates, making blood such a nourishing substance that some animals, including mosquitoes, can actually use it for food. The temperature of blood is very important to the proper functioning of tissues and organs, so it is carefully monitored by the body. A 150-pound person has about 5 quarts of blood in the circulatory system.

Lymph, which makes up about 2% of our body weight, is derived from blood that flows through the capillaries.

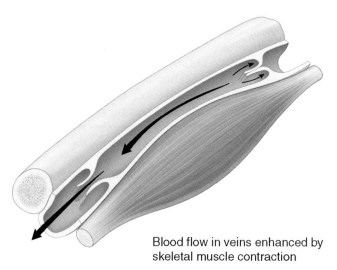

Blood flow in veins enhanced by
skeletal muscle contraction

FIGURE 3-4 ■ Skeletal muscle pump. (Reprinted with permission from Archer P. *Therapeutic Massage in Athletics*. Baltimore: Lippincott Williams & Wilkins, 2007, p 48.)

When blood, flows through the capillaries, some of its water is driven by hydrostatic pressure out of the capillaries and into the spaces around the cells. This water drains into the smallest lymphatic vessels, along with any bacteria, viruses, metabolic wastes, dead blood cells, large fat molecules, and leukocytes that are in the interstitial spaces. All of this together forms lymph. Drainage of lymphatic fluid removes excess proteins, bacteria, and wastes; prevents accumulation of fluid in the tissues; and can help fight local infections. Returning some of the water that escaped from the capillaries also maintains normal blood volume and pressure. Fluid is kept moving through the lymphatic vessels not only by muscle contraction and respiratory movements but by the contractions of the smooth muscle tissue of lymphatic vessels themselves. A 150-pound person has about 2 quarts of lymph in the circulatory system.

The circulatory system continually makes purposeful and coordinated responses when the body's equilibrium is threatened. However, no body system acts alone, and changes in the pipes and pumps of this system are usually a response to messages sent to it by the nervous system. For example, when a person is bleeding profusely, constriction of blood vessels in some parts of the body, such as the skin, will decrease their blood flow, making more blood available to vital organs such as the brain, heart, liver, and kidneys. The blood supply to the brain is protected above all because brain cells die in 4 to 6 minutes without blood flow.

SKIN

Human skin is a tough, supple, and complex organ with many important functions. Because hydrotherapy treatments are performed on the skin and rely on the skin's reactions for their success, it is especially important for anyone using them to understand these functions. Experienced hydrotherapist Agatha Thrash, MD, has stated, "Anyone fighting disease who will stimulate, cleanse, warm and protect the skin will have millions of robust allies in its versatile and talented structures." (2) Skin covers the entire body and consists of the epidermis on the surface, under that the dermis, and under that the superficial fascia (Fig. 3-5). In an average-sized adult, the skin covers about 18 square feet and weighs 10 pounds, which is roughly 7% of the body's weight. The skin is thinner in infants and children, reaches its full maturity in adulthood, and undergoes a number of degenerative changes in old age.

The epidermis is made up mainly of dead cells which have gradually moved upward from the dermis to the skin surface. The top layer of the epidermis, the stratum corneum, is constantly sloughing off dead cells, bacteria, and other pathogens. Below the epidermis lies the dermis. It is 100 times as thick as the epidermis, and it contains

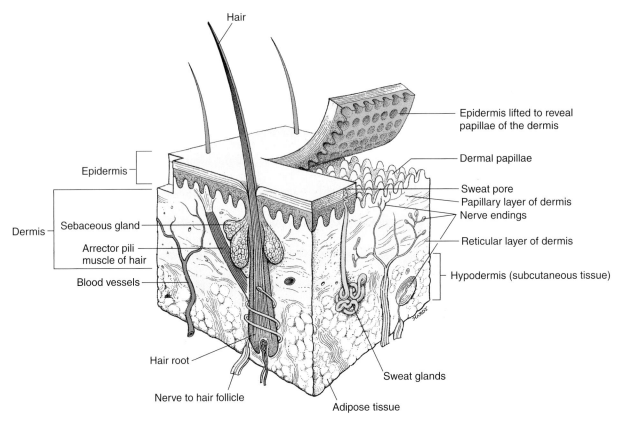

FIGURE 3-5 ■ Anatomy of the skin. (Reprinted with permission from *Stedman's Medical Dictionary*. 27th ed. Baltimore: Lippincott Williams & Wilkins, 2000.)

skin cells, hair follicles, blood vessels, sweat glands, various types of nerve receptors, many lymphatic vessels, nerve endings, and more than 50% of the immune system's killer T cells. All the nerve endings and hair follicles in the skin are supplied with nutrients by their own capillaries. The dermis contains so many blood vessels that when they are fully dilated, they can hold 25% to 30% of the body's blood supply at one time (Fig. 3-6). Under the dermis is the superficial fascia, made up of loose connective tissue. Nerves and blood vessels from the skin pass through this tissue, and tiny ligaments anchor the skin firmly to the soft tissues beneath.

The structures of the skin form a dynamic interface between our inner universe and the outer world. The skin, just by being intact, protects the delicate tissues of the body from sharp objects, harmful chemicals, extremes of hot and cold, and other dangers.

With its profusion of immune system cells, the skin is the first line of defense against many invading organisms. It also plays a vital role in controlling body temperature. Skin insulates the interior of the body and is a surface from which heat can be lost through vasodilation or retained through vasoconstriction. Body temperature can be raised 1° to 2°F through goose bumps (the contraction of the arrectores pilorum muscles in the dermis). Evaporative cooling through sweating is even more efficient at lowering core temperature than vasodilation.

Profuse sweating can actually remove 20 times the amount of heat that can be lost through the maximum vasodilation of the skin. The body contains about 3 million sweat glands, which are concentrated in areas that have large amounts of blood just beneath the skin, such as the face, neck, chest, palms, back, groin, and soles of the feet. Sweat glands are innervated by sympathetic nerve fibers, and if the hypothalamus is stimulated by excess heat, the message to sweat is transmitted via the autonomic pathways to the spinal cord and then to the skin.

The skin can also excrete metabolic wastes and toxins. During overheating, the sweat glands become very active, and toxins accumulated in the fatty layers under the skin can be metabolized and released. In general, the liver, colon, and kidneys are the organs most responsible for eliminating wastes, but when these organs cannot do their job, some of their wastes can be eliminated through sweat and sebum. In certain diseases, some toxic waste products are more readily handled by the skin than by the kidneys. Such toxic substances as solvents, nicotine, heavy metals, and amphetamines have been found in sweat. (For more on this topic, see section on Detoxification, Chapter 12.)

Just as the structure of the skin allows some substances to pass out of the body, its structure allows some substances to pass through it and enter the body. Because the dermis is so richly supplied with blood vessels, many fat- or water-soluble substances can penetrate the skin and

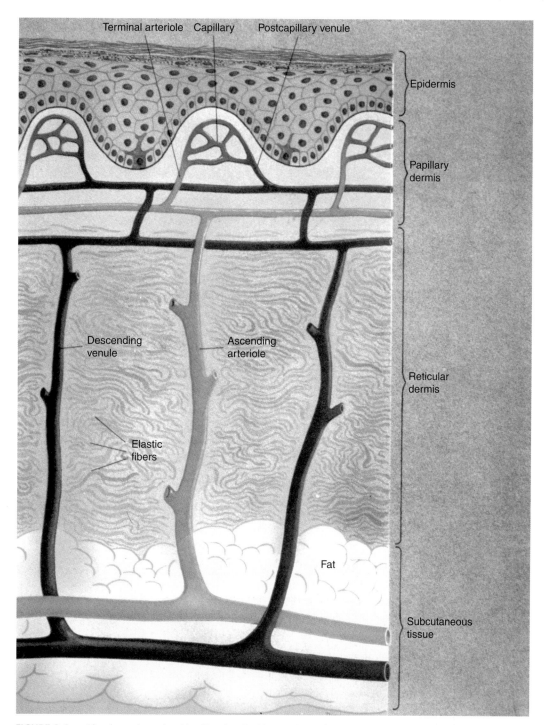

Terminal arteriole Capillary Postcapillary venule

Epidermis

Papillary dermis

Descending venule

Ascending arteriole

Reticular dermis

Elastic fibers

Fat

Subcutaneous tissue

FIGURE 3-6 ■ Blood supply to the skin. (Reprinted with permission from Rubin E, Farber JL. *Pathology*. 3rd ed. Philadelphia: Lippincott Williams & Wilkins, 1999.)

then easily enter the bloodstream through this network. These substances include the following:

1. Fat-soluble materials (vitamins A, D, and E)
2. Industrial chemicals, such as solvents (toluene), acetone, paint thinner, dry cleaning fluid, pesticides, chlorine, and heavy metals in a powdered form
3. Some minerals, such as magnesium sulfate (Epsom salts), if dissolved in water first

4. A variety of medications now administered with skin patches, including nicotine, estrogen, synthetic opioids, and nitroglycerine
5. Herbal preparations and essential oils

Perhaps the most important function of the skin is to keep the brain informed about the conditions of our external environment. Because it contains many specialized types of nerve endings which send the brain detailed information about the environment, the skin can detect a greater variety of sensations than any other of the body's tissues. Any kind of stimulation to the skin, from the tiny pressure of one raindrop falling on the face to the application of water with a high-pressure spray, is perceived and relayed to the brain in fractions of a second. Located about the thickness of a piece of paper beneath the surface of the skin, sensory receptors respond to stimulation by sending nerve impulses along sensory nerves to the **thalamus** (a part of the brain that receives sensory information, sorts out the information, then projects it to the sensory area of the cortex that is specific for that sense), where it is relayed to the brain's touch center in the somatosensory cortex.

Thermal receptors, which can detect warmth or cold, are one important kind of receptor. They tend to react more to changes in temperature than to actual temperature, and they respond to things that are hotter or colder than skin temperature (Box 3-2). For example, the skin can detect rapid changes in temperature of as little as

one-fiftieth of 1°F. This is one of the remarkably sensitive ways that the body's early warning system alerts the brain so that evasive action can be taken to avoid local injury (if tissue becomes too hot or cold) and to prevent dangerous changes in core temperature. In the body there are many more cold receptors, indicating that it considers cold more of a threat than heat. Heat-pain and cold-pain receptors respond to extreme temperatures. There are also many types of mechanical receptors, and they can detect light touch, tiny changes in pressure, fast and slow vibrations, and deep pressure. Some receptors for light touch cluster around the ends of hair shafts and respond to movement of the hair. This is why you can feel something that touches your hair even if it does not touch your skin. The input from hair follicles also helps you feel continuous movement across your skin.

Each type of sensory receptor is highly sensitive to only one type of stimulation. A tactile receptor will not respond to heat, and a pressure receptor will not respond to heat or cold. However, many sensations involve more than one

BOX 3-2 | *Point of Interest*

TEMPERATURE RECEPTORS CAN BE FOOLED

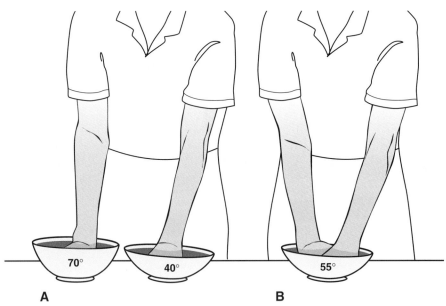

Temperature receptors can be fooled.

Put a bowl of hot water and a bowl of cold water on a table. Put a hand in each. After about 1 minute, put both hands in a bowl of neutral-temperature water. The hand that was in the hot water will feel that the water is cold, and the hand that was in the cold water will feel that the water is hot. This experiment shows that the receptors in the skin which sense temperature are better at sensing changes in temperature than absolute temperature. The receptors that were in the hot water got used to that temperature, so the neutral water felt cold; and the receptors that were in the cold water got used to that temperature, so the neutral water felt hot. This explains why when a person first gets in a moderately hot bath, it feels burning hot at first but soon feels comfortably warm—and why when a person first jumps in a cool (not cold) swimming pool, the water feels cold at first but soon feels comfortably cool.

receptor; for example, if someone touches you with something that is both hot and sharp, both heat and pain receptors respond. Or if someone touches you with something that is cold and heavy, both cold and pressure receptors respond. Many hydrotherapy treatments combine two types of stimulation to the sensory receptors of the skin. For example, a salt glow gives not only a mild thermal treatment from the water temperature, but a mechanical sensation from the sharp-edged structure of the salt crystals as they are rubbed back and forth over the skin. A cold whirlpool produces not only a thermal sensation from the water temperature but a mechanical sensation from the whirlpool jets.

NERVOUS SYSTEM

Composed of the central nervous system, the peripheral nervous system, and the autonomic nervous system, the entire human nervous system is sometimes likened to the control center for the body (Fig. 3-7). It is responsible for receiving a huge number of bits of information from the different sensory organs, then processing them in such a way that the appropriate motor response is made. For example, when a hand is placed in hot water, information from heat receptors is relayed to the brain, which determines whether the water is comfortably or dangerously hot and whether pulling that hand out of the water or plunging it in farther is the appropriate response; then the brain directs the muscles to perform that action. In addition, painfully hot or cold water can prompt a withdrawal reflex (the hand is pulled out of the water) before the signal even gets to the brain. Messages are constantly sent to the brain regarding the functioning of the circulatory system, and based upon that information, the brain monitors and adjusts the amount of blood being pumped by the heart, how hard it is being pumped, the temperature of the blood that vessels are dilated or constricted, the pressure in different blood and lymphatic vessels, and the chemical makeup of the blood. Fluids (blood and lymph) may be moved into one area and away from other areas. These kinds of corrections are sometimes achieved with direct nerve impulses to change the activity in an area, but often the brain directs secretion of a hormone which will cause the desired changes.

Central Nervous System

The brain and the spinal cord make up the central nervous system. The brain contains about 50 billion cells, and although it makes up only a small fraction of the body's total weight, it has very high metabolic needs and actually uses 20% of the body's oxygen and other nutrients. The brain is protected above all by the body's defense mechanisms, and receives first priority when it comes to available oxygen and nutrients. The spinal cord extends from the base of the brain to the base of the spine. It consists of gray matter (the cell bodies of nerve cells and their millions of dendrites) and white matter (nerve fibers that carry nerve impulses up and down the cord). Cranial nerves also bring to the brain sensory information such as tactile input, taste, sight, and smell.

Peripheral Nervous System

The peripheral nervous system is the part of the nervous system on the periphery, a network of small nerves that branch out from the brain and spinal cord and reach every part of the body. This includes the sensory and autonomic ganglia and plexuses through which the nerve fibers run. Spinal nerves, each with a sensory and a motor tract, branch out from the intervertebral spaces to various parts of the body. These nerves carry sensory information to the brain or carry motor signals out to the muscles. Information coming into the body from the periphery, which may tell the brain about pain, temperature, skin sensation, injury, or other conditions, can travel at about 300 feet per second. (In a 6-foot-tall person, this means a message can travel to the brain in one-fiftieth of a second!)

Autonomic Nervous System

The autonomic nervous system is the portion of the nervous system that controls the visceral functions of the body. It is made up of various parts of the brain, spinal cord, and peripheral nerves. Two of its major parts are the sympathetic chain ganglia, chains of large nerves running along each side of the spinal cord that link to many organs. The autonomic nervous system continually checks and adjusts conditions inside the body such as water balance, temperature, and blood chemistry. It helps control functions such as respiration, movement, secretion in the digestive tract, heartbeat, visual responsiveness, heart rate, blood pressure, and making energy available for life processes. This system can very quickly make adjustments. For example, when core temperature begins to rise, sweating can begin, the heart rate can double, and systolic blood pressure can increase or decrease dramatically in as little as 5 seconds. The two major subdivisions of the autonomic nervous system are the sympathetic and the parasympathetic systems. Most sympathetic nerve messages generally increase the activity of organs. For example, they can make the heart beat harder, the liver increase the release of sugar into the blood, or the pupils dilate. Parasympathetic messages generally cause organs to decrease their activity and work more slowly, causing changes such as a slower pulse, decreased release of sugar into the blood from the liver, or constriction of the pupils.

The **hypothalamus**, a small part of the lower front brain that is considered the central controller of the autonomic nervous system, contains an area that is specialized for monitoring and adjusting the body temperature. If blood flowing through this area is above or below the set point of 98.6°F, the hypothalamus adjusts the temperature

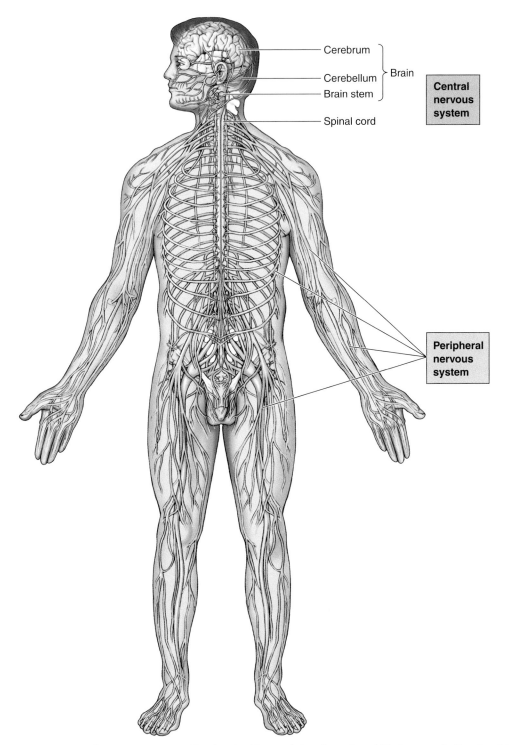

Cerebrum
Cerebellum } Brain
Brain stem
Spinal cord

Central nervous system

Peripheral nervous system

FIGURE 3-7 ■ The nervous system. (Reprinted with permission from Bear MF, Connors B, Paradiso M. *Neuroscience: Exploring the Brain*. 2nd ed. Baltimore: Lippincott Williams & Wilkins, 2002.)

through a combination of many defensive actions, such as increasing or decreasing the size of blood vessels and initiating sweating. There is also a thirst center that monitors the concentration of water in the blood. If the amount of water in the blood is too low, the hypothalamus sends signals which create a sensation of thirst.

Reflexes

A fascinating area of hydrotherapy is its use of **reflexes** to affect different areas of the body. Observant hydrotherapists have learned to take advantage of the body's reflex responses to enhance healing. Reflexes are body actions or movements that happen rapidly and automatically in response to possible danger (Fig. 3-8). When that danger is detected, sensory nerve impulses travel into the spinal cord faster than 300 feet per second. Once inside the cord, they pass directly to motor nerve cells, and a short circuit, or reflex arc, takes place. Motor nerve impulses go directly back to nearby muscles, quickly making them contract to carry out the defensive movement. Other impulses also travel up the cord to the brain, making the mind aware of what just happened but too late to stop the reflex action from taking place (Fig. 3-9). Our body functions rely upon a vast number of reflexes, most of which we are not even aware of. Common reflexes include the following:

1. The gag reflex
2. Blinking when something touches the eyeball
3. Flinching after touching something very hot
4. The knee-jerk reflex. That is, during a medical examination, when the kneecap is lightly tapped, the sensory signal from the quadriceps muscle spindle quickly produces a reflex twitch of the quadriceps muscle.

5. Blood vessel dilation in response to heat. That is, if the skin is exposed to a hot application such as a fomentation or a paraffin dip, heat receptors are stimulated and sensory nerves quickly carry impulses to the spinal cord, where motor nerves immediately branch back to the muscles of the skin blood vessels, causing them to dilate.

How does this information relate to hydrotherapy? Because the skin and the internal organs under it receive their sensory innervation from the same segment of the spinal cord, applications of heat or cold to skin areas reflexively related to the viscera can influence their function. Internal organs are usually reflexively related to the skin directly overlying them, but every part of the skin surface is also reflexively related to some internal organ or vascular area (Fig. 3-10). An application of heat or cold to the skin will affect the tissue directly under it to a much greater extent than the reflexively related organ. For example, an ice bag applied over the stomach may cause a brief change in the size of the blood vessels of the brain, but the greatest effect will be on the

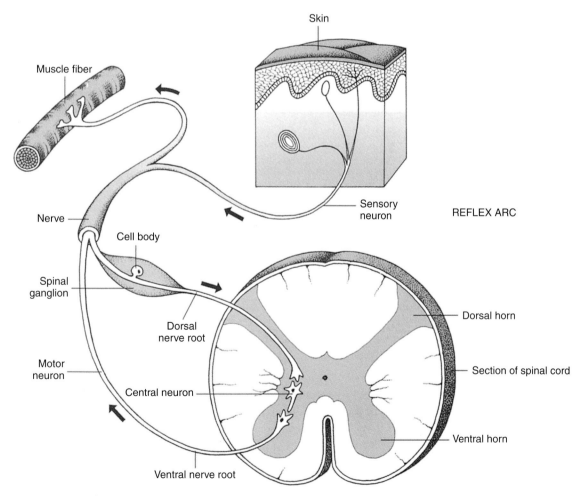

FIGURE 3-8 ■ Reflex arc. (Reprinted with permission from Werner R. *A Massage Therapist's Guide to Pathology*. 2nd ed. Baltimore: Lippincott Williams & Wilkins, 2002.)

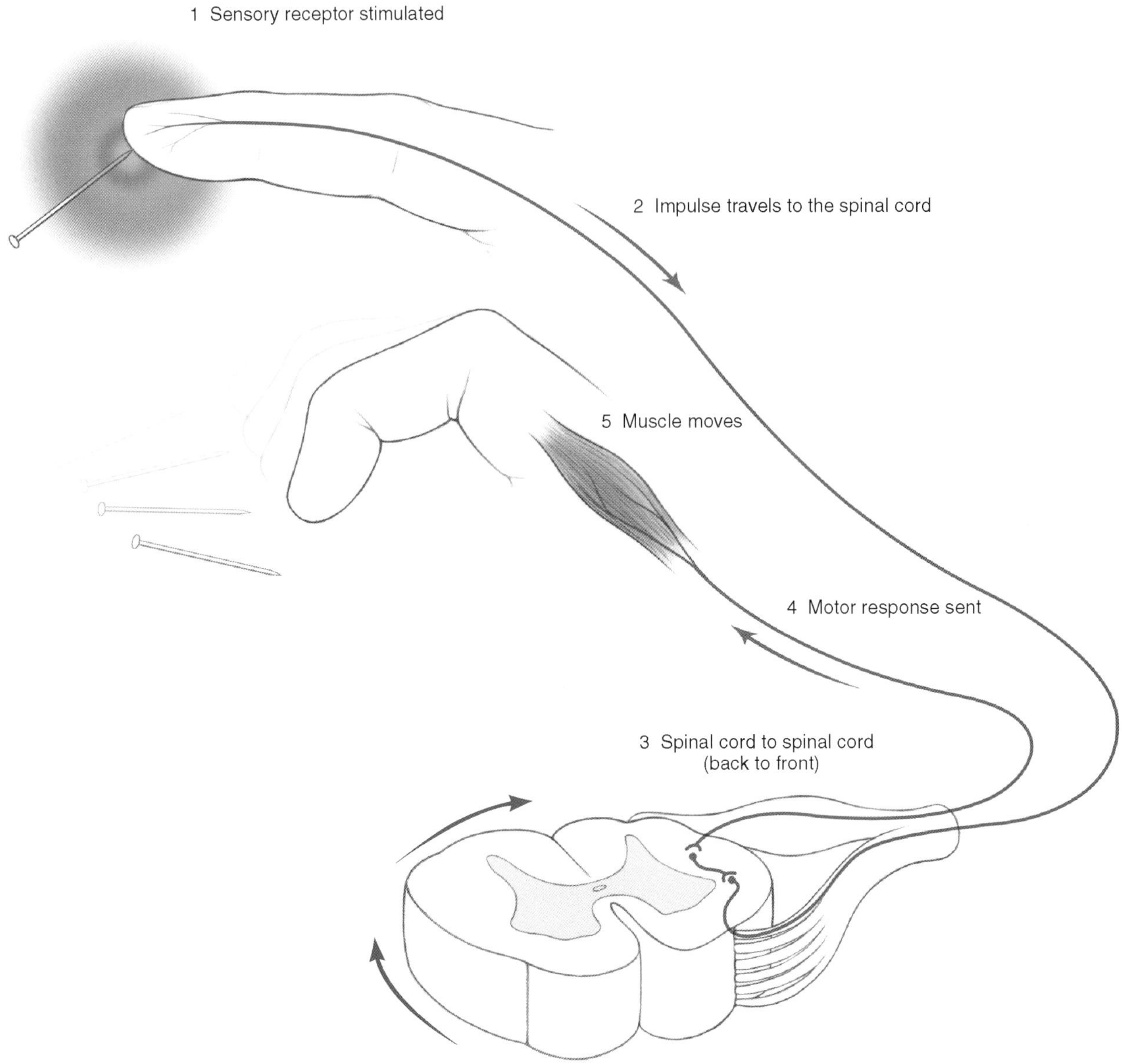

1 Sensory receptor stimulated

2 Impulse travels to the spinal cord

5 Muscle moves

4 Motor response sent

3 Spinal cord to spinal cord
(back to front)

FIGURE 3-9 ■ Reflex reaction. (Reprinted with permission from Dixon M. *Myofascial Massage*. Baltimore: Lippincott Williams & Wilkins, 2007, p 55.)

abdominal muscle directly under the ice. Although massage therapists will not be applying heat or cold for extended periods and do not treat problems in body systems other than the musculoskeletal, they need to understand how the body works as a whole and take advantage of the body's reflex relationships when performing hydrotherapy treatments.

PHYSIOLOGICAL EFFECTS OF HEAT AND COLD

Most hydrotherapy treatments are thermal; that is, they affect the body using temperatures above or below human body temperature. Heat and cold treatments cause dramatic changes in the blood vessels, chiefly **vasodilation,** widening of the blood vessels, or **vasoconstriction,** narrowing of the blood vessels (Fig. 3-11). Because blood vessels in local areas are still part of the circulatory system as a whole, changes in blood vessels in one area of the body can affect the entire circulatory system. For hydrotherapy purposes, it is helpful to picture the circulatory system as a closed system of pipes that hold a relatively constant amount of fluid, with pumps that move that fluid around. Anytime one or more pipes become larger through vasodilation or smaller through vasoconstriction, fluid must be redistributed within the system. For example, if the blood vessels in the feet are widely dilated by an application such as a hot foot soak, more blood will flow into them. If there are only 5 quarts of blood in the person's circulatory system and a large portion of that amount has flowed into the widely dilated vessels in the feet, blood

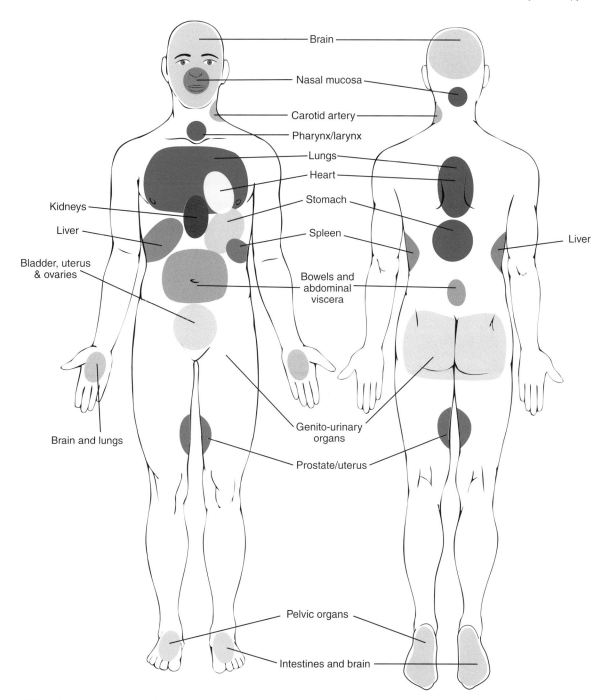

FIGURE 3-10 ■ Skin areas reflexively connected to specific organs and parts of the body.

flow in other regions of the body will be reduced. Another example of this fluid-shifting effect is immersion in a hot bath, which causes widespread dilation of blood vessels in the skin. As more blood flows to the skin, there is less blood available to the brain, so a bather may become light-headed. Still another example is an ice pack on the back of the head, which causes vasoconstriction and may relieve migraine pain by decreasing blood flow to swollen cranial vessels. Old-time hydrotherapists used this closed-system principle in many of their treatments; they termed these actions **derivation** (increasing blood flow in another area

of the body) or **depletion** (decreasing blood flow in another area of the body).

WHOLE-BODY HEAT

Whole-body heat treatments, such as hot baths, saunas, and steam baths, have a number of distinct effects on the body. These effects are often linked together in a chain of reactions. For instance, when a person is immersed in a hot bath, the skin temperature quickly begins to rise, which stimulates the heat receptors in the skin, causing

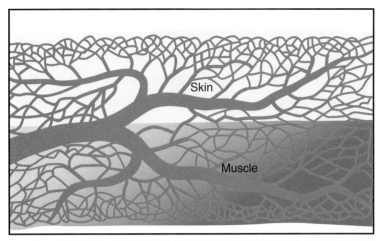

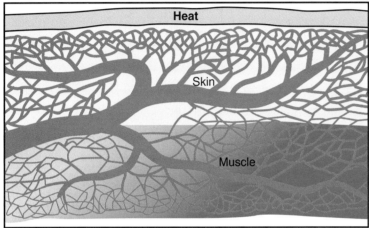

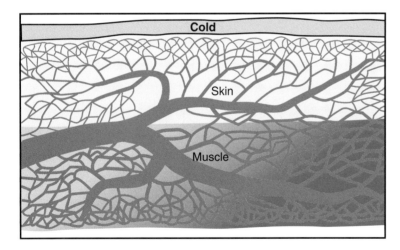

FIGURE 3-11 ■ The effects of hot and cold applications on the blood vessels of the skin and underlying muscles.

them to relay that information to the brain. (Although 98.6°F is the temperature of the vital organs [brain, heart, kidneys, and other viscera] deep in the body, normal temperatures are cooler nearer the surface of the body. Muscle tissues are about 94°F, subcutaneous tissues, about 92°F; and the skin itself, about 90°F.) The nervous and circulatory systems react quickly: the sympathetic nervous system causes vasoconstriction of the blood vessels under the skin, leading to a small, transitory rise in blood pressure. As the body begins to heat up, sympathetic

activity decreases and the blood vessels near the body's surface dilate. This creates more space for warm blood to flow to the skin, increasing heat loss through radiation. At the same time, constriction of the vessels of the viscera decreases blood flow there. With the skin blood vessels dilated and visceral vessels constricted, as much as two-thirds of the blood that the heart pumps may flow to the skin. When a person is in a neutral-temperature environment, the heart pumps approximately one-quarter of 1 liter of blood to the skin every minute, but when that same person becomes hyperthermic, that amount can increase to 6–8 liters per minute. When the response to possible overheating causes so many skin blood vessels to dilate, the available space within the circulatory system to hold the body's blood supply increases, which in turn decreases blood pressure. After a 10-minute immersion in a 104°F hot bath, blood pressure falls an average of 28 points systolic and 25 points diastolic.(3) At the same time, the heart rate increases: the heart beats faster to maintain perfusion (blood supply) to body tissues and to send more warm blood to the skin for heat loss.

If core temperature continues to increase, so does the heart's efforts to pump blood to the skin more quickly: for every single degree that core temperature increases, the pulse goes up about 10 beats per minute. In a hot environment, such as a hot bath, total cardiac output can increase by 60% to 70% over that of a neutral environment. During fever treatments, which involve periods of prolonged immersion in very hot water (104°–108°F), a person's heart rate may double as the core temperature climbs up to 102–104°F. As the heart pumps faster and faster, there is not time for it to refill completely after each beat, and so the amount of blood per beat (stroke volume) is reduced. One danger of hot baths is the possibility of becoming lightheaded: when a huge portion of blood flow is diverted to the skin, the brain may not receive its normal 20% of cardiac output.

Another effect of the increased body temperature is increased sweating. Although sweating can cool the body a great deal in most hot environments, it is not effective during immersion of the whole body, because the skin is surrounded by hot water and radiation off the skin is not possible. With the exception of the head, no heat can be lost through this mechanism.

In an attempt to eliminate heat through the lungs, breathing becomes faster. For every degree that the core temperature rises, the bather will breathe five or six more times per minute. Should the person begin to hyperventilate, the oxygen saturation in the blood will rise as well.

A rise in core temperature causes the number of white blood cells in the general circulation to increase significantly and remain increased for at least a few hours. This is the reason that whole-body heat treatments have been used for some immune system disorders (see Appendix C).

Connective tissue softens as it warms, and as skeletal muscles are penetrated by the warmth of the water, they relax. Musculoskeletal pain is often greatly reduced.

Very brief exposure to whole-body heat will not raise the core temperature much and thus will produce very different physiological effects than longer treatments. A summary of the physiological effects of both long and short whole-body heat treatments in presented in Table 3-1.

LOCAL HEAT

Applications of moist heat to small portions of the body are extremely effective not only for relieving muscle and joint pain but for softening muscles, joints, and other soft tissues before they are massaged or manipulated. Because hot packs, hot water bottles, hot local baths, hot compresses, hot moist towels, and hot moist heating pads are applied to the skin, their greatest heating effect is on the skin itself, while the subcutaneous tissues do not become as hot. If the application is hot enough, however, the muscle tissues underneath the skin and subcutaneous tissues will be warmed as well. (It takes at least 15 minutes for heat to fully penetrate the muscles.) Joints that are not covered with much soft tissue, such as the joints of the hands, may also be warmed. Effects may vary to some extent, depending upon skin temperature at the beginning, how hot the application is, and how long it is left on. For example, a hot fomentation, if it is put over an area that has been covered by an ice pack for a few

TABLE 3-1 THE EFFECTS OF LONG VERSUS SHORT WHOLE-BODY HEAT TREATMENTS

Effects	Long Treatment (>5 min)	Short Treatment (≤5 min)
Vasodilation	Complete	Not complete
Redness of skin	Present	Present
Heart rate	Increased	Decreases initially
Stroke volume	Decreased	No significant change
Systolic blood pressure	Normal or decreased	No significant change
Respiratory rate	Increased	Decreased
Muscle tone	Decreased	Increased
Blood flow	Up to 4 times faster	No significant change
Sweating	Profuse	No significant change
Migration of white blood cells	Increased	No significant change
Core temperature	Elevated	No significant change
Primary effect	Thermal, actual warming of the tissues	Stimulation of nervous system (tissue not significantly heated yet)
Physiological effect	Depressant and excitant	Depressant

The Hot Bath Homework Assignment

Sixteen students in a hydrotherapy class were given a homework assignment: to study the effects of a hot bath on their physical and emotional states. Each student recorded his or her pulse, respiratory rate, and oral temperature three times: before getting into a hot bath, after 20 minutes in the hot bath, and finally after getting out of the bath then having a cold shower and a 30-minute rest period. When the class assembled again, each student shared the experience, and the teacher wrote the change in vital signs on the board. Almost all reported that at the end of 20 minutes in the hot bath, their heart rate had increased significantly, their oral temperature rose at least 1°F, and their respirations were faster.

The only exceptions were students who were taking baths that were much cooler than their normal bath, students who were very cold when they got in the bath, and students who could not keep their bath water warm. Those students' heart rates, respirations, and core temperature did not rise because they were never sufficiently warmed by the bath water.

In addition to the information on vital signs, all except two students reported that afterward they felt much more relaxed mentally, and many fell asleep. The two who did not feel relaxed were the ones who could not keep their bath water warm and were chilled and tense when they left the bath.

Along with these similarities were some surprising differences. The preferred bath temperature varied widely among the students: one reported his comfortable bath temperature was 98°F, while another's was 108°F. One student felt so hot when he got out of the tub that he almost fainted, and the cold shower felt wonderful to him, while another student forgot to take the cold shower, cooled off rapidly in the cold air, and soon began to feel quite cold. The two who never became sufficiently warm in the bath found the cold shower extremely unpleasant.

Discussion Questions

1. Why did the student who forgot to take the cold shower cool off rapidly?
2. What does the case history tell us about the best way to help the client take a safe and effective hot bath?

minutes, will require more time to heat the tissues underneath than if that area was warm to begin with. Finally, the hotter the area becomes, the greater the reaction: every increase in temperature of 4°F doubles its blood flow, and oxygen and other nutrients are transferred from the blood to the tissues (Fig. 3-12).(4)

These reactions are caused by the local effects of temperature directly on the blood vessels and sweat glands, and by reflexes conducted from the skin receptors to the spinal cord and back to the same area. These reflexes help prevent excessive heat exchange from locally heated parts of the body.

The following are some of the body's protective reactions to local heat:

1. Dilation of skin blood vessels. When heat is applied to an area, sensory nerves are stimulated and cause local vasodilation. Increased blood flow to the area under the hot pack means that blood being warmed there will be carried off to other areas of the body, preventing that area from overheating to the point of tissue damage. (If the application is too hot, of course, even vasodilation will not prevent tissue damage).
2. Local sweating

3. Dilation of deeper blood vessels in muscle tissue as heat penetrates deeper. Local muscle blood flow can triple. Muscle tension is significantly decreased.
4. Reduction in muscle tone, muscle spasm, and muscle pain. For this reason, hot packs applied to trigger points can reduce pain during treatment.
5. Decreased muscular endurance in the heated muscle
6. Increased local metabolic rate
7. Increased oxygen delivery to tissues
8. Connective tissue becomes more elastic.
9. Heat applied to one limb causing vasodilation to the other limb. This is known as the **contralateral reflex effect**. The effect is not as strong in the limb that is not in direct contact with the heat.
10. Increase in core temperature if the application is very large or very hot
11. Reflex effects of prolonged heat on deeper organs. Prolonged applications of heat cause dilation of the blood vessels where the application is actually placed as well as in related viscera. Deep internal organs are more influenced by local applications of heat through their reflexive effects than by actual changes in the temperature of the tissues. For example:

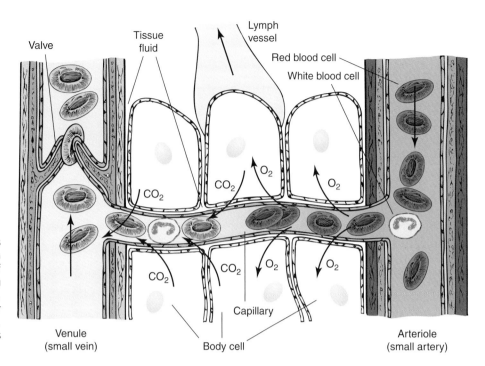

FIGURE 3-12 ■ Supplying the cells with nutrients. Red blood cells pass from the arteriole to the venule, dropping off oxygen and other nutrients and picking up carbon dioxide for elimination. (Reprinted with permission from Weber J, Kelley J. *Health Assessment in Nursing*. 2nd ed. Philadelphia: Lippincott Williams & Wilkins, 2003.)

Labels on figure: Valve; Tissue fluid; Lymph vessel; Red blood cell; White blood cell; CO_2; O_2; Venule (small vein); Body cell; Capillary; Arteriole (small artery)

- Prolonged heat to the abdominal wall causes decreased intestinal blood flow, decreased intestinal movement, and decreased production of stomach acid.
- Prolonged heat over the lower abdominal wall causes an increased production of urine.
- Prolonged heat to the chest makes breathing and expectoration easier.
- Prolonged heat over the kidneys increases production of urine.
- Prolonged heat over the pelvis relaxes the muscles of the bladder, rectum, and uterus; dilates their blood vessels; and can increase menstrual flow.
- Prolonged heat over the **precordium** increases the heart rate and decreases its force.

WHOLE-BODY COLD

The human body can endure heat far better than cold. At 82°F, an unclothed person who is resting generates exactly as much heat through metabolic processes as he or she loses through radiation, and no additional effort is needed to maintain ideal core temperature. The body has 20 times as many receptors for cold as for heat, showing that the body is more vigilant about core temperature being reduced than being raised. The body also reacts to cold temperatures more vigorously than to hot temperatures, which is why cold treatments are more stimulating than heat treatments. For example, a warm bath is far more relaxing than an icy-cold shower, but the strongest sensation of prolonged warmth afterward comes when the bath is followed by a cold shower, for the cold exposure has caused the body to increase its basal metabolic rate.

When a person first gets into a cold bath or shower and the skin over the entire body comes into contact with cold water, the cold receptors in the skin fire, and the nervous and circulatory systems quickly respond. Reflexes immediately increase the temperature of the body through inhibition of sweating, skin vasoconstriction, and shivering to increase the body's heat production. The sympathetic nervous system induces the blood vessels in the skin to constrict (reflex action), causing a rise in blood pressure, and the heart begins to pump out more blood with each stroke. Muscle tone is increased as well.

Should the person get out of the water after only one minute, he or she would feel invigorated. The generalized vasoconstriction floods the internal organs with nutrient-carrying blood, and the entire metabolism is stimulated. Reactive vasodilation of the blood vessels in the skin gives the person a prolonged sensation of warmth. These changes will last for a few hours. The person's body rose to the challenge of maintaining healthy core temperature by increasing many body functions, and the amount of time he or she was in the water was not long enough to cause any actual chilling. So with a brief exposure, cold immersion has been stimulating, not depressing.

Should one stay in the water longer, however, an entirely different reaction will take place. Vasoconstriction of blood vessels at the periphery of the body (skin and muscles of the arms and legs) keeps blood near to the body core, but the little that is coming back from the periphery is cold, which gradually reduces the core temperature. If the cold is beyond the body's ability to combat, core temperature decreases and the entire metabolism slows down. Breathing and heart rate slow, the muscles become clumsier and harder to move, the receptors in the skin do

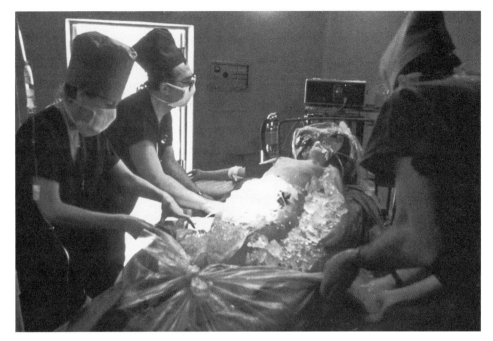

FIGURE 3-13 ■ Twelve-year-old girl being packed in ice before open-heart surgery in Novosibersk, Russia, 1994. As the ice cools this girl's body, her core temperature and heart rate will slowly drop, her metabolism will slow down greatly, and eventually her heart will stop beating altogether. When her core temperature has reached 84°F, her heart will be safely operated on without a heart-lung machine because her cells' demands for oxygen and other nutrients have been reduced to almost zero and, therefore, her brain and other vital organs can survive for an extended period without her heart supplying them with blood. (Photo by Heidi Bradner; Courtesy of Panos Pictures, London.)

not work as well, and thinking becomes muddied. (Clients who are in cold showers or baths too long may begin to chill and will be highly uncomfortable. Shivering and pale, they are likely to be tense, difficult to warm, and have an unsatisfactory massage experience.)

Should the person remain immersed, the body can become colder and colder, and an even more extreme reaction can happen. When the muscles in the blood vessels run out of oxygen and other nutrients, they dilate because they are unable to constrict anymore, the cold blood on the surface of the body returns to the body core, and real hypothermia sets in. Cold has been become a depressant. Interestingly, induced hypothermia has actually been used by Russian doctors as a way of depressing body

functions to allow open heart surgery without a heart-lung machine (Fig. 3-13). A summary of the physiological effects of long and short whole-body cold treatments is presented in Table 3-2.

LOCAL COLD

Applications of cold to small portions of the body are extremely effective in producing numbness, reducing edema, and preparing muscles, joints, and other soft tissues to be massaged or manipulated. These reactions are caused by the local effects of temperature directly on the blood vessels and sweat glands, and also by reflexes conducted from the skin receptors to the spinal cord and

TABLE 3-2 EFFECTS OF LONG VERSUS SHORT WHOLE-BODY COLD TREATMENTS		
Effects	**Long Treatment (>1 min)**	**Short Treatment (≤1 min)**
Vasoconstriction	Initially, but when completely chilled, muscles of blood vessels lack oxygen, cannot contract	Peripheral, followed by vasodilation
Circulation	Slows	Increases
Heart rate	Decreases	Decreases
Speed of nerve conduction	Decreases	Increases
Skin sensitivity	Decreases	Increases
Muscle effects	Sluggish and clumsy	Toned
Sensation	Cold	Warmth
Blood pressure	Decreases	Increases
Shivering	Begins once body is chilled, continues until too cold to continue	No shivering
Metabolism	Decreases	Increases
Migration of leukocytes through capillary wall	Decreases	No change
Physiological effect	Depressant	Stimulant
Core temperature	Decreased	Slight increase or no change

back. These reflexes help prevent excessive loss of heat from locally cooled parts of the body.

Because ice packs, ice massage, cold local baths, cold compresses, and cold iced towels are applied to the skin, their greatest cooling effect is on the skin itself, then on the subcutaneous tissues underneath the skin, and finally, if the application is cold enough, in the muscle tissues underneath that. Ligaments that are not covered with much soft tissue may also be chilled and deprived of blood supply.

These responses may vary to some extent, depending on how cold the skin is at the beginning, how cold the application is, and how long it is left on. For example, an ice pack, if it is put over a very warm area, will chill the area more slowly. Local cold penetrates far more deeply than local heat, as many of the small blood vessels are constricted and less warm blood from the heart can flow into the area to rewarm it. When tissues are cooled for a long time, vasodilation will occur intermittently. For example, when fingers are immersed in an ice water bath, skin temperature will decrease for 15 minutes, and then every so often it increases again. When the tissue becomes cold enough that it might become damaged—59°F—arterioles react to preserve the tissue by dilating long enough to raise the tissue temperature and supply the tissue with some nutrients. This is known as the hunting reaction, or reactive vasodilation. However, no cold treatment in this book will use cold applications that could cause this reaction, that is, extremely cold applications for long periods.

The following are some of the body's reactions to local cold:

1. Sympathetic nervous system stimulation occurs as a result of the cold input to the cold receptors in the skin, resulting in increased levels of norepinephrine, vasopressin, angiotensin, and other hormones.

2. Vasoconstriction occurs in many skin blood vessels, which shuts off much of the blood flow to local areas the way shutting off a faucet cuts off water flowing into a hose. Skin becomes pale and white because of the reduced blood flow, and metabolic rate is decreased for the same reason. A hand immersed in a 41°F water bath for 30 minutes will have a 78% decrease in blood flow.(5) Meanwhile, the internal blood vessels are filled and so dilate. This is an example of **depletion.**

3. Constriction of muscle blood vessels as cold penetrates the tissues. In the case of an immersed hand, reflex vasoconstriction will occur in the other hand as well. One study using the knee joints of dogs found that after 10 minutes of ice packs at 32°F, blood flow decreased by half.(6)

4. Cold applied to a limb will cause vasoconstriction in the other limb as well. This is known as the **contralateral reflex effect.**

5. When local cold treatments are given on a regular basis, such as a hand being regularly immersed in cold water, the blood vessels gain tone and begin to contract sooner and with greater force.

6. Reflex effects of cold applications occur in the area under the cold and in deeper organs and may be used for therapeutic effect. A short cold application to a reflex area has tonic and stimulating effects, as it causes active dilation of the blood vessels in the related viscera. A long, continuous application of cold affects both the skin and the underlying organs. The blood vessels constrict during the application and afterward, nerve conduction is slowed, and muscles are firmly contracted. Table 3-3 shows the reflex effects of both short and long applications of local cold on various parts of the body.

TABLE 3-3 REFLEX EFFECTS OF LONG AND SHORT LOCAL COLD TREATMENTS

Site of Local Cold Application	Reflex Effects of Long Cold Treatments	Site of Local Cold Application	Reflex Effects of Short Cold Treatments
Face, forehead, scalp, and back of the neck	Contraction of blood vessels of the brain	Face and head	Stimulates mental activity
Abdominal wall	Increases intestinal blood flow, intestinal movement, and production of stomach acid	Chest	First increases respiratory rate, then decreases and deepens it
Nose, back of neck, and hands	Contraction of blood vessels of nasal mucosa	Sacrum or feet	Dilation of the uterine blood vessels
Main trunk of artery	Contraction of the artery and its branches	Abdomen, hands, or feet	Constriction of muscles of the bladder, bowel, and uterus
Pelvic area	Stimulates muscles of pelvic organs	Over the liver	Increased liver activity
Precordium (anterior chest)	Slows heart rate, increases stroke volume	Stomach	Increased gastric secretion
Acutely inflamed joints or bursae	Contraction of blood vessels and provides pain relief	Over the precordia	Increases rate and force of heartbeat
Acute injuries such as bruises and sprains	Vasoconstriction and decrease of hemorrhage and edema		

TABLE 3-4   COMPARISON OF THE EFFECTS OF PROLONGED LOCAL APPLICATIONS OF HOT AND COLD

Effects	Long Local Heat Treatment	Long Local Cold Treatment
Local blood flow	Increased	Decreased
Muscle spasm, guarding	Decreased	Decreased
Local inflammatory response in acute injuries	Increased	Decreased
Joint stiffness in arthritis	Decreased	Decreased
Edema production	Increased	Decreased
Pain	Reduced	Reduced
Metabolic rate	Increased	Decreased
Nerve conduction velocity	Slowed	Slowed
Muscle strength	Reduced	Reduced
Tissue elasticity	Increased	Decreased
Joint stiffness	Decreased	Increased for a very short time, then decreased
Local sweating	Present	Absent

In addition to these protective mechanisms, the following effects stem from chilling of tissue and the lack of blood flow:

1. Decreased skin and muscle temperature. Skin temperature will decrease within a minute or less, followed by the subcutaneous tissue and finally the muscle itself. It may require as long as 30 minutes to cool muscle tissue to a depth of 4 cm using ice packs.
2. Decreased oxygen delivery to tissues
3. Muscle spasm decreased as a result of a reflex reduction in motor nerve activity caused by the increased activity of the skin's cold receptors.
4. Decreased blood flow to joints accompanied by a decrease in the mechanoreceptors sensitivity
5. Stiffer connective tissue
6. Decreased core temperature if the application is very large or very prolonged

Table 3-4 compares the effects of local cold treatments to local heat treatments.

CONTRAST TREATMENTS

Contrast treatments involve alternating heat with cold in a single treatment. They may be performed as whole-body or local treatments. Whole-body contrast applications consist of rapid alternations of whole-body hot and whole-body cold, such as a hot bath followed by a cold plunge, repeated three or more times. These applications combine the advantages of short hot exposures and short cold exposures and result in a dramatic increase in circulation, reflex stimulation of related tissues and organs, decreased musculoskeletal pain, and a strong feeling of invigoration.

Local contrast treatments consist of local heat applications (e.g., fomentation, paraffin dip, hot compress, hot local bath) followed by local cold applications (ice packs, cold compresses, cold baths or whirlpools, or cold mitten frictions) repeated three or more times. The circulatory effects of short hot applications (vasodilation) are combined with the effects of short cold applications (vasoconstriction followed by vasodilation) to produce a dramatic increase in local blood flow, at least double the resting amount.

When heat dilates arterioles, arterial blood has a tendency to slow down and congest tissues, but when cold is applied after heat, the muscles of the arteriole contract and push the increased blood flow through the capillaries and into venules and lymphatic ducts; this temporarily empties the arterioles and creates a suction effect, pulling more fresh blood into the arteries. Contrast baths therefore increase local circulation more than hot baths. A contrast footbath increases local circulation more than a hot footbath, and so does a contrast full-body shower compared to a hot one. These changes in circulation not only can be measured with a variety of instruments but can also be seen with the naked eye: the skin turns a much brighter red after a contrast treatment than after a warm application alone. This increase in blood flow is especially marked on the first change from hot to cold, suggesting that the muscles of the arterial walls can become fatigued.(7)

Contrast applications combine the advantages of heat and cold without their disadvantages. For example, while hot applications increase circulation, they can also promote congestion and edema, and while cold applications decrease edema, they also decrease local blood flow and deprive tissues of oxygen and other nutrients. However, when hot applications are combined with cold applications in a contrast treatment, local circulation is greatly increased without increasing edema.

While some of these circulatory changes may seem so transitory that they could not have any long-term effect, they can actually be significant for someone with a circulatory problem if performed on a regular basis. Patients with varicose veins who received alternating hot and cold showers to the legs for 25 days had significant improvements in the circulation to their legs, and this effect lasted a month or more.(8)

CASE HISTORY 3-2

Fluid-Shifting Effects of a Contrast Treatment to the Leg

Background

Janet was a healthy, athletic 57-year-old woman. She usually received massage once a month for chronic neck and shoulder tension and to improve general wellness. One day she went to her massage therapist with a specific problem: she had pain and edema in her left lower leg. She also had a reddish blotch, a discoloration about the size of a quarter, in her anterior left lower leg just medial to her left tibia. Her doctor had already evaluated her thoroughly, then approved massage and hydrotherapy. He ruled out bone disease, injury, and phlebitis and suspected a ruptured varicose vein that had leaked blood.

Treatment

The massage therapist noticed that the affected lower leg was noticeably larger than the right. Gentle pressure with an index finger along the left tibia left dents that remained for some time, a condition known as pitting edema. Janet's hamstring muscles were noticeably edematous to the touch. Janet lay prone, and the massage therapist performed 5 minutes of effleurage and pétrissage on her left hamstring muscles. The therapist checked her leg at this point and noted a slight reduction of lower leg edema and a distinct lightening of the color in the discolored area. Janet's hamstring muscles also felt less swollen. Another 5 minutes of massage was performed on Janet's gluteal muscles while she was still prone, followed by massage of her quadriceps muscles in supine position. The therapist checked her lower left leg again and noted another reduction of edema and lightening of coloring in the blotch, although not so pronounced as after the first 5 minutes. Clearly the massage had dilated the blood and lymphatic vessels in Janet's upper leg.

The massage therapist then began a mild contrast treatment of the lower leg. She heated a small gel pack in water in a slow cooker and placed it on the entire medial surface of the left tibia. It was covered with a dry towel to keep it from cooling off and left for 2 minutes. Then the therapist removed the hot pack and performed ice massage over the area for 1 minute. This round of heat followed by cold was repeated four times. When the therapist was not placing the gel packs or performing ice massage, she massaged Janet's head and neck.

Each time the hot or cold was changed, Janet's leg was evaluated again. The discoloration was slightly reduced after each application, and the entire area under the application gradually became pinker as the blood flow to the area increased. After the last hot-and-cold round, the area was a healthy pink, the ankle was back to its normal size, and the discolored area could no longer be seen. Janet felt no pain in the area. No hands-on massage was performed over the lower leg.

Discussion Questions

1. Explain the change in appearance of Janet's lower leg.
2. What does the case history tell us about the fluid-shifting effect of contrast treatments?
3. Why was a contrast treatment of the lower leg a better way to affect circulation than using massage techniques?

Almost everyone who receives a local contrast treatment reports a strong feeling of invigoration and relaxation in the area, and for many types of pain, great relief. Contrast treatments complement massage treatments, as both enhance circulation, relieve tension and musculoskeletal pain, and provide sensory stimulation.

NEUTRAL TREATMENTS

A neutral bath is one in which the water is 94° to 98°F. Neutral baths have traditionally been used for sedative purposes because they are very soothing and not stimulating, simply surrounding the entire body evenly. Water at a temperature approximating the core temperature

means there is no thermal stimulation, and any mechanical stimulation, such as friction, is contraindicated because it would also offer stimulation. Unlike a hot or a cold bath, the person's temperature and vital signs remain stable.

PHYSIOLOGICAL EFFECTS OF MECHANICAL AND CHEMICAL TREATMENTS

Mechanical and chemical treatments are less common than hot and cold treatments, but they provide an extra tool for the massage therapist to achieve therapeutic goals and are often much enjoyed by clients.

MECHANICAL TREATMENTS

There are two types of **mechanical treatments**, those that use friction on the skin and those that use water to strike the skin. Early hydrotherapists were accustomed to prescribing friction treatments to stimulate both nerve reaction and blood and lymphatic circulation, which increased the effects of heat and cold. For example, an overheated patient who was put in a cold bath might be rubbed vigorously with a cold wet cloth to bring blood to the surface, where it was in greater contact with the cold water. In this way, the person would be cooled faster than by the cold bath alone. Bedridden patients might be given a salt glow to stimulate the circulation of blood and lymph that they were not getting from physical exercise. Today, friction treatments such as salt glows, brushings, and cold mitten frictions are used and have an effect similar to that of tapotement and vibration strokes in massage, namely a very stimulating one.

Percussion treatments include jetted whirlpool tubs and showers. When something strikes the skin, the body reacts as if to a possible threat, increasing muscle tone and nerve reaction and dilating the blood vessels in the skin directly under the pressure or friction. John Harvey Kellogg described the mechanical effect of a strong stream of water on the skin:

[A]t the exact point upon which the column of water falls, the skin becomes instantly blanched, the color re-appearing as soon as the stream is allowed to fall on any other part. . . The blood-vessels are not only made to contract by the thermic impression of the water, but the weight of the stream of water, the force of the impact, compresses the tissues and forces the blood out of the vessels, leaving them free to dilate again as soon as the pressure is removed. Thus the tissues are alternately compressed and released. . . the thermic effect of the douche is thus materially aided by the mechanical or percussion effects of the moving water. . . A powerful reflex effect is produced by the stimulation of the various sets of nerves which recognize temperature, pressure, pain, and tactile impressions.(9)

The effects of mechanical treatments are difficult to measure and perhaps have to be felt to be truly appreciated. In general, mechanical treatments are most often performed to augment the thermal, fluid-shifting, and nervous system effects of hydrotherapy. If a hydrotherapy technique is used with hot or cold water, mechanical stimulation may also help warm or cool the tissue faster. For example, a cold mitten friction keeps the cold water in contact with the skin even better than simply laying a cold towel over the skin. The jets in a warm whirlpool keep the warm water more constantly in contact with the skin by continually bringing fresh warm water to it. These treatments also provide a great deal of sensory stimulation and

are appropriate for many massage clients who enjoy such stimulation. They are less appropriate for clients who are extremely body sensitive or tactile defensive. Examples of whole body treatments that rely on mechanical stimulation are whole-body cold mitten frictions, salt glows, and showers; examples of local treatments are salt glows and percussion douches to just one area of the body.

CHEMICAL TREATMENTS

Chemical substances can be dissolved in water and then applied to the skin through compresses, poultices, packs, ice massage, steam inhalation, local baths, or whole-body baths. Each chemical has a separate and distinct effect upon the skin or deeper tissues, and effects vary widely. These are a few of the most common substances used in hydrotherapy treatments, along with their effects:

- Oatmeal contains essential fatty acids and other chemicals that have a soothing and moisturizing effect upon the skin itself. It is used in full-body baths and body wraps.
- Essential oil of eucalyptus contains terpene alcohols, cineole, neral, geraniol, and other chemicals that give it anti-inflammatory, expectorant, and antiviral actions. Eucalyptus and other essential oils can be applied through local baths, steam inhalations, compresses, ice massage, and full-body baths. For more information about the use of essential oils in massage practice, see Martin L. *Aromatherapy for Massage Practitioners*. Baltimore: Lippincott Williams & Wilkins, 2006.
- Dried or fresh herbs contain a wide variety of chemicals and are used in steam inhalations, compresses, ice massage, and both local and full-body baths. Mustard seeds, ground to a powder, contain allylglucosinolates that cause dilation of the blood vessels of the skin, helping relieve muscular and skeletal pain. Mustard powder is used in local or full-body baths and in mustard plasters. Capsaicin, the pungent ingredient in cayenne pepper, binds to vanilloid receptors on nerve endings and causes both vasodilation and a sensation of heat. It is in used in compresses, fomentations, foot and hand soaks, and even full-body baths. For more information about the use of herbal preparations in massage practice, see Chapter 13.

CHAPTER SUMMARY

In this chapter, you have reviewed the anatomy and physiology of several body systems that are key to hydrotherapy. You have also learned how the body's natural skills at defending itself against possible threats can be used to clients' advantage. By making use of the body's own homeostatic mechanisms, hydrotherapy treatments help provide such benefits as overall relaxation, increased pliability of tissue, increased local circulation, pain relief, and reduction of muscle spasm. You have also learned how the body responds to hot and cold, mechanical and chemical treatments. In the next chapter, we move on to setting up and preparing for a wide variety of these treatments.

REVIEW QUESTIONS

Short Answer

1. Name six sensations for which there are separate receptors in the skin.

   _____

   _____

   _____

2. Explain the physiological effects of whole-body and local exposure to heat.

   _____

   _____

3. Explain the physiological effects of whole-body and local exposure to cold.

   _____

   _____

Fill in the Blank

4. Prolonged applications of heat can cause _____ of blood vessels in the area where it is actually placed, as well as in _____.

5. The brain must constantly receive a high proportion of the body's blood supply because it has high _____ needs and an inability to store _____.

6. A neutral bath is relaxing because of its lack of _____.

Multiple Choice

7. The circulatory system protects the body's
   a. Core temperature
   b. Skin temperature
   c. Blood supply to brain
   d. All of the above

8. The body's immediate response to a drop in skin temperature is
   a. Vasodilation of skin blood vessels
   b. Increased blood flow to the brain
   c. Vasoconstriction of skin blood vessels
   d. Sweating

9. Reflexes are useful because they increase the speed at which the body reacts to external threats such as
   a. Very hot objects
   b. Blood loss
   c. Object in the eye
   d. All of the above

10. An application of ice can relieve pain and muscle spasm by its effects on all except
    a. The skin
    b. The spinal cord and brain
    c. The digestive system
    d. The muscles

Matching

11.
___ 1. Artery	a. Toward heart
___ 2. Valve	b. Most plentiful vessel in body
___ 3. Lymph	c. Contains oxygenated blood
___ 4. Vein	d. Found in blood vessels going against gravity
___ 5. Capillary	e. Tissue fluid

12.
___ 1. Brain	a. Autonomic nervous system
___ 2. Reflex arc	b. Temperature center
___ 3. Parasympathetic	c. Central
___ 4. Peripheral	d. Far from center of body
___ 5. Hypothalamus	e. Shortcut

13.
___ 1. Mechanical	a. Absorption onto or through skin
___ 2. Thermal	b. Stimulation of skin and nerves
___ 3. Fluid shifting	c. Redistribution of blood or lymph
___ 4. Chemical	d. Warming or cooling of tissue

REFERENCES

1. Vogel S. *Vital Circuits: On Pumps, Pipes, and the Workings of Circulatory Systems*. New York: Oxford University, 1992.
2. Thrash A. *Home Remedies: Hydrotherapy, Massage, Charcoal and Other Simple Treatments*. Seale, AL: Thrash, 1981, p 16.
3. Shin TW, Wilson M, Wilson T. Real Risks or Made-Up Myths? The Truth About Hot Tubs and Saunas for Hypertensive Patients. *Hypertension*

4. Petrofsky J. et al. The use of hydrotherapy to increase blood flow and muscle relaxation in the rehabilitation of neurological and orthopedic patients. *J Neurol Orthop Med Surg* 2003;21(3):188.
5. Lee K et al. Influence of nicotine on cold induced vasodilation in humans [Abstract]. *Experiment Biol* 2004. Available at http://select.biosis.org/faseb/eb2004_data/FASEB007857.html.
6. www.caringmedical.com/sports_injury/rice.asp by Ross Hauser, MD, Accessed December 2005.
7. Fiscus KA. Changes in lower-leg blood flow during warm-, cold-, and contrast-water therapy. *Arch Phys Med Rehabil* 2005;86(7):1404.
8. Saradeth B et al. A single blind, randomized, controlled trial of hydrotherapy for varicose veins. *Vasa* 1991;20(2):147.
9. Kellogg JH. *Rational Hydrotherapy*. Battle Creek, MI: Modern Medicine, 1923, p 439.

RECOMMENDED RESOURCES

1. Buchman D. *The Complete Book of Water Healing*. New York: Instant Improvement, 1994, p 206.
2. Charkoudian, N. Skin blood flow in adult human thermoregulation: How it works, when it does not, and why. *Mayo Clin Proc* 2003;78:603.
3. Guyton A. *Textbook of Medical Physiology*. 8th ed. Philadelphia: Saunders, 1991.
4. Hayes B. *Five Quarts: A Personal and Natural History of Blood*. New York: Ballantine, 2005.
5. Kamler K. *Surviving the Extremes: A Doctor's Journey to the Limits of Human Endurance*. New York: St. Martin's, 2002.
6. Michlovitz S. *Thermal Agents in Rehabilitation*. Philadelphia: FA Davis, 1996.

PREPARING TO GIVE HYDROTHERAPY TREATMENTS

In the scientific use of water in the treatment of disease, elaborate apparatus is not essential for effectiveness. It is possible to secure the most valuable of the therapeutic advantages of water by the aid of sheets, towels, blankets, a pail, a bathtub and a thermometer, if coupled with the consummate skill that comes from long experience.

—John Harvey Kellogg, Rational Hydrotherapy

Chapter Objectives

After completing this chapter, the student will be able to:

- List the equipment needed for four levels of hydrotherapy treatments.
- Describe several considerations when selecting hydrotherapy equipment.
- Explain guidelines for sanitation of hydrotherapy equipment.
- Describe general cautions for giving hydrotherapy treatments to certain clients.
- Explain several contraindications to hydrotherapy treatments.
- Describe safety precautions to be used when giving hydrotherapy treatments.
- Explain factors that influence the body's response to hot and cold treatments.
- Describe additional questions that must be added to the standard massage therapist's health intake form if hydrotherapy treatments are to be given.
- Explain the basic guidelines for hydrotherapy.
- Describe the decision-making process for choosing which hydrotherapy treatments are best suited to individual clients.
- Explain how hydrotherapy can be used in a variety of environments.

In a single day, as you move from treating a chronically ill person in the home, to giving massages at a fair or sporting event, to treating clients in a nursing home or in your private office, hydrotherapy treatments can enhance each and every session (Fig. 4-1). Preparing to perform these treatments means selecting and maintaining the appropriate equipment, then choosing a treatment that is fine-tuned to the unique needs of each client. After reading this chapter, you will be able to select the hydrotherapy equipment that works for your individual practice, whether you are an independent practitioner in a one-person office or an employee of a chiropractic clinic, hospice, health club, or spa. You will also be able to determine which treatments are safe for which clients by taking a thorough medical history and taking note of cautions and contraindications. Basic guidelines that are relevant to all hydrotherapy treatments are explained, as well as how you can use them in settings as different as a private home, athletic event or nursing facility.

EQUIPMENT

A massage therapist who intends to make hydrotherapy an integral part of his or her practice can choose from a wide variety of modalities. Depending upon where you practice,

CASE HISTORY 4-1

Many Conditions Can Be Relieved by More Than One Hydrotherapy Treatment

Background

Susan, 45 years old, was being cared for by a county hospice service because she had widespread cancer, which began with breast cancer and then metastasized to her liver and the bones of her spine. Susan, who had a great deal of pain in her spine, enjoyed her massages very much and found that they reduced her nervous tension and temporarily relieved her back pain. Normally local heat is contraindicated for persons with cancer, but the hospice's supervising physician approved warm fomentations to Susan's spine before massage as a last-stage comfort measure. Susan has a hot tub in her back yard.

Treatment

Before each massage, the massage therapist placed a fomentation on Susan's back, then massaged her feet for a few minutes while the heat seeped into her spine. Then he removed the fomentation and gently massaged her back. After her massage, Susan was helped into her hot tub, where she remained for 15 to 20 minutes. At some of her appointments, Susan soaked in the hot tub before her massage. Because of the bone cancer, just being freed from the pull of gravity as she floated relieved some of her back pain and was tremendously soothing. This helped her to begin her massage in a relaxed state. The warm water also raised her core temperature slightly, which made it easier to keep her warm during her massage. At other sessions, Susan floated in her hot tub after a massage, which helped her feel more relaxed than with the massage alone.

Discussion Questions

1. What steps would you take to ensure that hydrotherapy treatments are safe for a patient such as Susan?
2. What other hydrotherapy treatment might help relieve her pain?

the access you have to running water and what types of clients you see, many different ways to incorporate hydrotherapy treatments are possible. This section will help guide you as you make decisions about what hydrotherapy equipment to purchase. This chapter presents four levels of investment in equipment and discusses factors to consider when shopping for equipment. Directions on sanitizing and maintaining your hydrotherapy equipment are also included.

LEVELS OF INVESTMENT

One of the strengths of hydrotherapy as a healing modality is that it can be performed with only a few basic items. If you plan to include simple hydrotherapy treatments in your sessions, only these basic items are needed. With planning and your equipment carefully laid out, you can add water treatments to every session without sacrificing hands-on massage time. You may want to purchase only simple equipment and try it before you go on to more expensive or elaborate items. Figure 4-2 shows a variety of simple hydrotherapy items. Then, if you plan to incorporate hydrotherapy treatments into a significant portion of your massage sessions or to perform advanced treatments, you may want to invest in more elaborate equipment. Some massage therapists use only one piece of hydrotherapy equipment in a variety of ways; for example, plastic dishpans can be used for hot, cold, or contrast baths of the hands or feet or to hold water for hot, cold, or contrast compresses over other body parts or for local salt glows. Simple, inexpensive,

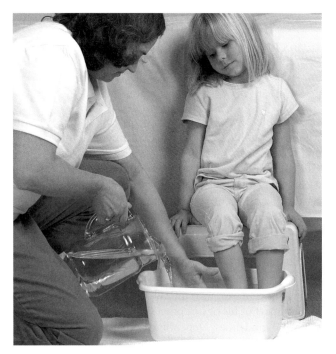
FIGURE 4-1 ■ Massage therapist providing a footbath for client.

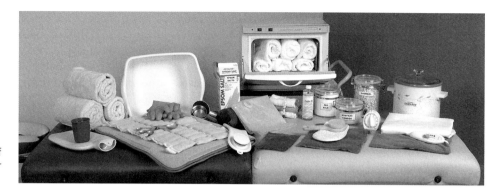

FIGURE 4-2 ■ Various kinds of hydrotherapy equipment suitable for local treatments.

and effective at a very modest price. Some other therapists become excited about more elaborate pieces of equipment. To help you determine what is ideal for your practice, descriptions of four levels of investment in hydrotherapy equipment follow.

Basic Equipment

With simple equipment and a modest investment you can easily give your clients a variety of local hydrotherapy treatments. With equipment for just one type of local heat and one type of local cold, you can give hot, cold, and contrast treatments; cold mitten frictions; and local salt glows. At this level, having running water in the therapy room is not absolutely necessary, but you will need a sink close at hand.

This is a list of basic equipment:

- Water thermometer, which is essential for safety. (Figure 4-3 shows both Fahrenheit and Celsius temperature scales.)
- Extra linens, including about 20 washcloths, 4 hand towels, and 4 bath towels
- Counter space or cart for hydrotherapy equipment
- Large tray to carry materials such as hot water bottles, pitchers of water, bowls, and used linens or other items to be cleaned. Brand-new cookie sheets, which are both sturdy and completely washable, work well for this purpose.
- Metal or plastic bowls that are 1-quart size. They may be used for water, ice cubes, salt for local salt glows, and so on. Two or more will be ideal.
- Pitchers, a 4-cup size and an 8-cup size
- Plastic tubs that can go underneath the table to hold used towels and can double as containers for local water baths
- One form of local heat. Choose a slow cooker, turkey roaster for hot water (useful for salt glows, hot compresses, silica gel packs, and hot water to pour into hot water bottles and hand and foot baths), a microwave oven (useful for heating fomentations and some types of hot gel packs), a hot towel cabinet (holds many hot moist washcloths), or a moist heating pad.

- Local cold options. Choose very cold water (useful for cold mitten frictions, cold compresses, and cold local baths), iced compresses, ice packs, or ice cups. Some kind of refrigeration is needed for all of these forms of local cold. A miniature refrigerator can hold all of these items comfortably. A small ice chest may also be used to hold ice packs and ice cups for the next session.
- Zipper closure bags of various sizes are useful for making ice packs and iced compresses and for heating fomentations in a microwave.
- Local friction treatment options. Choose Epsom salt and two washcloths for salt glows, cold water and two washcloths for cold mitten frictions, a loofah glove or mitt and two washcloths for loofah scrubs, or a soft natural-bristle brush and two washcloths for dry brushing.

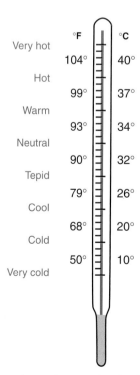

	°F	°C
Very hot		
	104°	40°
Hot		
	99°	37°
Warm		
	93°	34°
Neutral		
	90°	32°
Tepid		
	79°	26°
Cool		
	68°	20°
Cold		
	50°	10°
Very cold		

FIGURE 4-3 ■ General sensations associated with cold, neutral, and hot water.

- A plastic sheet may be put underneath cloth sheets to protect the massage table if desired. Towels are effective unless a large amount of water is spilled on the table.
- Floor covering. Anytime liquid water is being used for treatments, linoleum is a better floor covering than carpet because it is easier to clean. Many people do not care for the colder feel of linoleum, however. In that case, washable rugs can be put over the linoleum so that they can be easily removed and cleaned, but they should have a nonskid backing.

Basic-Plus Equipment

This level includes the same equipment as previously listed plus items for several additional local treatments. Simply by acquiring one more local heat treatment, you add many more options for adding hydrotherapy to your sessions. For example, one type of local heat treatment, such as a flat plastic hot water bottle, may be appropriate for warming a cold person and for increasing circulation to a person's entire back before massage, but it is too large for a hot or contrast treatment in a small body area and will not wrap around an area as liquid water will do. A paraffin bath is excellent for deep heating of the hands, feet, and face; for general body warming; and even for contrast treatments of the hands, feet, and face. However, it is not practical for someone with a stiff neck. Simply by adding one heat treatment, you can use hydrotherapy to help treat many more situations. Whole-body heat treatments, such as a hot blanket pack, may be provided with the equipment at this level without more expensive equipment, such as a steam cabinet or shower. One additional source of cold, an ice machine, makes it far easier to provide contrast treatments. Except for the handheld shower attachment, having running water in the therapy room is not absolutely necessary, but you will need a sink close at hand. Contrast applications with the shower attachment can be performed easily by your clients at home.

The following additional equipment is still relatively inexpensive:

- Equipment for one additional local heat treatment, such as a flat plastic hot water bottle, paraffin bath, hot towel cabinet, hydrocollator tank that holds four hot packs, or a hand-held shower attachment, which requires a room with a tiled floor or a bathtub
- Equipment for one additional local cold treatment, such as an ice machine or a handheld shower attachment, which requires a room with a tiled floor or a bathtub

Advanced Equipment

This level includes the same equipment listed previously along with equipment for one of the many kinds of whole-body heat treatments. A whole-body treatment can be as simple as a standard shower (which can be used for cleansing and for whole-body heating, cooling, or contrast treatments) or as elaborate as a soaking tub, steel whirlpool, steam room, sauna, or hot tub. Other facilities for whole-body treatments include individual steam canopies and cabinets. A large shower with a steam bath attachment is perhaps the most versatile of all for whole-body hydrotherapy treatments, because it can be used for steam baths, hot showers, cold showers, contrast showers, and whole-body salt glows.

However, many things are to be considered before purchase of any whole-body hydrotherapy equipment. Not only the added cash outlay but also the increased use of office space, water, energy and linens, plus the additional time needed to clean and sanitize everything after the client leaves, must be borne in mind. In a health club or a clinic with multiple practitioners, these added expenses may be more practical, since the cost can be divided among the practitioners. However, for an individual practitioner, the startup and maintenance costs may be prohibitive, and the amount of time the facility is in use may not justify the cost. In addition, consider that the cost must be passed on to the client. However, some practitioners feel so strongly about the value of a particular treatment that they are willing to invest in it. A therapist who invests $5000 to install a tiled sauna and shower or $20,000 to put in a Watsu pool in his or her own office will have to practice for some years to make back the original investment, yet for someone who feels passionate about this therapy, money is not the only consideration.

This is a list of equipment for a variety of whole-body treatments, in order of increasing cost.

1. Japanese soaking tub. This type of tub uses less space but more water (about 50 gallons) than a standard bathtub. Heating the water with gas or electricity is an ongoing cost. It may lose less heat than a standard bathtub, since the surface of the water—where heat radiates from—is smaller.
2. Standard bathtub. Standard tubs use about 30 gallons of water. Heating the bath water with gas or electricity is an ongoing cost.
3. Steam canopy, which can be laid over the client as he or she lies on the massage table. This item is highly efficient, using a maximum of 5 cups of water and the same amount of energy as a small kitchen appliance.
4. Standard tiled shower. Showers in general use less water than baths. Heating the shower water with gas or electricity is an ongoing cost.
5. Multihead shower panel. This can be added to a basic shower to make a multiple-spray shower. Because multiple-head showers use a great deal of water, heating the water with gas or electricity is more expensive than for a standard shower.

Installation of larger pipes needed to carry more water is another additional cost.

6. Individual steam cabinet. This uses little water but quite a bit of energy. A shower must also be provided.

7. Individual stainless steel whirlpool tub. Extremity whirlpools use approximately 50 gallons of water, whereas whole-body whirlpools use approximately 100 gallons, and Hubbard tanks use more than 400 gallons. The cost of installing plumbing must be taken into account. Energy to heat the water and to run the pumps which circulate the water is an ongoing cost.

8. Steam shower with steam generator. Upfront costs include plumbing, and heating the water is an additional cost.

9. Hot tub or spa. Upfront costs include plumbing, and heating the water is an additional cost. A shower must also be provided.

10. Dry sauna. A sauna—basically a small room with a heater—is a major investment that uses a lot of electricity. A shower must also be provided.

Spa-Level Equipment

This level includes the same equipment as listed previously plus spa equipment and facilities. Many spa treatments use very expensive equipment, such as specialty showers, special hoses for percussion treatments, and sophisticated hydrotherapy tubs. This level is not usually found outside of spas, since a tiled wet room is needed and the equipment is very expensive to install and maintain, takes up a great deal of space, and requires a great deal of maintenance. The increased costs for equipment, space, and maintenance also mean that clients who come there will have to pay considerably more for their treatments. In addition, if you as a therapist are doing these types of treatments, you will probably have less and less time for actual hands-on massage. However, it is still important that you know about these treatments because they have been practiced for centuries in both the United States and Europe and are still used in many modern spas. For more about these treatments, see *Spa Bodywork* by Anne Williams.

Below is a list of spa-level equipment.

1. A Swiss shower with 16 heads. About $5000 for the equipment itself, plus a minimum of $2000 for tiling a shower enclosure

2. Vichy shower. About $4000; also requires a wet room

3. A Scotch hose or percussion douche. About $4000; requires a wet room

4. Mud bath. About $5000 per bath to pay for the pouring of concrete for the tank and for extensive plumbing. Upkeep is very high.

5. Jetted hydrotherapy tub. $15,000. Not only must the tub be cleaned, sanitized, and dried between clients, the jets must also be flushed out.

6. Watsu pool. $10,000 to $30,000, depending upon whether the pool is part of an existing building or if a new building must be built for it

FACTORS TO WEIGH WHEN SELECTING HYDROTHERAPY EQUIPMENT

Selecting equipment is an important decision. Following are some key factors to consider as you make this decision.

Goals of Therapy

This answer will differ with the type of clients you treat. For example, a therapist who specializes in sports massage can use ice treatments with athletes to help them with sports injuries, while a therapist who specializes in working with the elderly can use warming treatments to help them tolerate being partially or completely undressed. The sports therapist does not need to help his athletic clients, who likely have excellent circulation, to stay warm, and the therapist for elders is not as likely to be treating his clients for athletic injuries.

Cost

To calculate this, figure the total cost of purchasing and installing equipment and upkeep, cleaning, and extra laundry. This is not a consideration with most local treatments, but for the whole-body heat treatments it is. For example, to do long hot treatments using multihead showers, steam baths, or many hot baths, a large hot water tank with large pipes is needed. Also, the more time and money you spend on equipment, the more money you must charge your clients.

Maintenance Time and Expense

Anytime your clients use a shower either before or after a massage session, it must be cleaned and dried before the next use. The shower may also need some type of periodic maintenance, such as replacing grout or cleaning the drainpipe. Local whirlpools must be sterilized after each use. A steam cabinet must be cleaned and dried after each use, whereas a steam canopy must merely be wiped off with cleanser and air-dried between clients. Parts may wear out and have to be replaced. These are just a few examples of maintenance issues that must be considered. Especially for large specialty equipment such as Vichy showers or saunas, be sure to ask, before purchasing them, who they have available in case something functions poorly or has to be replaced. An additional issue is how much time you, as a therapist, want to spend doing maintenance. Perhaps you would prefer to stay with a few simple local treatments that require little or no maintenance rather than be responsible for cleaning the equipment or repairs if breaks.

Water Consumption

Water consumption is important not only to keep costs low but also to conserve natural resources. Reducing water use means saving money and leaving more water in streams for fish and other aquatic life. Since getting water ready to use, distributing it, then collecting and treating it as waste water all require energy, water conservation also benefits the environment by reducing energy demands.

The amount of water used for various treatments varies widely. For example, while steam canopies use only a few cups of water for a treatment, standard-size bathtubs use about 30 gallons, Japanese soaking tubs and arm or leg whirlpools use roughly 50 gallons, and full-body whirlpools use about 100 gallons. A standard 10-minute shower uses about 25 gallons of water, while a 12- to 16-jet shower uses more than 10 times that much (for a 10-minute contrast shower, 175 gallons of hot and 175 gallons of cold). Perhaps the most water-wasteful of all hydrotherapy treatments are top-of-the-line showers complete with multiple jets and waterfall features, which use up to 80 gallons per minute.

Energy Consumption

Not only the cost of the water used in treatments but also the cost of heating or cooling it must be considered. The single biggest use of electricity in the average American home is to heat water, mostly for showers. Heating water with an electric steam boiler to do one Russian steam bath takes 68 kilowatts of energy. Making ice also uses a lot of energy, but not as much as using electricity to generate heat.

SANITATION PROTOCOLS

Just as with any other equipment used during a massage session, hydrotherapy equipment should be sanitized after each use. This protects your client's health and your own. Here are some specific directions on sanitizing your hydrotherapy equipment:

1. After a massage session, any surface that comes into contact with the client's skin, including floors, should be sanitized using an approved cleanser. All steam cabinets, showers, tubs, and other whole-body heating equipment must be cleaned with a bactericidal agent and then dried before another client uses them. Follow the manufacturer's specific instructions on how to clean them.

2. All bowls, lotion bottles, and other containers should be washed in hot soapy water and wiped with alcohol. Any substance that was used with the client that is in an open container, such as salt that was used for a salt glow, should be discarded if your hands touched it. If you removed the substance without touching it with your hands—for example, you used a spoon to remove Epsom salt from a container— the rest of it can be reused. The reason for this rule is that if you touched the salt with your hands, touched your client as you applied the salt, and then touched the salt again, that salt is contaminated and should not be used with anyone else. You may, however, give it to your client to use at home.

3. All cloth items, such as robes, sheets, towels, washcloths, and shower mats, must be washed in hot water with an appropriate detergent and then dried with heat. They must be stored on shelves, in compartments, or in cabinets that are at least 4 inches off the floor and used only for storage. Disposable shower caps, slippers, and other such items must be thrown away after being used.

GENERAL CAUTIONS AND CONTRAINDICATIONS

Hydrotherapy is generally very safe, and almost all of a massage therapist's clients can be safely treated with it. However, clients vary in their response to hydrotherapy applications. Before you give someone a hydrotherapy treatment for the first time, be sure to ask if he or she has had that treatment before and if so, what the response was. Anytime clients are receiving a whole-body heat treatment, such as a sauna, for the first time, their treatment time should be limited to 15 minutes. During the treatment, ask clients for feedback frequently and be ready to terminate any treatment that does not seem to be working. Signs of a poor reaction include nausea, headache, dizziness or lightheadedness, and complaints by the client of being of too warm or too cold. Tables 3-1 to 3-3 have further information on the physiological effects of hydrotherapy treatments. Table 4-1 shows generally whether a water temperature will be perceived as hot, warm, neutral, or cold. Below we discuss both cautions and contraindications to hydrotherapy.

CAUTIONS

When a caution is given, hydrotherapy treatments are not ruled out, but the special needs of the client must be carefully considered. Often a treatment may have to be milder, for example beginning with warm rather than hot water or using cool rather than ice water.

TABLE 4-1 THERMAL SENSATIONS

Descriptive Terms	Temperature Range (°F)	Temperature Range (°C)	Comments
Freezing	32	0	
Very cold	32–55	0–13	Painfully cold
Cold	55–65	13–18	Tolerable but uncomfortable
			Prolonged immersion in water <60°F may lead to hypothermia.
Cool	65–80	18–27	Produces goose flesh
Tepid	80–92	27–34	Slightly below skin temperature (92°F)
Warm or neutral	93–97	34–36	Comfortable
Hot	98–105	37–41	Tolerable, but parts turn red
Very hot	105–110	41–43	Tolerable for short periods
Painfully hot	110–120	43–46	Intolerable; this is likely to cause injury to diabetic feet.
Dangerously hot	≥125	≥50	Likely to burn skin
Boiling	212	100	

Attention Deficit Disorder

Many medications for attention deficit disorder promote vasodilation, so heat treatments should be avoided. All other treatments are fine.

Aversion to Cold

Clients who have a strong negative reaction to the idea of cold treatments can generally be accommodated by modifying the treatment. No treatment should ever be painful or unpleasant. For example, for a cold application, make the water warmer than usual. If the client's reaction is good, wait a bit and then add a few ice cubes to the water. For a contrast treatment, use water that is not as cold and increase the time of the treatment. For example, a contrast treatment of 2 minutes of heat followed by 30 seconds of cold could be changed to 2 minutes of heat followed by 1 minute of cool water. When treatments are going to be done in a series or if patients are going to do them at home, aversion to cold will probably decrease as they experience the good feelings at the end of the treatment.

Children

Compared to adults, children have thinner skin and a poorer ability to regulate their body temperature. In addition, children have more surface area for heat to escape from relative to their body mass, which means they can be chilled more easily. However, young children also heat up more easily than adults when exposed to heat.(1) Therefore, monitor them carefully when they are receiving hydrotherapy treatments. In general, make local hot and cold applications not quite so extreme, check their skin frequently, and ask them for more feedback than you would with an adult. Local salt glows are a good choice for children. Warm baths are very soothing and relaxing for children, most of whom love to play in water. Saunas and steam baths should last no longer than 10 minutes and should be supervised by a parent.(2) Also note that children tend to dislike cold applications, although individual responses can vary. For more information on hydrotherapy and children, see my book *Pediatric Massage Therapy*. Massage therapists should not perform hydrotherapy treatments with infants unless they have special training in this area.

Small Body Size

In general, small adults are more likely to become chilled by exposure to cold than larger adults. The U.S. army's research in environmental medicine has found that rates of peripheral cold injury in female soldiers are twice that of men because women have more surface area relative to their body mass than men do, so they lose heat faster during cold stress.(3)

Elders

Some of the physical changes associated with aging make it more difficult for older people to adjust to extremes of hot and cold. Loss of subcutaneous fat means it is easier for them to be burned by hot applications or chilled by cold applications. The muscles of the blood vessels often do not function as well, and so vasodilation and vasoconstriction are less efficient in controlling body temperature.(4,5) However, this does not mean that gentle hydrotherapy treatments are not appropriate. In a small study at

Kagoshima University in Japan, researchers studied the effects on elderly people of short (10-minute) hot baths. They found that 106°F baths improved exercise endurance on a treadmill, decreased fatigue, and also decreased leg pain in elders with and without heart disease. Researchers concluded that the hot water stimulated greater vasodilation, which caused more blood to flow to the skeletal muscles, and that made them better able to contract.(6) In general, be more vigilant with elderly people. Keep treatments shorter—no more than 15 minutes in a sauna, hot tub, or steam bath—and not as extreme in temperature. Also check their skin frequently, and ask them for more feedback than you would with a younger person.

HIV and AIDS

Because people with HIV or AIDS generally have a variety of body systems that are affected by the virus, hot baths or other whole-body heat treatments should be undertaken only with their doctor's approval. Hyperthermia (whole-body heating) is being studied for treatment of this condition. Researchers at John Bastyr College of Naturopathic Medicine found that a regimen of very hot baths that raised patients' temperatures to 102°F and kept it there for 30 minutes caused a significant inactivation of the HIV virus.(7)

Cancer

Both whole-body and local hydrotherapy treatments may be used for some people with cancer. Whole-body heat treatments have been given to strengthen the immune system (see Appendix C), and local heat, ice massage, and warm baths are sometimes used for pain. Massage is used by cancer patients to help them relax, promote general wellness, and ease discomfort and pain, so the massage therapist may be tempted to give hydrotherapy treatments for the same benefits. However, it is difficult to make specific recommendations here because the word *cancer* is used to describe more than 100 diseases. Also, cancers affect different parts of the body; the diseases have various stages; and different people receive vastly different medical treatments. Hydrotherapy treatments are also likely, at the very least, to affect the skin and challenge the circulatory system. For these reasons, although it is likely that the client's physician will approve hydrotherapy treatments, he or she should be consulted before giving them.

Pregnancy

Local treatments which do not raise the core temperature are safe for pregnant women, but do not place hot applications over the abdomen. Epsom salt hand and foot baths are a traditional treatment for local edema in the last stage of pregnancy, and so are neutral baths. There is concern that increased core temperature in the early months of pregnancy could harm a fetus, so prolonged hot baths, hot tubs, steam baths, and saunas are

contraindicated. One study investigated this risk and found that exposure to heat in the form of hot tub, sauna, or fever in the first trimester of pregnancy was associated with an increased risk of neural tube defects, with hot tubs having the strongest effect of any single heat exposure.(8)

Obese Clients

Because obese clients have thicker layers of fat covering their muscles, it may take longer for a local heat application to penetrate their tissues, and once that area is hot, it may take longer for the heat to dissipate. The same is true of cold applications. Because the thick layer of fat prevents heat loss, obese clients may also respond to whole-body heat treatments by heating up faster than thin clients and may not tolerate them as well. What this means for the therapist who wants to give them hydrotherapy treatments is that their medical history should be taken carefully to rule out any other contraindications and they must be carefully monitored during treatments.

Clients With Limited Mobility

Clients may have limited mobility because of conditions such as muscular dystrophy, severe arthritis, cerebral palsy, postpolio syndrome, partial paralysis from spinal cord injuries, Parkinson's disease, severe osteoarthritis, and even obesity. All of these clients may receive some types of hydrotherapy treatments, and indeed, bedridden people may find hydrotherapy treatments such as salt glows and contrast treatments effective and enjoyable. However, moving with difficulty means that they cannot get out of a hot bath quickly or remove a local application such as a hot pack. Be especially attentive to such clients and assist them as needed.

CONTRAINDICATIONS

Contraindications are special symptoms or conditions that make a procedure or other remedy risky. Below we discuss some specific conditions that rule out certain hydrotherapy treatments. Specific contraindications will also be given with the instructions for each hydrotherapy treatments. Avoid treating clients who are intoxicated from drugs or alcohol, are acutely ill, or have recently eaten a large meal. No hydrotherapy treatments should be given until at least 1 hour after eating a large meal.

Acute Local Inflammation

Heat applications are contraindicated, as they can encourage edema.

Artificial Devices

Do not apply heat over implants, pacemakers, defibrillators, medication pumps, or other artificial devices. Heat and cold may be safely applied over hip and knee replacements.

Asthma

Many people with asthma find whole-body heating and local moist heat very comforting, and it is safe to use. However, inhaling cold, dry air can contribute to asthma attacks, and even going from a sauna or steam bath into cold air can trigger an asthma attack in some people. Do not let a person with asthma become chilled for even a moment during or after a hydrotherapy treatment.

Circulatory System Conditions

High temperatures, such as a client may be exposed to in a sauna, steam bath, or hot bath, can create extra demands on the circulatory system, including significant changes in how fast the heart beats, how much blood the heart pumps with each beat, blood pressure, the size of blood vessels, and significant changes in local blood flow. In general, much more of the person's blood supply than usual will be shifted to the vessels of the skin. Even local applications that are quite large can challenge the circulatory system to adapt.(9)

Therefore, the following heart or blood vessel problems are contraindications for some hydrotherapy treatments unless approved by the client's doctor.

Whole-body heat treatments are contraindicated for patients with these conditions:

- High blood pressure. At the very beginning of a whole-body heat treatment, the blood pressure rises for a very short time, and this can be dangerous for some people. In addition, clients may be taking medications that change how the blood vessels react to heat and cold, such as beta-blockers and calcium channel blockers.
- Low blood pressure. Whole-body heat treatments, especially hot baths, may cause fainting.
- Heart disease, such as coronary artery disease or congestive heart failure. The client's heart may not be strong enough to meet demands of whole-body heating. In addition, clients with heart disease may be taking medications that alter heart function.
- Phlebitis. Local treatments are contraindicated.
- Varicose veins. Local treatments may be used with caution. Avoid extremes of hot and cold unless they are prescribed by the patient's doctor.
- Local cold is contraindicated for **Raynaud's syndrome**, a simple vasoconstriction disorder of the extremities which affects 5% to 10% of the general population. Spasm of the smallest arteries that supply the hands or feet can be triggered in situations which would not affect someone without Raynaud's. For example, as discussed in Chapter 3, constriction of blood vessels in the hands can accompany emotional stress in many people; however, in a person with Raynaud's syndrome, this vasoconstriction can trigger an episode of vasospasm. Exposing the hands or feet to even mild cold can have the same effect; the muscles of the arteriole walls spasm, drastically reducing blood flow, and the area turns blue and has either numbness or a tingling, burning sensation. The arteriole spasm does not go away readily, and it may last for an hour or longer. Soaking the hands or feet in warm water to rewarm them may stop an episode of vasospasm, but the area often throbs painfully when it is rewarmed. What all this means for massage therapy is that exposure to a local cold treatment such as a cold hand bath or an ice pack on the foot may trigger an episode of vasospasm in a person with Raynaud's.
- Local heat to the feet is contraindicated for these conditions:
  1. **Arteriosclerosis** of the feet and legs. Do not apply local heat to the feet in the form of hot footbaths or hot water bottles, heating pads, or paraffin dips.
  2. **Buerger's disease** is a rare disorder in which an inflammation of the entire wall and connective tissue around medium-sized arteries can result in clots, occlusions, and gangrene. Heat to the feet in the form of hot footbaths or hot water bottles, heating pads, or paraffin dips is contraindicated.

Diabetes

Because diabetes is becoming more and more common in the United States, it is important to know when hydrotherapy treatments can be used for clients with this condition. Diabetes can lead to cardiovascular disease, atherosclerosis in particular, and so anyone with diabetes may already have this problem. Therefore, hot baths are contraindicated. However, warm and neutral-temperature baths are a good choice for diabetics, as are whole-body salt glows.

Diabetes also affects the blood vessels of the legs and feet. The small blood vessels just under the skin become narrow and do not dilate normally in response to local heat. A local heat treatment such as a hot footbath leads to increased metabolism in the warmed tissues, which then require more oxygen and other nutrients. Because the blood vessels in the feet do not function well, they cannot supply enough oxygen and other nutrients, and this situation can lead to tissue death. Another potential problem is that diabetics often have little ability to feel pressure and temperature in their feet, so they may not be able to tell when hot applications are too hot and might burn their feet. Therefore, hot footbaths, heating pads, hot water bottles, paraffin dips, and hot moist packs are all contraindicated, along with steam cabinets in which the client sits upright and steam enters through the floor of the cabinet. However, footbaths of 102°F or less are safe for diabetics. Alternating footbaths are used under a doctor's supervision at several medical clinics in the United States to treat diabetic ulcers of the feet: alternating warm (102°F) and cold (55°F) footbaths promote circulation without dangerously high temperatures.

However, this treatment should never be performed without a doctor's permission.

Inability to Sense Heat or Cold

A variety of conditions can cause the loss of normal sensation, including arteriosclerosis, nerve injury, exposure to toxic substances, diabetes, and neuromuscular conditions such as spinal cord injury and multiple sclerosis. The potential danger in dealing with clients who cannot feel heat or cold very well is that they won't be able to tell you if a hot application is burning their skin or a cold application is freezing their skin. Therefore, hot and cold applications are contraindicated. Mild heat (no more than 102°F), cool water (but not ice), and neutral applications such as salt glows and neutral baths are safe.

Lymphedema

Lymphedema is an accumulation of lymph in subcutaneous tissues. It is most commonly seen after surgery for cancer that removes lymph nodes. Doctors advise patients with this condition to avoid exposure to heat. For example, patients with lymphedema of the arm are advised to wear a long insulated glove when removing something hot from the oven. Local heat to a limb with lymphedema will increase blood flow through vasodilation, leading to an increased amount of fluid leaking out of the capillaries and into tissue spaces. This is a normal process, and ordinarily the lymphatic system returns this fluid to the heart, but when lymphatic vessels or nodes are destroyed, surrounding tissues swell with fluid, sometimes dramatically, causing discomfort and possibly tissue damage. Therefore, such local treatments as hot fomentations, hydrocollator packs, hot water bottles, hot footbaths, and paraffin dips are contraindicated. Prolonged applications of ice should also be avoided, but ice massage and local treatments with warm (no more than 102°F) or cool water are safe. Doctors typically advise their patients to avoid hot showers, hot tubs, and any whole-body heat treatment, since the resulting vasodilation would include the affected limb. However, aquatic therapy in a 92°F pool can be an effective treatment to help move blood and lymph through an edematous limb.(10) Lymphedema patients should also not have prolonged (over 15 minutes) whole-body heat treatments. However, warm baths to 102°F are safe.

Multiple Sclerosis

Whole-body heat treatments and local applications of heat that are very large or are on the person's skin for a long time can raise core temperature. In clients who have multiple sclerosis, this can cause extreme fatigue, and so they are contraindicated. Neutral or cold treatments, including neutral temperature whirlpools, cold compresses, and exercise in cold water, are indicated. For more information, see the section in multiple sclerosis in Chapter 14.

Seizure Disorders

Seizures can be caused by a variety of factors, including head trauma, infection, and brain tumor, but for one-third of clients with seizures there is no known cause. When giving clients with seizure disorders whole-body treatments, extremes of hot and cold are contraindicated because they might trigger a seizure. Mild sedative treatments, such as salt glows, warm baths, neutral baths, and wet sheet packs taken to a neutral stage are indicated; however, someone must be present at all times in the unlikely event of a seizure.

Skin Infections and Rashes

Do not apply any hydrotherapy treatment over skin that is infected or has a rash except with a doctor's permission.

Thyroid Disorders

Whole-body heat treatments affect metabolic rate and thyroid activity in ways that are not yet fully understood. Very frequent heat treatments are contraindicated for patients who have low thyroid activity, or hypothyroidism. (A one-time heat treatment will have little effect on a thyroid condition, but regular saunas, hot tubs, or other heat treatments may have a depressing effect.) Conversely, very frequent whole-body cooling treatments are contraindicated for clients who have overly high thyroid activity, or hyperthyroidism. (A one-time cold treatment will have little or no effect on a thyroid condition, but regular cold baths may have a stimulating effect.)(11)

Nerve or Crush Injuries to the Extremities

Sometimes clients with nerve or crush injuries are permanently hypersensitive to cold. If the sensation of cold is very uncomfortable, cold treatments are contraindicated. In this case, contrast treatments may be more successful in increasing circulation, as a brief cold immersion will not actually chill the tissue. Water temperature should be tailored to the person, so begin with cool, not cold water, and if the client tolerates it, water temperature may be lowered gradually. Salt glows at a mild temperature may be even more effective.

Prescription Medications

Clients who are taking certain medications should not receive hydrotherapy. Cold treatments that promote vasoconstriction should not be combined with medications

Choosing the Right Treatment for a Patient with Nervous Tension and Sciatic Pain

Background

Gene, a 70-year-old woman, was referred to a massage therapist by a friend. She noted on her intake form that she had a hip replacement 6 months before and explained that although she healed very well from the surgery, she had had "sciatica" ever since. She was also experiencing severe emotional stress. She explained that she had sciatica a long time ago but had gone many years without it until after her hip replacement surgery. She commented to the therapist that she is often colder than the people around her. Gene was seeking massage to help her relax her whole body and hoping it could also relieve her sciatic pain.

Discussion Questions

1. What additional questions should the therapist ask Gene when interviewing her?
2. Some traditional hydrotherapy treatments for sciatica include ice massage (see Chapter 14). Is it safe to perform any of these hydrotherapy treatments with her? What steps should the therapist take to determine this?
3. If approved, which of the hydrotherapy treatments would be appropriate and effective for her?

that promote vasoconstriction, such as migraine headache medications that include caffeine. Heat treatments that promote vasodilation should not be combined with medications that promote vasodilation, such as decongestants and migraine headache medication. Clients with high blood pressure should not be treated hot or cold, it is especially dangerous if they are taking medications that lower blood pressure. Neutral baths are safe for them.

SAFETY PRECAUTIONS

A few simple safety precautions should be observed during hydrotherapy treatments:

1. Since some hydrotherapy treatments involve immersing a part of the client's body in water, it is possible that some water could be spilled on the floor. Mop up any spills immediately so that there is less chance of anyone slipping.
2. Exercise caution when handling hot packs, using metal tongs or gloves, so your hands are not burned (Fig. 4-4).
3. If a client has had a massage before going into a hot tub, steam room, or sauna, he or she should be sure to wash off the massage oil or lotion thoroughly before going in. This prevents bath water from being contaminated, and there will be no slippery film left on floors or benches. However, in most cases, if the client is going to have a whole-body heat treatment, it is better to have it before the massage session to make the massage more effective. Then the client begins the session already

relaxed, with more pliable soft tissue and greater joint range of motion.

4. Clients should not be barefoot, especially if they have just had a massage. Oily feet should not be on the floor of your facility, and if a client is going to walk to a sauna or hot tub or shower, he or she could slip. Clients should have socks on at the end of the massage and then wear shoes with nonslip bottoms.
5. As seen in Figure 4-5, grab bars in showers or whirlpools and next to hot tubs may help stabilize

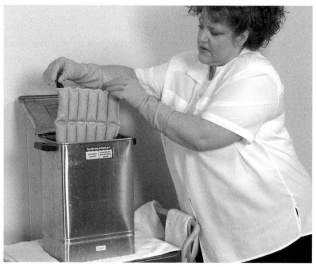

FIGURE 4-4 ■ Use of gloves to protect the hands while handling hot packs.

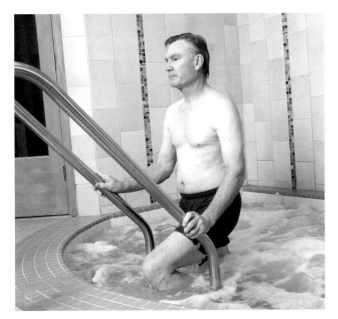

FIGURE 4-5 ■ Client using grab bars.

someone who is obese, unsteady on his or her feet, or lightheaded from overexposure to heat.

6. Clients are more likely to complain of cold after baths in the winter: indoor air is generally very dry then, and so the small amount of water on the skin evaporates rapidly and cools them more than if the air were not so dry. To prevent chilling, make sure that clients are wrapped in a towel or dry clothing as soon as they get out of a bath or other whole-body immersion.

7. To prevent burns, saunas should always have a wood railing or fence around the heater.

FACTORS AFFECTING THE BODY'S RESPONSE TO HEAT AND COLD

When you give a hydrotherapy treatment during a massage, you are hoping that the person's system will respond strongly. For example, when ice is put on the skin, the goal is a powerful constriction of the client's blood vessels. When a client is put in a hot bath, the goal is a strong stimulation of the circulatory system. However, because clients are unique, a treatment that is appropriate for one person may be wrong for another. Some factors affect how well a person responds to a treatment, and while we cannot always predict how an individual will respond, being aware of these factors can help guide you in choice of treatment.

BODY COMPOSITION AND GENETICS

Just as individuals vary widely in their response to tactile stimulation, they also vary widely in their tolerance of heat and cold. One client may feel comfortable receiving a massage with the windows open, no heat turned on in the massage room, and minimal draping, while another client in the same room at the same season of the year feels comfortable only when the windows are shut, room heat is turned on high, warming devices (such as hot water bottles or hot fomentations) are placed on the body, and he is covered with extra blankets. People are also very different in their responses to water temperatures. Over many years, hydrotherapy students in classes I taught have reported their "ideal" bath temperature as everything from 98° to 110°F. (Figure 4-3 on p. 67 shows generally whether a water temperature will be perceived as hot, warm, neutral, or cold.)

These individual differences are a combination of many factors, such as percentage of body fat and genetic inheritance. Someone with a low percentage of body fat will feel cold much more acutely than someone with a high percentage. Because fat is a good insulator, people who are obese cannot dissipate heat as well thin ones and can overheat more easily. Differences in the body's response to temperature have been found in groups such as Eskimos, Asians, African-Americans, and whites. These differences reflect the different climates where their ancestors originated.(12–15) The client's ability to generate body heat and to cool off by sweating and the extent to which the blood vessels react to cold are genetically influenced. Some people actually have thinner skin than others, and their thermal receptors are closer to the skin surface, so local applications of heat and cold will feel different to them than to someone with thicker skin.

However, as therapists, our first responsibility is to rely on our client's feedback as we give them treatments, not on assumptions or stereotypes. Since each client is an individual, it is not always possible to predict how they will respond, and responses to treatments vary widely. Listening to their past experience with heat and cold, then paying close attention to how they respond, is the best guide to the appropriateness of the treatment.

SEASONAL CONSIDERATIONS

Clients who are regularly exposed to very hot or cold temperatures tend to respond better to extremes of hot or cold. Because keeping core temperature at 98.6°F is crucial to our well-being, as the seasons change our bodies quickly adjust to outside temperatures. Over days or weeks many subtle adjustments are made. For example, when the temperature climbs in summer, the amount that we sweat increases and the amount of salt we lose in our sweat decreases. People who work in severe cold develop an increased ability to tolerate any cold exposure, and even repeated exposure to a cold hand bath causes the blood vessels of the hand to react more and more strongly. What this means for hydrotherapy treatments is that your clients may react better to a treatment if their system has been recently exposed to hot or cold temperatures than if not.(16–18)

In addition, the client who comes in on a hot day already overheated is not likely to enjoy a hot fomentation, which usually feels wonderful in the dead of winter, just as a client who enters your office on a cold winter's day already chilled is not likely to be receptive to ice massage unless his or her body has been thoroughly warmed first. One of the most effective ways you can use hydrotherapy treatments in your office is to maintain your clients' body temperature so they are neither chilled nor overheated. For example, a client who needs a heat treatment as part of his or her massage session but who is already very warm can receive a cooling treatment at the same time and not become overheated. On a hot day I have used hot moist packs before stretching particular areas while using a cold footbath to prevent the client from becoming overheated. For more on this topic, see Boxes 4-1 and 4-2.

PHYSICAL CONDITION OF THE CLIENT

Healthy people are stronger and react to hydrotherapy faster than those who are weak or unhealthy. The very old, the very young, those with major health problems, inactive people, obese people, and those with generally low resistance are likely to respond more weakly. For example, a young, vigorous person may be able to tolerate a cold plunge after a hot bath and then enjoy the prolonged feeling of warmth that the cold plunge usually gives. A weaker person, however, may become chilled during the plunge and never warm up.

TEMPERATURE OF THE CLIENT'S SKIN AND BODY CORE BEFORE A TREATMENT

If the client's skin is very cold or hot at the beginning of a treatment, he or she will probably have a slower or weaker reaction. If the skin is very hot, it will take longer

---

BOX 4-1 *Point of Interest*

USING HYDROTHERAPY TO COOL THE CLIENT DURING A SESSION

1. When clients enter your office on a hot day, a simple way to help them cool down before massage is a brief cold foot soak. Even 5 minutes of soaking can reduce their body temperature. Soaking can be performed with clients seated or lying supine on the massage table with knees bent.
2. A cool shower before or after the massage session will reduce body temperature.
3. A flat plastic bottle filled with cold water may be placed on the therapy table, then covered by the sheet the client will lie on.
4. A washcloth or round cotton pads dipped in ice water can be used to cool the eyes and upper face. Miniature ice packs with a thin layer of cloth underneath or a cooled gel mask specifically for the eyes are also effective.
5. Ice packs can be used for almost any part of the body if they are the right size: small ones can go over the eyes, long narrow ones can go behind or around the neck or on any other part of the body, and larger ones may be used on areas such as the upper thigh or back. Caution must be observed to protect the skin with a thin layer of cloth directly on it.
6. Chilled gloves (loofah gloves or even very thin wool or cotton gloves) for the hands or chilled cotton socks for the feet provide cooling that may be more acceptable for some clients than cold nearer the center of the body. Both the gloves and the socks are soaked in water, wrung out, and kept in the freezer until they are needed. Then they are thawed slightly until they are limp but still cold and put on the client's hands or feet. When they warm up, they can be dipped in ice water or iced herbal tea and applied.
7. A hot water bottle filled with ice water may be used on any part of the body.

8. A large towel dipped in ice water and wrung out well is effective for cooling the back. Massage may be done through the cold towel.
9. To cool the chest and abdomen, use a slightly smaller towel dipped in ice water and wrung out. Massage may be done through the cold towel.
10. Spray ice water from a mister bottle over the client's body. This is especially effective if you have a fan blowing cool air over the client's body. Some therapists use a few drops of cooling essential oils, such as peppermint. Do not spray the face.
11. Wash each portion of the body with a washcloth dipped in ice water as you finish massage. This is especially effective if you have a fan blowing cool air.
12. Apply a salt glow with ice water on individual areas of the body or the entire body. Ice water is used to moisten the salt and to wash the client before and after the salt application.
13. Use ice massage on individual areas.
14. Apply an iced sheet wrap, using a sheet wrung out in cold water, then put in the freezer for 10 minutes or in an ice chest half-full of ice cubes for 10 minutes or in the refrigerator for 20 minutes. A sheet can also be soaked in a large container of very cold water (made with plenty of ice cubes) and used right away. The iced sheet is placed on the massage table, and the client lies on the iced sheet, is wrapped, and then receives massage on face, hands, and feet before the sheet is removed.
15. Cold plunges are extremely cooling. After a massage session, clients should shower first to remove massage oil or lotion.

Reference
1. Bruder L, Cooling Down Your Sessions. Available at http://www.spamassagealliance.com2003/issue 104/cool.html.

BOX 4-2 | *Point of Interest*

USING HYDROTHERAPY TO WARM THE CLIENT DURING A SESSION

1. Hot foot soak prior to massage. This can be done with the client sitting in a chair or lying supine on the massage table.
2. A hot shower, hot tub, sauna, steam bath, or hot bath in a bathtub prior to massage. Extra care should be taken that clients do not become chilled between getting out and getting on the massage table.
3. A flat plastic bottle filled with warm water may be placed on the therapy table, then covered by the sheet the client will lie on. When the massage table is warm at the outset of the massage, the client is likely to relax quickly.
4. Warmed gel eye mask, moist, round cotton pads or washcloth dipped in hot water, or small ice packs with layers of cloth underneath to warm the eyes and upper face.
5. Washcloths or round cotton pads that are dipped in warm water can be used to cool the eyes and upper face. Warmed gel masks specifically for the eyes are also effective.
6. Moist local heat applications. These include hydrocollator packs and hot fomentations, hot hand

towels kept in a cooler after having hot water poured over them, and washcloths that are either heated in a slow cooker with a small amount of water in the bottom or dipped in hot water and then wrung out before being applied to the client's skin.
7. Paraffin treatments of the hands or feet. These are effective at warming the whole body, especially if prolonged.
8. Hot water bottles of various sizes filled with warm water.
9. Large towels dipped in hot water and wrung out may be used to warm the entire back or front of the body. They will cool off rapidly, however, and when cold should be replaced with another warm towel. As soon as the last towel is removed, the client should be dried thoroughly and covered immediately with a drape.
10. Hot wash to remove massage oil or lotion. Wash each portion of the body with a washcloth dipped in hot water as you finish massage. Dry the skin immediately and cover the client to keep the area warm.
11. Full-body wrap during massage of the feet or head using warm wrap equipment.

for a cold application to chill it, and if the skin is very cold, it will take longer for a hot application to warm it.

Core temperature is also important: if a client is cold before a cold immersion, he or she is likely to react weakly.(19) Clients should be thoroughly warm but not overheated before a treatment begins. Keep the treatment room at about 70°F.

PART OF THE BODY TREATED

Different areas of the body have different amounts of warm and cold receptors, so some parts are more sensitive to temperatures. For example, an ice pack laid upon the chest is likely to chill the client far more than the same ice pack laid upon the foot.

TREATMENT TEMPERATURE

The hotter or colder the hydrotherapy, the faster and stronger the client's reaction. A neutral-temperature shower, which is at the person's own body temperature, will create much less of a reaction in the skin, nervous system, and circulatory system than a very hot or very cold shower. Because the body is constantly defending its core temperature and neutral temperature water will not warm or cool the body, much less response is required to maintain normal 98.6°F temperature. For this reason, neutral temperatures have a more calming and sedating effect than hot or cold.

ABRUPTNESS OF TREATMENT

The more sudden the application of a hot or cold treatment, the greater the client's reaction. For example, if a person is standing in a warm shower and the water temperature is gradually changed to cold, the reaction will not be as strong as if the water temperature is changed from warm directly to cold. The more abrupt the change, the more stimulating the treatment will be.

DURATION OF TREATMENT

In general, the less time the application lasts, the more stimulating it is to the circulation. For example, a short hot bath is more stimulating than a long hot bath, and a short cold shower is more stimulating than a long cold shower. A short hot application, such as a hydrocollator pack laid on an area for 2 minutes, is more stimulating to the circulation than a longer hot application, and ice massage, with which the cold continually moves to new areas, is more stimulating to the local circulation than an ice pack, which remains in one place for many minutes.

PROPORTION OF THE BODY THAT IS EXPOSED TO THE TREATMENT

All other factors being the same, the client's reaction is directly proportional to the size of the area covered: that is, the larger the application, the greater the reaction. A client who lies on a bed of three warm fomentations that contact her skin from her knees to her neck will have a much stronger reaction than a client who has a small warm compress over her eyes.

USE OF FRICTION OR PRESSURE

Adding mechanical stimulation to a hot or cold treatment speeds up or increases the body's response: it stimulates the nerves to a greater extent, which causes the blood vessels in the skin to react more strongly. Rubbing or pouring also keeps the water in greater contact with the skin, so that the heat or cold in the water will be continually warming or cooling it. A cloth wrung out in ice water and simply laid over a small area of the body will cause a far weaker reaction than if you lay it on the skin, then rub the area briskly through the cloth. Rubbing not only stimulates the blood vessels in the skin to dilate, it keeps the cold water moving over the skin.

BODY TEMPERATURE AFTER A WHOLE-BODY TREATMENT

Chilling of the body immediately after the treatment will undo much of its positive effects. A client who takes a short hot bath, for example, will not have increased the temperature of the body core, but the blood vessels in the skin will have dilated to radiate heat off the skin, and the body will actually begin losing heat as soon as the client steps out of the water. Therefore, a client who goes immediately to receive a massage is more likely to lie on a treatment table shivering than relaxing. However, a very short cold shower or a cold mitten friction after the hot tub causes the blood vessels of the skin to constrict, giving a prolonged sensation of warmth, and the client will be far more comfortable once on the treatment table. It is important to be aware of clients' body temperature after they have taken any kind of whole-body heat or cooling treatment. Being chilled or overheated can prevent clients from relaxing, as their body may be expending energy trying to normalize their body temperature, and they may be uncomfortable.

AVERSION TO HEAT OR COLD

Some people have an intense dislike or fear of heat or cold, possibly stemming from a bad experience with hot or cold applications in the past, making them unwilling to try a hydrotherapy treatment. *Pediatric Massage Therapy* quotes a woman who was physically abused when she was a child. Growing up, she had many welts and bruises from the abuse, and hot baths always made them sting. Even though as an adult her skin was intact, she still avoided taking baths.(20) As a very young

child, Suzanne Pike was admitted to Warm Springs Rehabilitation Institute at Warms Springs, Georgia, for treatment of her clubfeet. Pike regularly received painfully hot paraffin footbaths followed by painful massage and manipulation on her clubfeet. At age 73, she confessed that because of that childhood experience, she had been afraid of medical treatments and doctors all of her life, and just the idea of heat on her extremities was unpleasant to her.(21) If your client has such an aversion to a particular treatment, it may be better to use a different one that will achieve the same end. For example, if your client has an aversion to a local heat treatment such as a fomentation, local circulation can be enhanced by a salt glow with neutral-temperature water instead. Sometimes if you explain the purpose of a treatment the client may be willing to give it a try, but never coerce anyone to have a particular treatment.

CLIENT'S HEALTH HISTORY

If your client is going to receive a hydrotherapy treatment along with massage therapy, taking a careful health history will alert you to any conditions that might contraindicate hydrotherapy treatments. (An interview with a client is seen in Figure 4-6.) Additionally, at the end of the form, several questions are included that can help you explore how the client may feel about certain treatments. (Figure 4-7 gives a sample health history form.) Take a few minutes to discuss the history with your client and address any particular health concerns. Should there be any question about a treatment that the client would like to have but that you know is unsafe, take time to explain your concerns to the client. For example, a client with lymphedema may not be aware that she should not enter a sauna just because her friends are all going in together. You may wish to read her the information from this book or another source to make your concerns really clear.

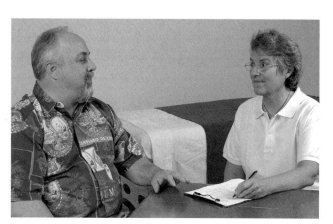

FIGURE 4-6 ■ Interviewing the client.

Health History

Name: _____   Today's date: _____

Address: _____   Phone #: _____

1. How is your health in general? _____

_____

2. Do you have any conditions that are being monitored by a healthcare practitioner? _____

_____

3. Please check if you now have or have had any of the following conditions:

_____ arteriosclerosis   _____ migraine headaches

_____ arthritis   _____ multiple sclerosis

_____ artificial devices   _____ nerve or crush injury to an extremity
          (joint prosthetics, implants,
          pacemaker, or other)   _____ phlebitis

_____ asthma   _____ pregnancy

_____ bursitis   _____ Raynaud's syndrome

_____ cancer   _____ seizure disorders

_____ diabetes   _____ skin disease

_____ heart disease   _____ stroke
          (history of heart attack, congestive heart
          failure, coronary artery disease)   _____ tendonitis

_____ hepatitis   _____ tension headaches

_____ HIV/AIDS   _____ tension or soreness in a specific area

_____ high blood pressure   _____ thyroid conditions

_____ joint pain or swelling   _____ whiplash injuries

_____ loss of feeling in any part of the body   _____ other conditions

_____ lymphedema   _____ other pain

Comments: _____

_____

_____

_____

4. Operations in your whole life: _____

_____

_____

_____

_____

5. Traumatic injuries such as bruises, sprains, broken bones, dislocations and concussions: _____

_____

_____

_____

_____

FIGURE 4-7 ■ Client's health history.

6. Any recent injuries, hospitalizations or illness? _____

7. Are you taking any medications? _____

8. How much stress have you been under recently? _____

9. How much stress have you been under for the last few years? _____

10. Where do you tend to store stress? _____

11. What do you do to relax?_____

12. How well can you relax when you are under stress? _____

13. Who is your family doctor? _____

14. What is your main goal for receiving massage today? _____

Hydrotherapy-related questions:

1. *If a local heat treatment will be used:*

   How do you usually react to heat on your skin? _____

   Do you enjoy intense heat on your skin? _____

2. *If a local cold treatment will be used:*

   How do you usually react to ice or very cold water on your skin? _____

   Do you enjoy cold on your skin? _____

3. *If a whole-body heating treatment will be used:*

   How do you usually react to hot baths, saunas, steam baths or hot tubs? _____

   Do you enjoy the feeling of being very warm? _____

4. *If a whole-body cold treatment will be used:*

   How do you usually react to cold showers or cold baths? _____

   Do you have a strong dislike of cold?_____

5. *If a whole-body wrap (hot blanket pack, wet sheet wrap) will be used:*

   Have you ever had a whole-body wrap? _____ If so how did you like it? _____

   Some people love being wrapped up in blankets, and find it warm and cozy, but some people may feel too confined.

   Do you ever feel claustrophobic? _____

6. *Do you know any medical reason why you shouldn't have hot or cold t reatments on your skin?*

7. *Do you know any medical reason why you shouldn't have hot or cold t reatments on your whole body at once, such as*

   a hot tub or cold shower? _____

I understand that massage/body work is not a substitute for medical examination and treatment. I further understand that a massage practitioner does not diagnose or treat illness, rather that massage is for the basic purpose of relaxation, release of muscular tension and the enhancement of health through increasing circulation and energy flow.

Client's signature _____

FIGURE 4-7 ■ *(Continued)*

BASIC GUIDELINES FOR HYDROTHERAPY

Following these basic guidelines will ensure that you give your client a safe and effective treatment:

1. Check the temperature of hot or cold applications before putting them on your client's skin. Check hot applications, such as steam packs, against your own skin. When you use water in a treatment, always use a thermometer to check its temperature.
2. When using a hot application, always tell your clients, "Let me know if this starts to feel too hot." Even if you have given your clients the same hot application many times before, remind them that you want to know if it is too hot.
3. While you are giving the hydrotherapy treatment, explain to the client what you are doing and why. This may be as simple as telling your client, "Now I'm going to put an ice pack over your bruise; it will feel cold at first, but it will help relieve the swelling and discomfort" or "I'm going to put this hot pack over your lower back. It will help relax those muscles before I massage them."
4. During treatments, carefully observe the client. Check occasionally under a hot application to see what the skin looks like, especially during the first 5 minutes, when a hot pack is at its hottest. Also ask the client how it feels. For example, with either a hot pack or a cold pack you could ask, "How does this feel on your skin now?"
5. Make sure your clients are comfortable during any hydrotherapy treatment. For example, if they are not entirely comfortable with ice, reassure them that you will make sure the rest of their body is extra warm. Drape carefully around areas where you are doing ice massage to keep trickles of ice water from going into sensitive areas. Preserve their modesty by carefully draping them if parts of their body are going to be exposed during treatments.
6. Never start or end treatment with a chilled client—always warm the client before treatments if necessary. A cold client will not be able to relax during a massage. A client should never leave your office with wet hair or damp clothing.
7. Observe all contraindications.
8. Instruct clients to follow safety rules. For example, in a facility such as a health club, clients should take seriously the warning on the sauna door prohibiting those with hypertension or cardiac problems from entering.

SESSION DESIGN

Choosing which treatments to give your client during a massage session is not difficult. Taking a good history at the first session (including any experience with hydrotherapy), listening carefully to your client's concerns, and getting feedback on the treatments makes it easy to pick the right one. Hydrotherapy applications should always complement massage techniques and work toward the same goals. For example, when your client arrives, try to determine whether he or she is interested in relief from stress, needs help with a musculoskeletal issue, or simply needs to be touched. If relief from stress is the help he or she needs, ice massage is probably not called for: a more soothing treatment would be a warm bath, hot shower, or body wrap followed by massage. If the client has a musculoskeletal injury, ice massage or a contrast bath may be the best treatment to increase circulation and relieve discomfort in the injured area without touching it, and afterward massage techniques may also be applied around the injured area. If the client is seeking massage to receive nurturing touch, perhaps a local salt glow to provide additional stimulation to the skin would complement your touch.

Some specific examples:

1. A client arrives for an appointment that was scheduled a month ago, only to tell you that she was in a car accident yesterday. She was evaluated at the emergency department of a nearby hospital and found to be free of major musculoskeletal injuries. However, most of her body except her hands and feet still hurt too much to be touched. In addition, she is emotionally upset by the accident. Any vigorous massage is obviously contraindicated. A simple, comforting session could include first soaking three small bath towels in water with Epsom salts dissolved in it, then wringing them out and placing them gently on her trunk, abdomen and legs, then covering each with a warm fomentation or a thin sheet of plastic and a heating pad. (Hydrocollator packs would be too heavy for her sensitive tissue.) Then the client could receive massage on her hands and feet or energetic techniques. This hydrotherapy treatment not only helps with her pain, it also allows her to have a relaxing session.
2. A client with a painful shoulder arrives straight from her doctor's office. Her doctor has ruled out a sprained shoulder, bursitis, or rotator cuff syndrome and diagnosed muscle strain: she is a nurse and lifted a heavy patient that morning. A session that meets her needs could consist of a contrast treatment on her shoulder, using a moist hot pack followed by ice massage, followed by gentle massage around the shoulder. This will desensitize the area somewhat, improve circulation, and help relieve pain.
3. A client arrives with a severe lower back spasm; in fact, his back is in such severe spasm that he almost has to be carried in by a friend. He has come directly from his chiropractor, who found the client's muscles too tense for an adjustment and recommended massage. A salt glow of the lower back followed by ice massage helps increase circulation, relieves pain, and decreases muscle spasm, making the massage much more effective. Another possibility in a facility that

has steam cabinets or full bathtubs would be a steam bath or hot Epsom salt bath followed by local ice massage over the back muscles, then hands-on techniques. Still another method would be to place a towel soaked in Epsom salt water on his back, then cover the towel with a thin piece of plastic and a hydrocollator pack, fomentation, or hot water bottle. After a 15- to 20-minute application, his back muscles will be far more relaxed and ready for massage. During this time, massage could be performed on related muscle groups, such as gluteals, piriformis, and spinal erectors proximal to his lower back. A study of 117 people who were hospitalized for lower back pain found that patients with chronic back pain had shorter hospital stays when treated with ice massage, and patients with acute back pain had shorter hospital stays when treated with moist hot packs.(22)

When working with clients to determine the best hydrotherapy treatment to meet their needs, it is helpful to follow a standard three-step process. Step 1: review the client's medical history. Step 2: interview the client. Step 3: select the appropriate treatment. The following are two examples of how to use this process, one for a relaxation massage and the other for a therapeutic massage.

CHOOSING HYDROTHERAPY TREATMENTS FOR A RELAXATION MASSAGE SESSION

Step 1: Review the Client's Medical History

- Does the client have any contraindications to hydrotherapy treatments?
- Has the client had hydrotherapy treatments before, and if so, how did he or she respond to them?

Step 2: Interview the Client

- In what part of the body does the client tend to store stress?
- Which of the client's muscles particularly tight?
- What type of massage does the client prefer: light touch techniques such as energy work or gentle Swedish massage, or deep pressure techniques such as myofascial release or deep Swedish massage? A highly sensitive person who prefers light touch techniques is more likely to prefer a hydrotherapy technique which is not highly stimulating, such as a warm compress. A less sensitive person who prefers deeper techniques may enjoy, and tolerate well, such highly stimulating techniques as contrast applications and sprays and showers.

Step 3: Select the Appropriate Treatment

- Decide which hydrotherapy treatments are options for this relaxation massage session. Of course, the

treatments you can give are also determined by the hydrotherapy equipment in your office.
- Review contraindications.
- Choose a treatment that is safe and appropriate.
- Obtain the client's permission.

CHOOSING HYDROTHERAPY TREATMENTS FOR A THERAPEUTIC MASSAGE SESSION

Step 1: Review the Client's Medical History

- What soft tissue condition or conditions does the client have?
- Is this condition acute or chronic?
- Does the client have any contraindications to hydrotherapy treatments?
- Has the client had hydrotherapy treatments before, and if so, what was the response to them?

Step 2: Interview the Client

- In what part or parts of the body is the client's pain or discomfort?
- Does anything increase or decrease the pain or discomfort?

Step 3: Select the Appropriate Treatment

- Determine which part or parts of the body to treat
- Decide which hydrotherapy treatments are options for this therapeutic massage session. Of course, the treatments you can choose from are determined by the hydrotherapy equipment in your office.
- Review contraindications.
- Choose a treatment that is safe and appropriate.
- Obtain the client's permission.

ADAPTING HYDROTHERAPY TREATMENTS TO DIFFERENT SETTINGS

Most of the discussion of hydrotherapy in this chapter has been directed to a massage therapist working in an individual practice or sharing an office with other massage therapists. However, individual hydrotherapy treatments can be performed in many other environments. Remember that treatments in any setting offer positive sensory stimulation along with their physiological benefits. Following are some examples of settings and how hydrotherapy treatments can be adapted for use there.

OUTDOOR SPORTS EVENT

A massage practitioner working outdoors at a sports massage event can take bags of ice and bottled water in a cooler, along with extra towels and washcloths, plastic dish tubs for foot soaks, and Epsom salt. If a hose or other source of running water is nearby, many more athletes can be treated. With these few simple tools items, you can perform the following:

- Ice massage to relieve sore and aching muscles
- Local salt glows of the back, legs, and feet to increase circulation and relax those areas
- Ice-cold foot soaks for aching and burning feet and to cool down on a hot day
- Epsom salt foot soaks for tired and aching feet. Water does not have to be hot for these foot soaks; even tepid water will be effective. Perhaps athletes who are waiting for a massage would like to soak their feet while they wait.

HOSPITAL

An individual massage practitioner working in a hospital setting may see patients who have access to a whirlpool. For example, some hospitals that offer whirlpool baths for women during labor may have them available after the birth to help with perineal and low back discomfort. Massage therapy for new mothers after a whirlpool bath is a wonderful complement to this service. With the permission of the nursing staff, warm, moist towels may be used with any patient to provide mild local heat and to wash off massage lotion at the end of the massage. These treatments are very comforting for patients and practical if they are in bed. See Box 4-3 for an example of a hospital that incorporates hydrotherapy and massage extensively in the care of its patients.

BOX 4-3 | *Point of Interest*

HYDROTHERAPY AND MASSAGE IN A HOSPITAL SETTING

Wildwood Hospital in Wildwood, Georgia, operated by the Seventh Day Adventist Church, is an acute-care hospital, outpatient clinic, and health education center. The entire facility, including the hydrotherapy department, was built in 1942 and has treated patients continuously since then. Hydrotherapy treatments are an integral part of the hospital's care of both sick patients and of participants in health education programs.

Hospitalized patients receive hydrotherapy treatments and massage as part of the hospital's philosophy of using natural treatments to promote health and provide an alternative to the use of prescription medication. Each patient's case is reviewed by staff physicians (medical doctors), who prescribe treatments. I have observed hydrotherapy treatments at the hospital for patients with liver cirrhosis, cancer, high blood pressure, asthma, diabetic ulcers, varicose ulcers, musculoskeletal complaints, and diseases of the immune system. After surgery, when their doctor has determined that the danger of bleeding is past—generally after 36 hours—many patients receive contrast treatments over their incision to reduce pain and speed healing. Generally the incision is covered with a sheet of plastic to keep it dry, then warm fomentations are alternated with cool cloths or even iced cloths, for a total of three changes.

At Wildwood, whole-body treatments are performed using large whirlpools, multiple-jet showers, and Russian steam baths. Local treatments are performed using small whirlpools, sitz baths, hot fomentations, and ice. Many of the patients receive a contrast shower at the end of their other treatments. Patients who are strong enough to walk or be taken by wheelchair have their treatments in the hydrotherapy department of the hospital. However, if they are too weak or have too many intravenous lines, monitors, or other equipment to be moved, they receive treatments in their room. In that case, nurses or specially trained therapists generally use hot fomentations and ice to perform treatments. Fomentations are heated in the hydrotherapy department, placed in a large cooler, and taken in a rolling cart to the patient's room along with a supply of ice cubes.

The hydrotherapy department, which is managed by a physical therapist, is a heavily used area of the hospital. It has separate

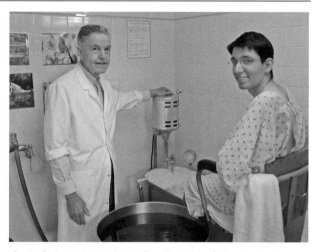

Physical therapist Earl Qualls, director of the hydrotherapy department, gives a contrast leg bath to a patient. Hot whirlpool is on the right; cold pool is on the left. Qualls graduated from physical therapy school in 1951 and was still practicing as a physical therapist and supervising the hydrotherapy department at Wildwood Hospital in 2007. (Photo courtesy of Wildwood Hospital, Wildwood, Georgia.)

men's and women's sides, each containing a multiple-jet shower, Russian steam bath, linen storage area, and five treatment rooms. These rooms contain treatment tables where patients may receive massage therapy after their water treatments. A common area used by both men and women contains porcelain sitz baths and large and small steel whirlpools (photo). The entire hydrotherapy department is tiled from floor to ceiling, and its walls have many built-in niches with shelves for gloves, massage oils, and other small items.

Those who are staying at Wildwood for their health education program also receive hydrotherapy treatments, either in the hydrotherapy department or in a nearby bathhouse equipped with showers, a whirlpool, and a sauna.

CHIROPRACTIC OR PHYSICAL THERAPY CLINIC

An individual massage practitioner working in a chiropractic office or physical therapy clinic almost always has access to a hydrocollator unit with multiple hydrocollator packs. These hot, moist packs are highly effective in relieving muscle tension and increasing local circulation and are easy to place on one part of the body while massage is being performed on another part. Ice massage is also very useful in this setting, where many clients have severe musculoskeletal pain.

ASSISTED LIVING FACILITY

Clients who are seen in assisted living facilities generally receive massage in their own rooms, which contain a small kitchenette, and so here you have access to running water and ice. (Kitchen staff at assisted living facilities have ice machines and may be willing to give you larger quantities of ice).You may wish to bring containers for water, such as plastic tubs or buckets, but you may also find them in the kitchenette.

A simple, effective, and much-loved treatment in this setting is a warm footbath that incorporates a salt glow of the feet and lower legs. Place a large towel on the floor, place a chair on top of it and then have the client sit in the chair. Sitting on the floor in front of the client, treat each lower leg and foot in turn. One foot may be taken out of the footbath and an Epsom salt glow performed with the foot resting on the edge of the tub or bucket. Then put that foot back and repeat with the other foot and lower leg. Rinse off with clean water, cooler if possible; dry the feet; and finish with hands-on massage techniques.

NURSING HOME

Clients are generally given massages in their own rooms, which are smaller and have no kitchenette; however, they always have a bathroom adjacent to their room. With the hot and cold water coming out of the tap, simple treatments such as the local salt glow are feasible, and washing off massage lotion is simple. A hot cloth on the forehead on a cold winter day or a cold cloth on a hot summer day is easy and very comforting. You may wish to bring a container for water or obtain one from the nursing staff.

HEALTH CLUB OR SPA

Generally, any health club or spa that offers massage has at least one hot tub, shower, steam room, or sauna. After doing a health history, if there are no contraindications, you can suggest that clients use those facilities before or after massage sessions. Many clubs and wellness centers have patrons sign a form that lists contraindications, such as these:

- Do not use the hot tub or sauna under the influence of alcohol or drugs.
- Do not use hot tub or sauna if you have an infectious disease, high or low blood pressure, or very low blood sugar, as this can decrease your tolerance to heat.
- Understand your own heat tolerance and do not exceed 15 minutes in the heat without a cool-down.

In addition, there is often a sign on the door of commercial saunas that lists contraindications. At The Barefoot Sage, a spa in Portland, Oregon, that offers primarily foot treatments including foot soaks, paraffin dips and mud applications, followed by foot massage, their notice to clients reads as follows:

Any person with diabetes, nervous system or cardiovascular disorders, skin conditions, or cancer (including chemotherapy and radiation therapy) that may affect the sensation, circulation, or health in the feet may need a physician's release before some therapies can be provided. If you neglect to inform us of such conditions you do so at your own risk.

The point is that a health club that offers hydrotherapy treatments must ask clients to waive liability, whether you have seen them before that time or not.

CLIENT'S HOME

With a little preparation, a practitioner who gives a massage to a client at his or her home can do many basic treatments. Figure 4-8 shows the contents of a portable hydrotherapy kit. Here are some items that can be kept together as a kit for home visits:

1. Water thermometer
2. Ice chest to transport ice to your client or to hold preheated moist towels, hydrocollator packs, or fomentations
3. Heat-resistant gloves
4. Resealable plastic bags, 1 quart and 1 gallon, to make ice packs from ice cubes and to microwave fomentations
5. Moist hot packs (fomentations or hydrocollator packs) with towels for wrapping them
6. Washcloths, small towels, and bath towels, if linens are not available at the client's home
7. Epsom salt
8. Plastic bag for used linens
9. If running water is not available, take a plastic gallon jug with fresh water and a bag of ice. If hot running water is not available, you can make it by mixing boiling water with cold water as follows. Begin by boiling water on a stovetop. Mix in the proportions listed below to obtain the desired temperature, and always check the water with a thermometer before using it.

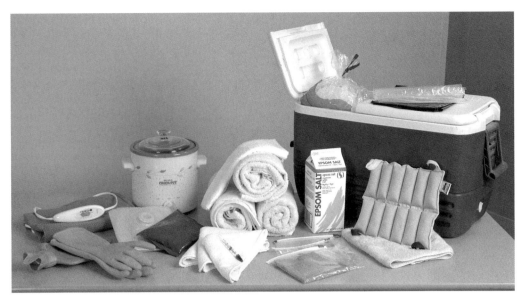

FIGURE 4-8 ■ Portable hydrotherapy kit.

- 1 quart of boiling water plus 4 quarts of cold tap water equals 5 quarts at 85°F.
- 1 quart of boiling water plus 3 quarts of cold tap water equals 1 gallon at 92°F.
- 1 quart of boiling water plus 2 quarts of cold tap water equals 3 quarts at 106°F.
- As the water cools off, if you want to maintain it at the same temperature, you can take out 1 cup of the cooled water and replace it with 2 cups of boiling water. Take the client's limb completely out of the water while you do this. Check the temperature again before putting the limb back in the water.

10. Hot water bottles. In a pinch, any clean plastic bottle may be used for a hot water bottle.
11. Optional: portable steam canopy in carrying container, as described earlier in this chapter. This weighs 20 pounds, can be set up on any comfortable towel-covered surface, and requires only electricity and a little water.
12. Optional: slow cooker or turkey roaster to heat water
13. Optional: plastic garbage bag, cardboard box, and sturdy tape to construct a local bath, such as an arm bath or sitz bath

CHAPTER SUMMARY

In this chapter, you have learned how to select and maintain hydrotherapy equipment, take proper cautions and recognize contraindications for hydrotherapy treatments, and to obtain a thorough health history from the client. You have also learned some basic treatment guidelines, how to design a session to meet your client's unique needs, and how to adapt hydrotherapy treatments to various situations. Equipped with this knowledge, you can use water treatments and your own creativity to help your clients, using water in a variety of ways that are fine-tuned for their individual needs. In the chapters to come, we will explore many hydrotherapy treatments in far more detail and deepen your understanding of their potential.

REVIEW QUESTIONS

Short Answer

1. Name six factors that affect a person's response to a hydrotherapy treatment.

   _____

   _____

2. Describe the additional questions you must add to a standard health intake form if you are going to give a hydrotherapy treatment.

   _____

   _____

3. Describe the physical changes that might cause a client to become lightheaded or nauseous during a whole-body heat treatment.

   _____

   _____

4. Discuss the factors you need to take into account to select a hydrotherapy treatment for a client.

   _____

   _____

Multiple Choice

5. Some hydrotherapy treatments are contraindicated for all but which one of the following?
   a. Chilled person
   b. Multiple sclerosis
   c. Lymphedema
   d. Inactive person
   e. Raynaud's syndrome

6. All of these factors related to the client could cause a poor response to some hydrotherapy treatments *except*
   a. Sedentary lifestyle
   b. Cold skin at the beginning of the treatment
   c. Chronic illness
   d. Distracted client
   e. Emotional stress
   f. Chilling after treatment

7. All of these people might be easily chilled *except*
   a. One with a hypothyroid condition
   b. One from a family in which everyone gets cold easily
   c. One who is small and thin
   d. One who is obese
   e. One who is not accustomed to cold

8. All of these are effective ways to conserve water when you perform hydrotherapy treatments *except*
   a. Avoid letting water run to get it to the desired temperature
   b. Use appliances that do not waste water
   c. Flush trash down the toilet
   d. Choose hydrotherapy treatments that use relatively little water
   e. Warm the client, not the air

9. Which heat treatment is the most expensive?
   a. Paraffin bath
   b. Sauna
   c. Hot footbath
   d. Steam canopy
   e. Homemade fomentation

True/False

_____ 10. Local cold is contraindicated in Raynaud's syndrome.

_____ 11. Intense heat to the feet is safe for people with diabetes.

_____ 12. Salt glows can be used to improve skin circulation and provide sensory stimulation for bedridden people.

_____ 13. The most important hydrotherapy tool is one basic heat treatment.

_____ 14. After a massage session, all cloth items should be washed in hot water and hung up to dry.

Matching

15.
_____ 1. Crushing injuries   a. No heat to abdomen
_____ 2. Asthmatics   b. Thicker insulation
_____ 3. Limited mobility   c. Thinner skin
_____ 4. Obesity   d. No cold dry air
_____ 5. Pregnancy   e. Difficult movement
_____ 6. Children   f. No local cold treatments

16.
_____ 1. Scalding   a. 92°F
_____ 2. Very cold   b. 60°F
_____ 3. Neutral   c. 110°F
_____ 4. Very hot   d. 97°F
_____ 5. Cold   e. 125°F
_____ 6. Tepid   f. 212°F
_____ 7. Boiling   g. 32°F

17.
_____ 1. Mops   a. Prevent falling onto heater
_____ 2. Gloves   b. Prevent chilling
_____ 3. Grab bars   c. Prevent slipping in a puddle
_____ 4. Towels or dry clothing d. Prevent falling
_____ 5. Fences inside sauna   e. Prevent burning the hands

18.
_____ 1. Local heat   a. Steam bath
_____ 2. Whole body cold   b. Ice massage
_____ 3. Hot air bath   c. Sauna
_____ 4. Local cold   d. Paraffin
_____ 5. Whole-body hot water application e. Wet sheet pack

REFERENCES

1. Tsuzuki-Hayakawa K et al. Thermoregulation during heat exposure of young children compared to their mothers. *Eur J Appl Occup Physiol* 1995;72(1-2):12.
2. Jokinen E. Children in sauna: Hormonal adjustments to intensive short thermal stress. *Acta Physiol Scand* 1991; 142:437.
3. www.usareim.army.mil. Prevention and Treatment of Cold-Weather Injuries. TB Med Bulletin 500. Accessed September 2005.
4. Proctor D, Koch D, Newcomer S, et al. Impaired leg vasodilation during dynamic exercise in healthy older women. *J Appl Physiol* 2003;95:1963.
5. Inoue Y, Kuwahara T, Araki T. Maturation and aging-related changes in heat loss effector function. *J Physiol Anthropol Appl Human Sci* 2004;6:289.

6. Norton A. A Nice Warm Bath May Be Good for the Heart. *Reuters Health Information*, November 3, 2002.

7. Standish L, Calabrese C, Galantino ML. AIDS and Complementary & Alternative Medicine: Current Science and Practice. St. Louis: Churchill Livingstone, 2002.

8. Milunsky A, Ulcickas M, Rothman KJ, et al. Maternal heat exposure and neural tube defects. *JAMA* 1992; 268:882.

9. Smith E. The cold pressor test: Vascular and myocardial response patterns and their stability. *Psychophysiology* 1993; 30:366.

10. Rymal C. Can patients at risk for lymphedema use hot tubs? *Clin J Oncol Nurs* 2002;6:369.

11. DeLorenzo F et al. Haemodynamic responses and changes of haemostatic risk factors in cold-adapted humans. *Q J Med* 1999; 92:509.

12. Charles K. Fanger's Thermal comfort and draught models. Institute for Research in Construction, National Research Council of Canada, Ottawa, October, 2003.

13. Kelsey R, Alpert B, Patterson S, Barnard M. Racial differences in hemodynamic responses to environmental thermal stress among adolescents. *Circulation* 2001;101:2284.

14. Marino FE, Lambert MI, Noakes TD. Superior performances of African runners in warm humid but not in cool environmental conditions. *J Appl Physiol* 2004; 96:124.

15. Nguyen MH, Tokura H. Sweating and tympanic temperature during warm water immersion compared between Vietnamese and Japanese living in Hanoi. *J Hum Ergol (Tokyo)* 2003;32:9.

16. DeLorenzo F et al. Haeomodynamic responses and changes of haemostatic risk factors in cold-adapted humans. *Q J Med* 1992:509.

17. Geurts C. Local cold acclimation of the hand impairs thermal responses of the fingers without improving hand neuromuscular function. *Acta Physiol Scan.* 2005;183:117.

18. LeBlanc J et al. Autonomic nervous system and adaptation to cold in man. *J. Appl Physiology* 1975; 39:181.

19. Belanger A. *Evidence-Based Guide to Therapeutic Physical Agents.* Baltimore: Lippincott Williams & Wilkins, 2002, p 269.

20. Sinclair M. *Pediatric Massage Therapy.* Baltimore: Lippincott Williams & Wilkins, 2004, p 157.

21. Pike S. Interview with author, Warm Springs, Georgia, Feb 23, 2005.

22. Lander BR. Heat or ice for relief of low back pain? *Phys Ther Rev* 1967; 47:1126.

RECOMMENDED RESOURCES

1. Kandel R. *Water from Heaven: The Story of Water from the Big Bang to the Rise of Civilization and Beyond.* New York: Columbia University, 2003.

2. Michlovitz S. *Thermal Agents in Rehabilitation.* Philadelphia: FA Davis, 1996.

3. Pielou EC. *Fresh Water.* Chicago: University of Chicago, 1998.

4. Qualls E. *Hydrotherapy.* Wildwood, GA: College of Health Evangelism, 1985.

5. Thrash A, Thrash C. *Home Remedies: Hydrotherapy, Charcoal, and Other Simple Treatments.* Seale, AL: Thrash, 1981.

6. www.epa.gov/watrhome/you/chap3.

7. Williams A. *Spa Bodywork.* Baltimore: Lippincott Williams & Wilkins, 2006.

HOT PACKS, FOMENTATIONS, COMPRESSES, AND OTHER LOCAL HEAT APPLICATIONS

5

She [Catherine Parr, queen of England] would herself remain on her knees beside him [King Henry VIII] for many hours, applying fomentations and other palliatives to his ulcerated leg.

— Agnes Strickland, *Lives of the Queens of England*

Chapter Objectives

After completing this chapter, the student will be able to:

- Describe the effects of local heat treatments.
- Explain the contraindications for local heat treatments.
- Name and describe the local hydrotherapy treatments, including local applications of moist heat, mustard plasters, and castor oil packs.
- Perform local heat treatments using the procedure included with each treatment.

This chapter covers various treatments that heat one part of the body. Because they are relatively simple and inexpensive, they are more accessible to the average massage therapist than many whole-body treatments, which require installing more elaborate and expensive equipment. They are also versatile and can be used in a variety of ways (Fig. 5-1). How can applying local heat treatments improve a massage session? Here are some examples. Before working with an area that needs concentrated stretching, deep heat from a hydrocollator pack, fomentation, hot compress, moist heating pad, hot water bottle, mustard plaster, or castor oil pack makes tissues far more pliable and stretchable. Local heat relaxes both skeletal and smooth muscles. (Hot fomentations, hot sitz baths, and even electric blankets can relieve kidney stone pain, which is caused by a spasm of the smooth muscle that lines the ureter.) Local heat also makes myofascial trigger points less painful to pressure while they are treated, and reduces muscle soreness from trigger point treatment when it is applied immediately afterwards. It improves local circulation and relieves the joint stiffness and discomfort of osteoarthritis. Hot applications can be combined with cold ones to form contrast treatments to stimulate local circulation and relieve pain. Finally, the soothing and nurturing feel of local heat helps reduce nervous tension.

While many local heat treatments—such as dry heating pads, hot water bottles, and rice-filled microwaveable bags—can be administered without the use of water and have many of the same effects, water is more efficient at transmitting heat than dry materials. For example, even if heated, dry cloth packs do not warm the body as much as heated moist cloth packs. Moist applications also have a soothing "watery" quality.

The advantages of any type of hot application must always be weighed against two major disadvantages: hot applications can burn and so must be carefully monitored, and prolonged application of heat to the body surface can raise body temperature.

Because heat applications are so soothing and relaxing, they are used not only in almost every kind of medical setting but also in spas that offer creative and enjoyable ways to integrate them into massage sessions. For example, El Monte Sagrado Spa in Arizona offers a whole-body massage session called a *hot towel infusion massage*. In this massage, for each part of the body, first an essential oil is applied to the skin and then a heated towel is placed on top of that. Next, massage is performed through the hot towel. Then another dry towel is placed on the skin, and on top of that a hot **silica gel pack,** a pack made of canvas, filled with silica gel, and heated in water. As each

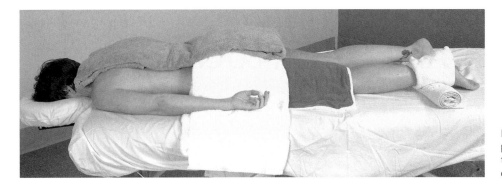

FIGURE 5-1 ■ Client with silica gel pack on the posterior thigh, fomentation on the entire back, and hot compress on the ankle.

new part of the body is massaged, a fresh hot silica gel pack is warming the area that has just been massaged, and the total effect is one of warmth and deep relaxation. This use of hot towels and silica gel packs is only one way local heat treatments can be used; there are many more.

Indications are similar for all heat applications:

1. Muscle spasm, including infant colic caused by muscle tightness
2. Poor local circulation
3. Musculoskeletal pain (muscle soreness, stiff joints, arthritis pain, chronic back pain)
4. Muscle tightness
5. Warming of tissue to make it more pliable and stretchable before massage, especially for athletic persons with very dense tissue or areas with sensitive scar tissue
6. Soreness after deep massage
7. Menstrual cramps
8. Active trigger points
9. When derivation (a tissue-shifting effect) is desired— moving blood toward the hot application and away from congested areas. Useful for migraine headache.
10. Nervous tension
11. Chilled local area
12. Chilled client

Local contraindications:

1. Loss of sensation (lack of feeling), which can be caused by spinal cord injury, diabetic neuropathy, other medical condition, or the use of some medications. These conditions can render the person unable to feel the pain of a too-hot application. Never put a hot application on a numb area.
2. Rash or other skin condition that could be made worse by heat
3. Inflammation
4. Swelling
5. Broken skin—burn, wound, sore, cracked skin from eczema or severe chapping
6. Malignancy
7. Implanted device such as cardiac pacemaker, stomach band, and infusion pump

8. Diabetics should not receive hot applications to the legs or feet.
9. Peripheral vascular disease, including diabetes, Buerger's disease, and arteriosclerosis of the lower extremities
10. Sensitivity to heat, especially in those with thin skin, such as the elderly and small children, who might burn more easily

Cautions:

1. Elderly (over 60 years old)
2. Children

SILICA GEL HOT PACKS

Silica gel–filled hot packs, marketed under such names as Hydrocollator and Thermollator, are one of the most popular ways for hands-on therapists to apply heat to the body. Because they are easy to heat up and to apply to the client, silica gel packs are the most commonly used hot moist application in chiropractic offices and physical therapy clinics. They provide a simple way to help clients relax, ease muscle tension before hands-on treatment, and warm cold clients. In offices with multiple practitioners, it is common to see the hot pack heater turned on throughout the day and packs being used, returned to the heater to rewarm, and used again. Usually only one pack per person is used, but on occasion multiple packs are used. Packs are available in various sizes and shapes, from large ones that cover the entire back to small ones that fit over the hand.

Silica gel packs cause the greatest temperature elevation in the skin and the subcutaneous tissue. Properly used, they can raise the temperature of the skin as much as 20°F and that of the subcutaneous tissue as much as 15°F. However, even the temperature of the muscle tissue underneath that can increase up to 6°F. The joints of the hand, foot, wrist, and ankle can also be significantly warmed with the application of these packs. As tissues warm, muscles relax, joint stiffness decreases, and collagen fibers become more stretchable. (The tissue must be stretched when it is still hot, however, to have this effect.) Combining silica gel pack applications with gentle prolonged stretching produces greater long-term improvement in flexibility than stretching alone. Silica gel packs, however, may not always be the best choice when applying moist heat, because they don't conform to body curves as well as fomentations or hot compresses, are too heavy to be applied to very sensitive areas, and cannot be applied underneath the body. The client should not lie on the pack for three reasons: (1) They are bumpy and uncomfortable; (2) the client's body weight could squeeze water out of the pack and possibly cause a burn; and (3) the skin cannot be continuously monitored without rolling the client to one side to examine it.

The packs are made of canvas and filled with silica granules, which can absorb a great deal of water and then form a gel-like substance which holds heat very well. They are heated on racks in special metal containers with electrical heating elements. Once the metal container is filled with water and turned on, the water will reach a temperature of 160° to 166°F in 1 to 2 hours. The gel-filled packs lie in the hot water and absorb its heat. Or the container can be left on overnight, and then the packs will be hot and ready to use right away. The packs can be taken directly out of the hot water, wrapped in towels, and applied to clients. They can also be taken from the hot water, wrapped in towels, and kept hot in an ice chest for 20 minutes.

If you are going to use only one silica gel pack at a time and you are not using them more or less continuously, it may be more economical to buy individual silica gel packs and heat them for 20 minutes in simmering water on a hot plate or stovetop. Hot pack water heaters require a fair amount of energy; the heater in the smallest container, which holds four silica gel packs, uses 1000 watts (the same as ten 100-watt light bulbs). However, there are some simple strategies for reducing the amount of energy you use. If you use your hot silica gel packs for just a few hours every day, it may save both energy and money to empty the container in the morning and fill it with hot tap water rather than reheat cold water. The water will heat to the proper temperature far more quickly. For the smallest metal containers, an insulating foam wrapper may be used to reduce heat loss from the tank (NAIMCO, 425-648-7730). Tanks that hold more than four packs use more energy when turned off at night and reheated in the morning than left on overnight so the water in the tank stays hot.

The following discusses a step-by-step procedure for using a silica gel pack on the upper back, but gel packs can be adapted to treat almost any area of the body. They can also be combined with cold applications to create contrast treatments.

Temperature: Silica gel packs are heated in water that is 160° to 166°F, and they come out of the hot water at that temperature. They begin to cool off as soon as they are taken out of the water but will present a burn danger until they have cooled off considerably.

Packs cool at various rates depending upon how hot they are when they come out of the water and how thick the towels are, so it is not possible to say exactly how fast they will cool off. Assume they have the potential to burn clients throughout the treatment and monitor them at all times.

Time Needed: 15 to 20 minutes on the skin for a relaxing sedative effect.

Equipment Needed: Metal hot pack container, hot pack, tongs or gloves to remove hot pack from the container, enough towels to make four to six layers of towel between the client's skin and the hot pack. Specially made terry cloth covers may be purchased from manufacturers of the packs, but at least one layer of towel is still needed between the cover and the client's skin.

Effect: Primarily thermal

Cleanup: Return hydrocollator pack to container, dispose of used towels. Water in the tank should be changed periodically, depending upon how frequently it is being used, as the water in the tank will become contaminated with small silica particles.

Procedure
1. Check with client to make sure there are no contraindications to the use of local heat.
2. Explain the use of local heat to client and get his or her consent.
3. Check the water temperature, which is displayed on the lower part of heater.
4. Remove the silica gel pack from the hot water with tongs, or put on gloves and pick up the pack by the loops on the edges (Fig. 5-2A).
5. Wrap it in one or more towels. You may fold a large bath towel in half and wrap the hot pack in it or use several smaller towels. The layers of towel will protect the client's skin from burning and prevent the pack from cooling off too fast. Silica gel packs generally require four to six layers of towels, but keep extra towels on hand to use if needed. Specially made terry cloth covers may also be used. More towels may be needed for an elderly person or a child (Fig. 5-2B).
6. Check to make sure the pack is not too hot by feeling it with your own hand or wrist (Fig. 5-2C).
7. Warn the client the hot pack is going on, and say, "Be sure to tell me right away if this feels too hot."
8. Check the area visually before applying towel-wrapped pack (Fig. 5-2D). This allows you to see what the client's skin normally looks like.
9. Place the hot pack on the client's lower back (Fig. 5-2E).
10. Check the skin every 2 or 3 minutes at first: lift the pack and check the tissue. It will be bright pink due to increased blood flow, which is normal, but check for any signs of blistering or burning.

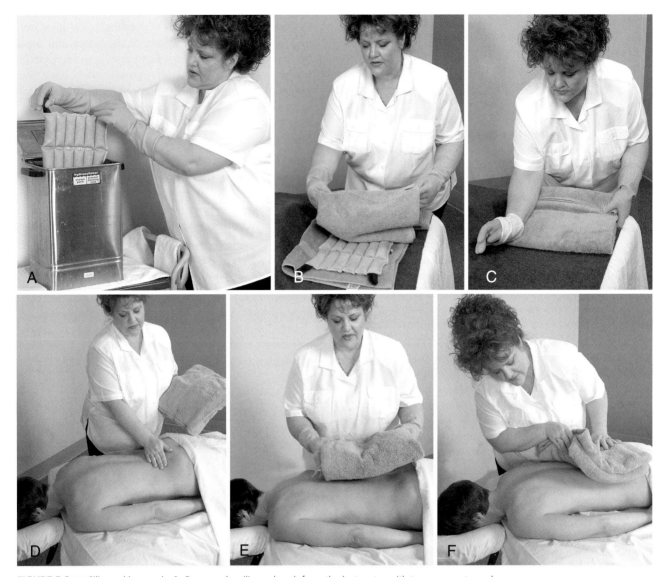

FIGURE 5-2 ■ Silica gel hot pack. **A.** Remove the silica gel pack from the hot water with tongs, or put on gloves and pick the pack up by the loops on the edges. **B.** Wrap it in one or more towels. **C.** Check to make sure the hot pack is not too hot by feeling it with your own hand or wrist. **D.** Check the area visually before applying towel-wrapped pack. **E.** Place the hot pack on the client's lower back. **F.** Check the skin every 2 or 3 minutes at first: lift the pack and check the tissue.

Also ask the client how it feels. Add more towels to protect the skin if needed. The hot pack will stay warm for about 20 minutes but will begin to cool off right away, so that danger of burning decreases as time goes on (Fig. 5-2F).

11. As the hot pack cools off, you may wish to remove a layer of towels to keep the area warm and continue to monitor the client's skin.
12. Remove the hot pack if there are any signs of damage to the skin or if the client tells you the area is too hot.
13. Dry the skin, apply oil or lotion, and begin massage. You will find the client's tissue warm, pink, and pliable.

FOMENTATIONS

A **fomentation,** from the Latin word *fomentum*, which means soothing application or poultice, is any warm, moist application that delivers heat to the body for healing. This book refers to fomentations as the large pads specially made for moist heat applications, composed of many layers of thick laundry flannel, toweling, or other thick material that can absorb hot water and hold heat effectively. (Box 5-1 has directions for making fomentations.) Like other moist heat applications, fomentations raise local tissue temperature, improve local circulation, relax and soften muscles and fascia, and relieve many kinds of musculoskeletal pain. Fomentations have been used in various forms by many ancient medical traditions.

BOX 5-1 *Point of Interest*

HOW TO MAKE FOMENTATIONS

Fomentations are relatively easy to make, and a miniature fomentation can be made on the spot from a few simple ingredients. Directions are included for making both a miniature and a full-size fomentation.

MINIATURE FOMENTATION

Equipment needed: Boiling water, protective gloves, kitchen sponge, hand towel, and microwave oven

Effect: Thermal

Cleanup: Wash hand towel.

Procedure

1. Lay the sponge on the hand towel.
2. Using gloves, wet the sponge with a small amount of boiling water.
3. Now fold the towel around the sponge to make a small pack, and pick it up by the dry ends of the towel.
4. Microwave it for 30 seconds.
5. Remove it from the microwave by holding the dry ends of the towel.
6. Check the temperature of the miniature fomentation against your skin before applying it to your client's skin,

and monitor the skin carefully, as with all hot applications.

STANDARD SIZE FOMENTATION WITH COVER

Once you have made the fomentation, follow the directions in this chapter for preparing and applying it.

Equipment needed: 1 yard of heavy cotton laundry flannel, terry cloth material, or a thick towel for the fomentation and 1 yard of wool or polar fleece for the cover

Procedure

1. Cut the fabric into a piece measuring 25 × 40 inches.
2. Fold it in half and then in half again, so the finished size is 10 × 25 inches.
3. Sew the pack together around the edges (a serger is good for this) or make about six quilting stitches through all the layers to hold them together.
4. Cut the wool or polar fleece material so it measures 30 × 32 inches, which is large enough to overlap the fomentation on all sides.

For purchasing information, see Appendix D.

In the twentieth century they were used extensively in water cure institutions, for rehabilitation of wounded soldiers during the World Wars I and II, and during many polio epidemics (Box 5-2).

Some practitioners prefer silica gel packs to fomentations, and each has its advantages. Silica gel packs can be wrapped only in towels, whereas fomentations necessitate a layer of wool and a layer of towels. Fomentations may initially be more intensely hot, but preparing them takes more time than for silica gel packs, and they cool off faster. Fomentations can cover larger areas and drape to fit body curves, whereas silica gel packs are smaller and are not flexible.

Because they are very hot when ready to use, fomentations are generally wrapped in wool felt, which retains heat well, and then in additional layers of towels which protect the client's skin. Once applied, fomentations may be kept warm longer if they are covered with a waterproof material (such as a sheet of heavy plastic) and then an electric heating pad. Hot fomentations can be wrapped and then put into a cooler and will stay warm for 10 to 20 minutes.

To prepare fomentations, first soak them in water to wet them all the way through, then wring them out so that they are thoroughly wet but not dripping (Fig. 5-3A). Then heat them. Here are four options for heating a fomentation:

- Wet the fomentation, then place it inside a gallon-size resealable plastic bag and heat in a microwave oven, approximately 5 minutes for a standard-wattage microwave, longer for a low-wattage one.

- Wet the fomentation, roll it up in heavy-grade aluminum foil, and heat in a 425°F oven for 25 minutes.
- Wet the fomentation. Roll it up and stand it rolled end up in the steamer basket of a spaghetti cooker. Put the steamer basket over simmering water for about 20 minutes. Use a pot that holds 2 gallons of water or more.
- To make a large homemade fomentation when none is available, you will need protective gloves and a large bath towel. Put on the gloves, then carefully twist the towel, dip it in boiling water, and twist it again to squeeze out excess water. A hot, wet towel can go directly against the client's skin rather than being wrapped in wool and dry towels if you use common sense. First check the hot, wet towel against your own skin to make sure it is not too hot and then monitor the client's skin carefully for burning. Hot towels lose heat faster than ready-made fomentations, but they can be covered with a waterproof material and then an electric heating pad to keep them warm longer.

Below is a step-by-step procedure for using a hot fomentation on the anterior thigh. Fomentations can be adapted to treat almost any area of the body. They can be especially useful when the client is in a side-lying position, over the chest muscles, or if you wish to apply heat to the front and back of the body at the same time.

They can also be combined with cold applications to create contrast treatments. For an example, see the section in this chapter on the full-body treatment using three local treatments.

BOX 5-2 | *Point of Interest*

FOMENTATION AND STRETCHING TREATMENT FOR POLIO

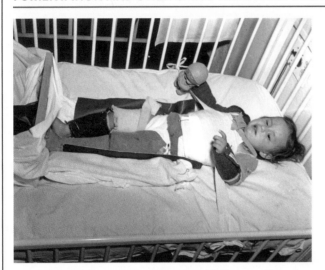

Girl with polio in hospital crib, wrapped in fomentations. San Angelo, Texas, June 1949. (Photo courtesy of March of Dimes Birth Defects Foundation.)

In the 1930s an Australian army nurse named Elizabeth Kenny developed a treatment for polio victims that began with wrapping the limbs of acutely ill polio patients with hot fomentations to reduce muscle spasms and the pain they caused. "Foments" were made of wool blankets, individually cut to fit each patient.

Wool was used because it retained heat well. The wool pieces were heated in very hot water, removed with tongs, run through a wringer twice, and then placed on the patient. During the acute phase, hot packs were applied once per hour around the clock. (In the nearby photo, the young girl in the acute phase of polio is shown receiving this treatment.) Even though the fomentations gave relief to tight, painful muscles, they were very hot, and burns sometimes occurred. As soon as the initial fever receded, nurses and physical therapists began to work with patients by applying fomentations and moving limbs passively to maintain range of motion. Later, the fomentations were again applied to relax tight spasmodic muscles prior to massage, stretching, and active exercise, which were all designed to restore muscles to their full function.

Kenny's regimen was quite different from the standard medical treatment for polio patients, which consisted of prolonged bed rest and immobilization of the limbs with splints and casts. The standard treatment actually did more harm than good, as it caused atrophy and contractures in limbs which were already weak. The medical profession grudgingly accepted Sister Kenny's techniques, and they had became standard treatment for polio victims by the mid-1940s. Sister Kenny became a household name, and in 1946 a movie was made about her life, with Rosalind Russell in the title role (see Recommended Resources list at the end of the chapter).

References

1. Campion M. *Hydrotherapy in Pediatrics*. Rockville, MD: Aspen Systems, 1985, p 236.
2. Wilson D. *Living with Polio: The Epidemic and Its Survivors*. Chicago: University of Chicago, 2005.

Temperature: Properly heated fomentations are very hot. Although they begin to cool off as soon as they are removed from the heat source, whether that be a microwave oven, regular oven, or steam bath, they present a burn danger until they have cooled off considerably. Fomentations cool off at varying rates depending upon how hot they are when they come out of the water and how thick the covering towels are, so it is not possible to say exactly how fast they will cool off. Assume they have the potential to burn clients throughout the treatment and monitor them at all times. When checking the client's skin, slide your hand under the wrapped fomentation and feel the client's skin as well as checking it for signs of blistering or burning.

Time Needed: 15 to 20 minutes for a relaxing, sedative effect

Equipment Needed: Protective gloves, fomentation, wool felt, one or two towels, and a heat source, such as a microwave oven, regular oven, or a canner with a rack has can be placed over boiling water

Effect: Primarily thermal

Cleanup: Hang the fomentation and the felt cover up to dry. Because they never touch the client's skin, they

do not have to be laundered except occasionally. The towels must be laundered after each use, just like sheets and any other linens that touch the client's skin.

Procedure

1. Check with client to make sure there are no contraindications for the use of local heat.
2. Explain the use of local heat to client and get his or her consent.
3. Soak fomentation and wring it out (Fig. 5-3A).
4. Place in zipper closure bag and heat in microwave (Fig. 5-3B) or roll up and stand in steam basket over boiling water.
5. Carefully remove the fomentation from its heat source (microwave oven, steamer, oven) using gloves (Fig. 5-3C).
6. Wrap the fomentation in a layer of wool felt or polar fleece (Fig. 5-3D) and then in towels (Fig. 5-3E). You may double a large bath towel and wrap the fomentation in it. The towels will protect the client's skin from burning and prevent the fomentation from cooling off too fast. Fomentations generally require about four layers of towels, but keep extra towels on hand to use if needed. Work quickly to prevent the fomentation from losing too much heat.

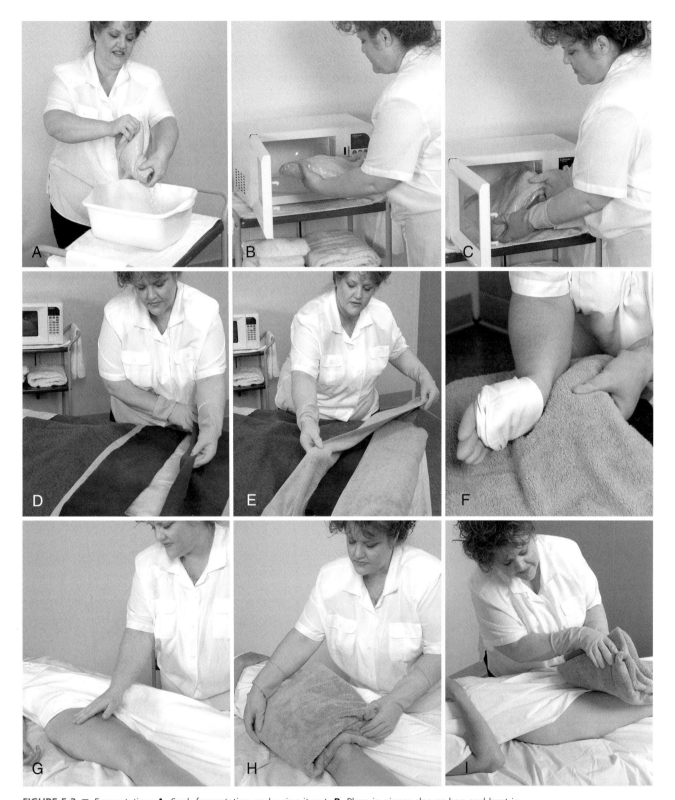

FIGURE 5-3 ■ Fomentation. **A.** Soak fomentation and wring it out. **B.** Place in zipper closure bag and heat in microwave oven (shown) or roll up and stand in steam basket over boiling water (not shown) or roll up in aluminum foil and heat in oven (not shown). **C.** Remove the fomentation from its heat source (microwave oven, steamer, oven) using gloves. **D.** Wrap the hot fomentation in a layer of wool felt, or polar fleece. **E.** Wrap the hot fomentation in towels. **F.** Check to make sure the fomentation with its covers is not too hot by feeling it with your own hand or wrist. **G.** Check the area visually before applying towel-wrapped fomentation. This allows you to see what the client's skin normally looks like. **H.** Place the fomentation on the client's thigh. **I.** Check the skin every 2 or 3 minutes at first: lift the pack and check the tissue.

A Hot Fomentation for a Painful Muscle Spasm

Background

Rebecca was a 65-year-old retired secretary in good health. She had received a massage from the massage therapist only once before, but now called to say she had hurt her back hiking yesterday and would like a massage for that reason. She arrived in severe pain, half-carried by her husband. Any movement was excruciating for Rebecca, and getting up on the massage table or even undressing was impossible for this reason. Her mid back, where the pain was located, was also very sensitive to the touch. Her chiropractor would later diagnose the cause of her muscle spasm as a protective reaction to a torn sacral ligament, which became injured the day before, when she took a very long walk for which she was completely unconditioned.

Treatment

Rebecca was able to sit straddling a chair, and so the massage therapist draped a hot fomentation around her mid back and secured it in place with an elastic bandage while listening to her history. Although her mid back was still very painful and getting on the massage table was impossible, the fomentation reduced Rebecca's pain slightly after just a few minutes. She remained seated on the chair, however, and her husband helped her to remove her shirt. Then the therapist proceeded to massage Rebecca's back above and below the area still covered by the fomentation. Rebecca's pain gradually began to decrease, although it was still severe. After 15 minutes of massage above and below the painful area, the therapist removed the fomentation, and with her husband's assistance Rebecca was able to get on the massage table so that the therapist could give more specific massage to the painful muscles. Her mid back area was pink, pliable, and ready for treatment.

Discussion Questions

1. How did the fomentation relieve Rebecca's pain?
2. What other local heat or cold applications could have been used in this situation?

---

7. Check to make sure the fomentation with its covers is not too hot by feeling it with your own hand or wrist (Fig. 5-3F).
8. Warn the client the fomentation is going on, and say, "Be sure to let me know if this ever feels like it is too hot."
9. Check the area visually before applying the towel-wrapped fomentation (Fig. 5-3G). This allows you to see what the client's skin normally looks like.
10. Place the fomentation on the client's thigh (Fig. 5-3H).
11. Check the skin every 2 or 3 minutes at first. Lift the pack and check the tissue (Fig. 5-3I). It will be bright pink due to increased blood flow, and this is normal, but check for any signs of blistering or burning. Also ask the client if it feels too hot.
12. The fomentation will stay warm for about 20 minutes but will begin to cool off right away, so danger of burning decreases as time goes on. As the fomentation cools, you may wish to remove a layer of towels to keep the area warm, but then you must keep checking the skin.
13. Remove the fomentation if there is any sign of damage to the skin, if the client tells you the area is too hot, or if he or she is uncomfortably hot.
14. Dry the skin, apply oil or lotion, and begin massage. You will find the client's tissue warm, pink, and pliable.

COMPRESS

A hot **compress**—a folded cloth dipped in water—is a milder form of the intense moist heat of the silica gel pack or the hot fomentation. An advantage to using hot compresses over silica gel packs or fomentations is that hot compresses may be easily made and applied with simple items.

All the massage therapist needs to make a hot compress is hot water, cloths to use for the compress, and gloves to protect the hands when wringing out the cloths. A disadvantage to hot compresses is that they cool off faster than silica gel packs or fomentations. Historically, hot compresses have been used to apply countless substances to the skin by soaking the cloths in hot water mixed with herbs, essential oils, minerals and salts, to name just a few. They have also been combined with various cold applications to create contrast treatments.

You can make compresses to suit the individual client quite easily. For example, a tiny hot compress to cover the eyes may be made by soaking a washcloth in hot water and then wringing it out. Small or medium-size hot compresses may be made with a few layers of cloth or with small towels. Large hot compresses that can cover the entire back can be made with a large bath towel. There are many ways to prepare hot compresses. Water for compresses can be heated on a stovetop, in a slow cooker or turkey roaster on a low setting, in a microwave, or even from tap water if the water heater is set quite high. You can soak cloths in a bowl of hot water and then wring them out, or you can roll them up in the shape of a sausage, place them in an ice chest, and pour boiling water over them. Wet washcloths can also be heated in a resealable plastic bag in a microwave oven for a short time. The amount of time will vary depending upon the wattage of the microwave. Commercial heating cabinets marketed under such names as Hot Towel Cabi not only heat small and medium-size cloths that you have wrung out in water, they also keep them warm until needed.

To make sure the compress does not burn the client, as always, check the compress with your own hand or wrist, monitor the client's skin, and let the client determine whether the hot compress is uncomfortably hot. Compresses must never be allowed to burn the client or feel unpleasantly hot.

An overview of treatment details and a sample procedure using the forearm follows.

Temperature: Hot (110–120°F)

Time Needed: 10 to 20 minutes, depending upon the size of the compress and whether more than one is to be used. Small compresses cool off faster than large ones.

Equipment Needed: Water thermometer, hot water, towels of appropriate size, gloves to protect hands

Effect: Primarily thermal

Cleanup: Clean and sanitize water container and launder used towels.

Procedure
1. Check with the client to make sure there are no contraindications for the use of local heat.
2. Explain the use of local heat to client and get his or her consent.
3. Check the water temperature and adjust if it is not within 110° to 120°F (Fig. 5-4A).
4. Wearing gloves, wring out the cloth in hot water (Fig. 5-4B).
5. Check to make sure the cloth is not too hot by feeling it with your own hand or wrist (Fig. 5-4C). If it is, let it cool to a safe temperature.

6. Warn the client the compress is going on, and say, "Be sure to let me know if this ever feels like it is too hot."
7. Check the area visually before putting on hot application. This allows you to see what the client's skin normally looks like.
8. Place the hot cloth on the client's skin (Fig. 5-4D). A small sheet of plastic may be put on top to help prevent heat from escaping.
9. Monitor the client's skin, and ask for feedback occasionally.
10. Replace with a new hot cloth every 2 minutes if a heating pad is not used. If a heating pad is placed over the sheet of plastic (Fig. 5-4E), the compress need not be replaced and can stay on 10 to 20 minutes.
11. When you remove the compress for the last time, gently dry the area with a dry cloth. You will find the client's tissue warm, pink, and pliable.

MOIST HEATING PAD

Electric heating pads are one of the options you may consider when you feel the client will benefit from a warm or hot application. They take no preparation time, as they are hot with the flip of a switch; they are easy to take with you; and they are very flexible and can be draped around almost any part of the body. Because they do not have to be wrapped in layers of towels, they are less bulky and easier to work around than silica gel packs or hot fomentations, for example when you wish to warm the lower back while massaging the upper back. However, heating pads lack the penetrating intense heat of silica gel packs and hot fomentations, and they cannot be used without electricity (such as at an outdoor sporting event). Also, once the pad is plugged into a nearby outlet, the therapist must work around the electrical cord. Heating pads can also be combined with various cold applications to create contrast treatments, although the client's reaction will be milder because the heat is not intense.

There are two kinds of commercial electric heating pads, moist and dry ones. Moist heating pads are electric heating pads with outer covers that draw humidity from the air and retain it. When the pad is turned on, the moisture is heated, then forced out of the cover and onto the area being treated. Any dry electric heating pad can be made into a moist heating pad by laying a wet cloth over the area to be treated, covering that with a thin sheet of plastic, and then putting a dry heating pad on top of that. Moist heat is preferred to dry because it penetrates deeper. A hazard of both wet and dry pads is falling asleep with them on; burns can then occur. Many heating pads now come equipped with an

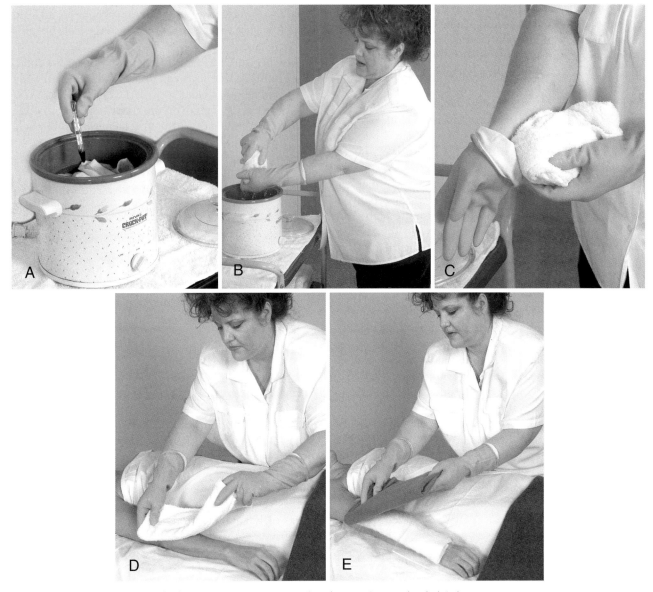

FIGURE 5-4 ■ Hot compress. **A.** Check water temperature. **B.** Wearing gloves, wring out the cloth in hot water. **C.** Check to make sure the cloth is not too hot by feeling it with your own hand or wrist. **D.** Place the hot cloth on the client's skin. **E.** Place a heating pad over the sheet of plastic (optional).

automatic shutoff feature: after a period of minutes or hours, they turn off automatically. Not all heating pads have automatic shutoff features, so a client who is using one at home should always check whether this feature is available and should not fall asleep on the heating pad. It is dangerous for persons with reduced sensation, such as those with diabetic neuropathy or spinal cord injury, to use a heating pad, since they cannot feel when the pad might burn them.

Next is an overview of treatment details and a sample procedure using the abdomen. When the client is receiving a massage, a thin layer of cloth or a sheet of plastic is placed between the client's skin and the heating pad for hygienic reasons.

Temperature: Settings vary from low heat (78°F) to high (125°F).

Time Needed: 15 minutes or longer, depending upon the condition

Equipment Needed: Heating pad in cloth cover, small sheet of plastic or cloth

Effect: Primarily thermal

Cleanup: Anything that has touched the client's skin should be sanitized. If a layer of cloth was put between the heating pad and the skin, it should be laundered, and if a sheet of plastic was used, either wash it with hot water and soap or throw it away.

Procedure

1. Check with the client to make sure there are no contraindications to the use of local heat.
2. Explain the use of local heat to client and get his or her consent.
3. Inspect heating pad (Fig. 5-5A).
4. Plug in heating pad and turn on to desired setting (Fig. 5-5B).
5. Warn the client before applying the heating pad, and say, "Be sure to let me know if this ever feels too hot."
6. Check the area visually before putting on the heating pad (Fig. 5-5C). This allows you to see what the client's skin normally looks like.
7. Place the heating pad on the abdomen (Fig. 5-5D).
8. Check the skin every 5 minutes: lift the pad and check the client's tissue (Fig. 5-5E).

HOT WATER BOTTLES

Often people take a drug which risks injury of the health for all future time, when a hot water bottle would have been more effective, more economical, and entirely safe.

—*Agatha Thrash, MD, Home Remedies*(6)

Hot water bottles are another ancient tried-and-true hydrotherapy treatment. Used by many cultures before the advent of plastic or rubber, hot water bottles were most often made of earthenware, with a cork stopper. They were used to warm cold beds before people got in them to sleep and for all manner of aches and pains. Extremities could be kept warm with them too—some ceramic water bottles were even made with indentations

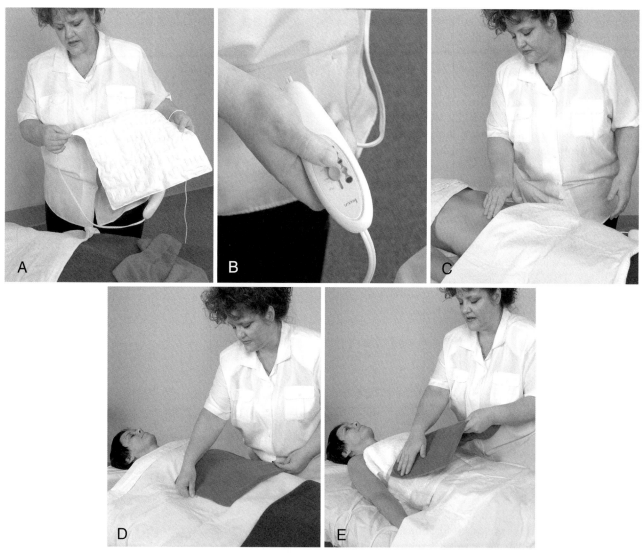

FIGURE 5-5 ■ Moist heating pad. **A.** Inspect heating pad. **B.** Plug in heating pad and turn on to desired setting. **C.** Check the area visually before applying heating pad. **D.** Place the heating pad on the client's abdomen. **E.** Check the skin every 5 minutes at first by lifting the pad and checking the tissue.

for the feet—and miniature water bottles once were put in muffs to keep the hands warm.

Today, hot water bottles are made of rubber or plastic and are a simple, cheap, and versatile way to use local heat in your massage sessions. They can be used to heat a massage table or warm a cold client. They can also be put on an aching part of the body while another part of the body is being massaged, or laid on top of fomentations or compresses to keep them warm longer. Hot water bottles are readily available, come in a variety of sizes, and can be made from any plastic bottle, such as a water bottle or a detergent bottle. A disadvantage of rubber hot water bottles is that they do not cover large areas. An advantage of hot water bottles over electric heating pads is that they cool off gradually, so if someone falls asleep on them, there is less potential for burns.

RUBBER HOT WATER BOTTLE

A rubber hot water bottle can be put over or under any part of the body. When air is expelled from it and the right amount of water is put in, it becomes flexible, so it conforms to different parts of the client's body. For example, a small hot water bottle can be placed under the chin, atop a small area of the arm, on the abdomen with the client supine, or on the back of the neck or behind a knee with the client prone. A larger one may be placed on the chest, abdomen, or legs of a supine client, or on the back or legs of the prone client. During a massage, a hot water bottle placed over the chest or abdomen gives the client a convenient place to warm his or her hands, whole warming the body core at the same time.

Do not put weight or pressure on a hot water bottle. To extend its life, never fill it with boiling water, check it before using to make sure there are no splits in it, and do not fold it.

Below is an overview of treatment details and a sample procedure using an application to the lower back.

Temperature: Hot (110–120°F)

Time Needed: 10 to 30 minutes

Equipment Needed: Water thermometer, hot water bottle, thin cloth to wrap the hot water bottle in

Effect: Primarily thermal

Cleanup: Launder cloth. Empty the water bottle and hang it upside down for storage. Keep in a cool, dry place.

Procedure
1. Check with the client to make sure there are no contraindications for the use of local heat.
2. Explain the use of local heat to the client and get his or her consent.
3. Fill bottle about one-half to two-thirds full of hot water from the tap (Fig. 5-6A). Use the thermometer to ensure the water is 110° to 120°F. Expel the air and check to make sure the top is properly seated and firmly closed so it does not leak (Fig. 5-6B).
4. Place a thin cloth on the client's back or wrap the hot water bottle in a cloth or pillowcase to protect the skin (Fig. 5-6C).
5. Warn the client the hot water bottle is going on, and say, "Be sure to let me know if this ever feels like it is too hot."
6. Check the area visually before putting on the hot water bottle. This allows you to see what the client's skin normally looks like.
7. Place hot water bottle on the lower back (Fig. 5-6D).
8. Even though burns are uncommon with rubber hot water bottles, be sure to monitor the client's skin.

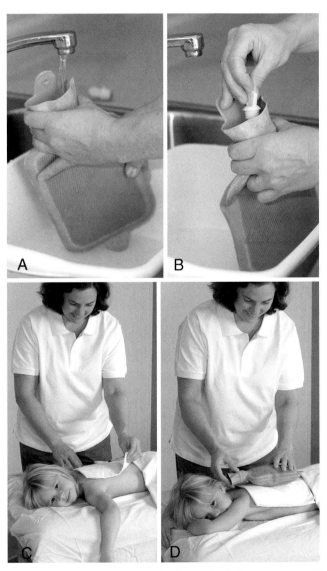

FIGURE 5-6 ■ Rubber hot water bottle. **A.** Check the temperature of the water at the tap, then fill the bottle about one-half to two-thirds full with it. **B.** Expel the air and check to make sure the top is properly seated and firmly closed so it does not leak. **C.** Place a cloth or pillow case on the client's back. **D.** Place the hot water bottle on the cloth on the lower back.

FLAT PLASTIC HOT WATER BOTTLE

When filled with hot water at the appropriate temperature, a flat plastic hot water bottle is safe to lie on. (It can also be laid on the upper surface of the body.) When laid flat on a massage table before a session begins, it warms the table. During the session it can keep the client's entire body warm and can warm and soften local areas before they are massaged. It will stay warm for up to 2 hours. An advantage of this particular hydrotherapy treatment is that it is inexpensive and fairly low tech: all the therapist needs is the bottle and hot water. Once filled with hot water, it may even be used with two clients if it is put in a cooler to retain its heat after the first session. It can also be combined with various cold applications, including another bottle filled with chilled water, for contrast treatments. An important consideration with a large hot water bottle is that it may heat a large portion of the client's body, and so it has even more potential for raising the core temperature.

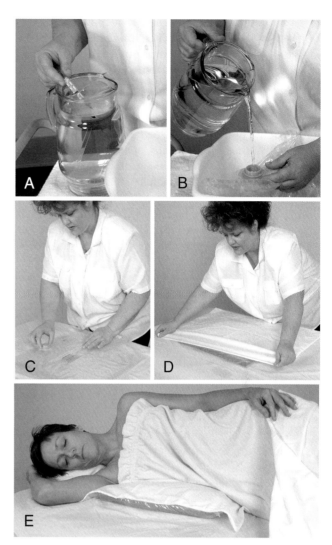

FIGURE 5-7 ■ Flat plastic hot water bottle. **A.** Check the temperature of the water. **B.** Fill the bottle about one-half to two-thirds full. **C.** Expel the air, snap the lid on, and check to make sure the lid is firmly closed and water does not leak out. **D.** Cover the hot water bottle with a pillowcase. **E.** Client lying on hot water bottle.

Temperature: Very hot (water at 108–113°F)

Time Needed: 5 to 30 minutes. The client's tissue will begin to warm after about 5 minutes.

Equipment Needed: Water thermometer, hot water bottle, thin cloth to cover or wrap the hot water bottle (a pillowcase is ideal)

Effect: Primarily thermal

Cleanup: Launder cloth. Empty the bottle and lay it flat with the lid off so the last drops of water will evaporate. Then it can be folded for storage.

Procedure

1. Check with the client to make sure there are no contraindications to the use of local heat.
2. Explain the use of local heat to the client and get his or her consent.
3. Use a thermometer to ensure the water is 108° to 113°F (Fig. 5-7A). Fill bottle about one-third full of hot water. (Fig. 5-7B). About 6 cups of water will be needed for a large 18 × 24 inch bottle.
4. Carry the open bottle carefully to the massage table, lay it flat on the table, use your hand to expel the air bubbles, and check to make sure the top is snapped on securely so it does not leak (Fig. 5-7C).
5. Cover it with a cloth or pillowcase or place it inside a pillowcase (Fig. 5-7D).
6. As the client lies on the cloth-covered hot water bottle, say, "Be sure to let me know if this ever feels like it is too hot" (Fig. 5-7E).
7. Even though burns are highly unlikely if the correct water temperature is used, be sure to monitor the client's skin and ask for feedback. The area will warm up more slowly than if a silica gel pack or fomentation is used.

MUSTARD PLASTER

A **plaster** is a pastelike mixture, usually of herbs, that can be spread upon a cloth and applied to the body. Ground mustard seeds contain chemicals and enzymes that, when combined with water, liberate compounds that encourage blood flow to the surface of the skin. The plaster also functions as a **counterirritant,** a substance that stimulates nerve endings on the skin, distracting the central nervous system from deeper-seated pain and relieving it. Plasters made with ground mustard are used to warm muscle tissues, especially deeper tissues, and to treat chronic aches and pains, such as those of arthritis.

Mustard was used in Europe for centuries for both medicinal and culinary purposes and was brought to this country by European settlers. Mustard seed was once listed in the *U.S. Pharmacopeia* (list of approved medications) and was included in baths, liniments, plasters, and massage oils. Mustard preparations were widely available commercially, and mustard powder was one of the medicines used by the U.S. Army. Use of plasters became less common in the last half of the twentieth century, and they are now seen chiefly as a home remedy. Originally mustard plasters were thought to draw out "bad humors." Practically speaking, however, the plasters were used to provide soothing heat, increase local circulation, relieve arthritis pain, and treat respiratory ailments such as chest colds and bronchitis by deeply warming the chest. Today's massage therapist may wish to use a mustard plaster before massage to ease a painful muscle or joint and to bring heat to a deeper muscle before it is massaged.

Mustard plasters are indeed very hot and can even cause blistering, so you must monitor the skin underneath them carefully and take the plaster off at the recommended time.

Below is an overview of treatment details and a sample procedure using the anterior shoulder area.

Indications
1. Poor local circulation
2. Painful muscles that will be massaged after the plaster is removed
3. Frozen shoulder
4. Gout
5. Acute lower back pain of muscular origin
6. Chronic back pain
7. Arthritis pain

Contraindications
1. Sensitive skin
2. Allergy to mustard seed
3. Open skin (e.g., wound, rash, eczema)
4. Any area where heat is contraindicated, such as in diabetic neuropathy or spinal cord injury

Temperature: Hot (110°F)

Time Needed: 15 to 30 minutes

Equipment Needed: 1 tablespoon of mustard powder, 4 tablespoons of wheat flour, and enough tepid water to make a paste; spoons for measuring and stirring the paste; thin cotton cloth, approximately 10 × 12 inches; piece of plastic that is slightly larger; a small towel; fomentation, hot water bottle, or heating pad to keep plaster warm; small tray

Effect: Primarily chemical from the ground mustard, but also thermal due to the application of heat over the plaster

Cleanup: Dispose of plaster and plastic sheet, launder thin cloth and towel.

Procedure
1. Check with the client to make sure there are no contraindications for the use of local heat.
2. Explain the use of local heat to client and get consent.
3. Mix mustard powder, flour, and water to make a paste that can be spread on the cloth but is not so thin that it will run (Fig. 5-8A).
4. Place the cloth on a tray (Fig. 5-8B).
5. Spoon the mustard mixture onto the cloth, and spread it out, leaving enough dry cloth to fold over well on all four sides. Only one thin layer of cloth will be between the skin and the plaster (Fig. 5-8C).
6. Warn the client before applying the plaster, and say, "Be sure to let me know if this ever feels too hot."
7. Check the area visually before applying the plaster (Fig. 5-8D). This allows you to see what the client's skin normally looks like.
8. Place the plaster on the client's anterior shoulder (Fig. 5-8E).
9. Cover it with the piece of plastic (Fig. 5-8F).
10. Cover the plastic with a small towel.
11. Place a source of heat on top of the plaster, plastic, and small towel (Fig. 5-8G).
12. Leave the plaster on for 20 minutes.
13. Monitor the client's skin carefully. If the skin becomes very red before the 20 minutes is up, the reaction is finished and the plaster may be taken off. If the client feels any stinging or burning, remove the plaster immediately.
14. To clean the skin, apply a tissue or small cloth dipped in vegetable oil and wipe off the mustard (Fig. 5-8H).

CASTOR OIL PACK

Castor oil is a thick, clear oil extracted from crushed castor beans. Because the castor plant grows well in many parts of the world, the oil is easy to obtain. It has been used medicinally for centuries in both Ayurvedic medicine and European folk medicine, and today it is commonly sold in drugstores. It has a high concentration of fatty acids, especially ricinoleic acid. Castor oil packs have long been used for increasing local circulation of blood and lymph, relaxing smooth muscle, softening scar tissue, relieving muscle and joint pain, and helping relax specific areas. Vasodilation from hot applications laid over the packs increases absorption of chemicals in the oil and creates the effects of local heat.

Some practitioners of natural medicine prescribe months-long regimens of daily castor oil packs because they are believed to have strong detoxifying properties; however, no research has been done to investigate this claim. More important for the massage therapist is the

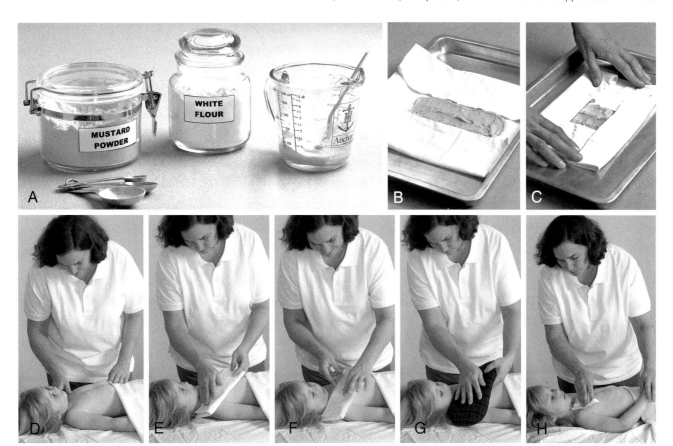

FIGURE 5-8 ■ Mustard plaster. **A.** Mix mustard powder, flour, and water to make a paste that can be spread on the cloth but is not so thin that it will run. **B.** Place the cloth on a tray. **C.** Spoon the mustard mixture onto the cloth and spread it out, leaving enough dry cloth to fold over well on all four sides. Only one thin layer of cloth should be between the skin and the plaster. **D.** Check the area visually before applying the plaster. **E.** Place the plaster on the client's anterior shoulder. **F.** Cover it with the piece of plastic. **G.** Place a source of heat on top of the plaster, plastic, and small towel. **H.** At end of treatment time, remove pack, apply a tissue or small cloth dipped in vegetable oil, and wipe off the mustard.

use of castor oil packs to soften fibrotic nodules and adhesions. Castor oil packs may be applied at the beginning of a massage session to prepare these tissues for treatment and then taken off after 30 minutes or longer.

Rather than using castor oil packs during massage sessions, an alternative is to cover the area to be treated with a thick application of castor oil, cover it with plastic wrap, and apply heat on top. Remove after 30 minutes, cleanse the area, and begin massage. Below is an overview of treatment details and a sample castor oil pack procedure using the calf, showing you how to incorporate it into a massage session.

Indications
1. Muscle pain, including menstrual cramps
2. Tight, fibrous tissue which is going to be treated with massage, including fibrotic knots, scar tissue, tight iliotibial bands, and adhesions
3. Arthritis

Contraindications
1. Any area where heat is contraindicated, such as in diabetic neuropathy, or where there is local inflammation
2. Broken skin
3. Tumors
4. Ulcers
5. Lower abdomen in pregnant women

Temperature: Warm (from heating pad)

Time Needed: 45 minutes to an hour

Equipment Needed: Flannel cloth (wool is preferred, but cotton may be used); bottle of castor oil; metal pan or tray large enough to hold the flannel; piece of plastic wrap or a thin sheet of plastic cut from a garbage bag that is slightly larger than the flannel; local heat source to keep the pack warm, such as a fomentation, hot water bottle, or heating pad; washcloth; soap or ½ tsp of baking soda to be added to 1 cup of water to cleanse the skin after the pack is removed

Effect: Primarily chemical from the action of the castor oil itself but also thermal from the application of heat over the entire pack

Cleanup: Dispose of plastic sheet, wash metal pan with soap and water, launder washcloth. If desired, the oil-soaked flannel can be taken home in a plastic bag and reused by the client up to 10 times if it is kept in a plastic container in the refrigerator between uses: otherwise, it should be thrown away. No one else should use the flannel.

Procedure

1. Check with the client to make sure there are no contraindications for the use of local heat.

2. Explain the purpose of the castor oil pack to the client and get consent.
3. Cut or fold the flannel to the appropriate size so there will be three layers of cloth, and place it on a metal pan or tray.
4. Pour castor oil over the flannel and leave it until it is well saturated. The cloth should be wet but not dripping (Fig. 5-9A).
5. Warn the client before applying the flannel, and say, "Be sure to let me know if this ever feels too hot."
6. Check the area visually before applying the flannel. This allows you to see what the client's skin normally looks like.

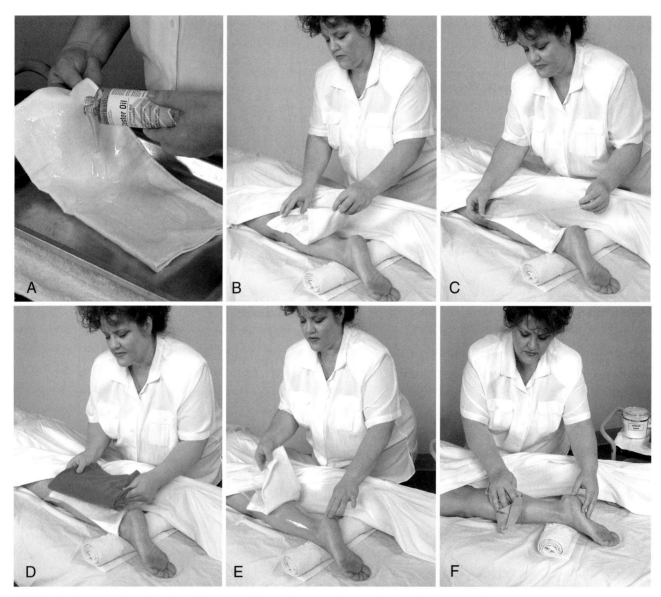

FIGURE 5-9 ■ Castor oil. **A.** Soak flannel in castor oil. **B.** Apply to skin. **C.** Cover flannel with plastic. **D.** Cover plastic with heating pad or water bottle. **E.** Remove treatment. **F.** Clean skin with 1 cup cool water mixed with ½ tsp of baking soda.

7. Apply the flannel to the calf (Fig. 5-9B).
8. Cover it with the piece of plastic (Fig. 5-9C).
9. Apply heat on top of the plastic-covered flannel. Use a heating pad on the highest setting that can be tolerated. A high setting is preferable, but a medium setting is acceptable. Or use a hot water bottle (Fig. 5-9D).
10. Proceed with massage on other areas of the body.
11. Remove pack after 30 to 90 minutes (Fig. 5-9E).
12. Clean skin with 1 cup cool water with ½ tsp of baking soda added to it (Fig. 5-9F) or use soap and a washcloth.
13. Proceed with local massage.

COMBINATION TREATMENT

This whole-body treatment is actually a combination of three local treatments that stimulate local circulation and warm the entire body. A contrast treatment to the chest using a hot fomentation and ice rub is combined with a hot fomentation to the back and a hot footbath. Combining three heat treatments causes the core temperature to rise rather quickly. At the end of the treatment, clients generally feel soothed and stimulated and find that their breathing is more relaxed.

Because it promotes good circulation in the chest, the full combination treatment is a classic treatment for chest congestion in colds, influenza, pneumonia, and bronchitis. Heat helps liquify chest secretions so that they can be expelled, eases breathing, and pulls white blood cells into the area to help fight infection. This treatment has also been used for problems in internal organs, such as cirrhosis of the liver. It has also been used after abdominal surgery—under doctor's supervision only—with an additional hot fomentation over the organ. A direct application of heat to the chest followed by a cold application (contrast treatment) is given to increase circulation to the chest, and both the fomentation to the back and the hot footbath are given to draw congestion away from the chest and/or abdominal organs.

Massage therapists do not treat any of these problems; however, sometimes this combination of treatments is useful within our scope of practice. This treatment, especially if the fomentations are given very hot for brief periods and followed quickly by short, very cold applications, can be a tonic and stimulating treatment for the circulation. It is also excellent to relieve musculoskeletal discomfort, such as soreness in the chest muscles from prolonged coughing, deep tension in the chest muscles, or arthritic pain in the back. Fomentations that are moderately warm and are applied for a longer period provide a more sedative, relaxing treatment which can relieve nervous tension, insomnia, and muscle spasm. This treatment is well suited for a client who would benefit from a warm bath or other full-body heat treatment but cannot get in and out of a tub, such as someone with severe arthritis or Parkinson's disease. At the end of this treatment, the massage therapist can begin a massage with a relaxed client who has enhanced circulation and warm tissue. By combining three simple treatments, the massage therapist can do the entire procedure without expensive hydrotherapy equipment.

Indications
1. Relief of musculoskeletal pain, including arthritis pain, muscular pain, and rigidity of Parkinson's disease
2. Scalene, intercostal, or pectoralis major muscles which are sore or tight after a great deal of coughing caused by allergy, pneumonia, bronchitis, asthma, or emphysema. Nervous tension or poor breathing habits can cause habitual patterns of tightness as well.
3. Muscle spasm and muscle soreness
4. Nervous tension
5. General tonic
6. Insomnia

Contraindications
1. Diabetics should not have heat applied to the feet.
2. Lack of sensation
3. Any condition that specifically contraindicates whole-body heating, such as cardiovascular problems, diabetes, hepatitis, lymphedema, multiple sclerosis, and seizure disorders, unless treatments are specifically prescribed by a doctor.
4. Great obesity
5. Pregnancy
6. Ingestion of alcohol or drugs
7. Inability to tolerate heat

Temperature: Hot, combining hot fomentations and hot footbath (110°F) with cold mitten frictions, cold compress to forehead, and cold water poured over the feet

Time Needed: 30 minutes

Equipment Needed
Water thermometer
Kitchen timer
Table or counter space to hold equipment
Rubber gloves to protect your hands when handling fomentations
Plastic bed sheet or thick towels to cover the massage table
Cotton sheets
A blanket
Footbath (a rectangular plastic dishpan works well)
Two pitchers
A drinking glass with straw
About six towels

Three fomentations with fabric covers
Two washcloths for cold applications to the forehead
Basin for ice cubes
Hot water for the fomentation
Cold water for the cold compress to the forehead
Ice cubes and cold water for the cold friction
Drinking water for the client

Effect: Primarily thermal, some mechanical

Cleanup: Clean and put away all equipment and launder used linens.

Procedure

1. Wet the fomentations by soaking them in a container of warm water and wringing them out (Fig. 5-10A).
2. Heat the fomentations in the microwave in a resealable plastic bag for 5 minutes or over boiling water on the rack of a canner for 15 minutes (Fig. 5-10B).
3. While the fomentations are heating, prepare a place for the client to lie during the treatment. Cover the surface of a massage table with a blanket, cover that with the plastic sheet, and cover that with one cotton sheet (Fig. 5-10C).
4. Using rubber gloves, wrap the first hot fomentation in its cover. Lay it down on the sheet where the client's back will be, and cover it with one or two towels (Fig. 5-10D).
5. Have the client quickly get on the table and lie supine, and make sure that the pack is warming the entire back from sacrum to shoulders (Fig. 5-10E). (A flat plastic hot water bottle filled with water at 110°F may also be used.) Should it feel like it is going to burn the client's skin at any time, add another towel or two over it. Be sure to ask the client for feedback, especially in the first 10 minutes, before the fomentation cools at all, and if it feels too hot, add another layer of towel.
6. Fill the dishpan with hot water (110°F) and place the client's feet in it. The client's knees should be bent and feet flat on the surface. Check with the client to make sure the water temperature is tolerable (Fig. 5-10F).

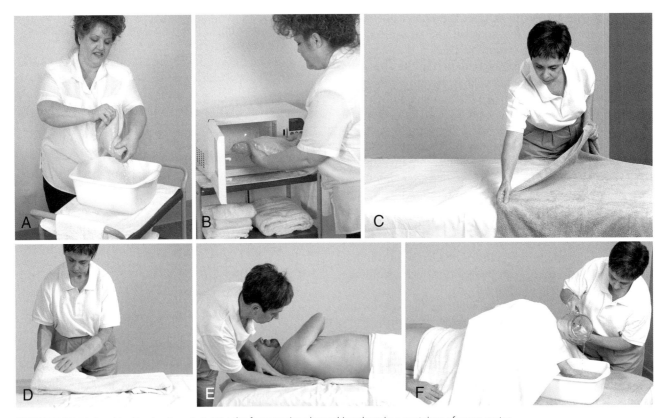

FIGURE 5-10 ■ Combination treatment. **A.** Wet the fomentations by soaking them in a container of warm water and wringing them out. **B.** Heat the fomentations in the microwave in a resealable plastic bag for 5 minutes or over boiling water on the rack of a canner for 15 minutes. **C.** While the fomentations are heating, prepare a place for the client to lie during the treatment. Cover the surface of a massage table with a blanket, then the plastic sheet, then a large bath towel, and finally a cotton sheet. **D.** Using rubber gloves, wrap the first hot fomentation in its cover. Lay it on the sheet where the client's back will be and cover it with one or two towels. **E.** Have the client quickly get on the table and make sure that the pack is warming the entire back from sacrum to shoulders. **F.** Fill the dishpan with hot water (110°F) and place the client's feet in the bath. (*continued*)

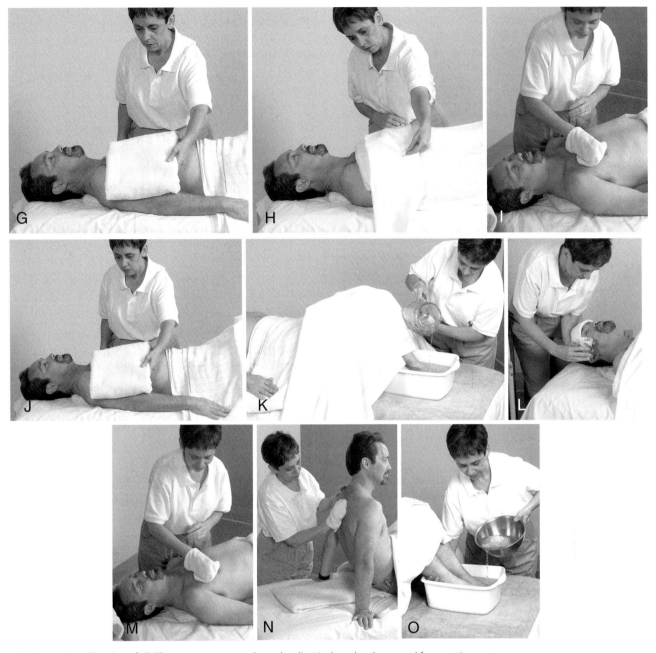

FIGURE 5-10 ■ (*Continued*) **G.** Place one or two towels on the client's chest, lay the second fomentation on top, then lay one more towel on top. **H.** Cover the client with a sheet and then a blanket. **I.** When the timer rings, rub the entire chest briskly for 30 seconds with a washcloth or terry cloth mitt wrung from ice water. **J.** Place another hot fomentation on the chest. Set the timer for 5 minutes. **K.** Add hot water to the footbath if needed. **L.** Provide water to drink as needed, and place a washcloth wrung out in ice water on the forehead. **M.** Remove the fomentation on the chest and rub the chest with ice water as before. Dry the chest thoroughly. **N.** Remove the fomentation and rub the entire back briefly with ice water. Dry the back. **O.** Take the client's feet out of the hot water, pour ice water (left from the cold application to the chest) over them, and dry them off.

7. Place one or two towels on the client's chest, place the second fomentation on top, then place one more towel on top. Again check with the client to make sure it is not going to burn the skin (Fig. 5-10G).

8. Cover the client with a sheet and then a blanket. Set a timer for 5 minutes. During this time you may perform a brief facial massage (Fig. 5-10H).

9. When the timer rings, rub the entire chest briskly for 30 seconds with a washcloth or terry cloth mitt

wrung from iced water (Fig. 5-10I). Do not apply this friction over a woman's breasts. Alternatively, a small towel may be wrung out of ice water, laid over the entire chest, and rubbed for 30 seconds. This may be more appropriate for a woman, as then the breasts will not be exposed. To minimize exposure, slide the ice-cold towel onto the chest from above just as you pull the fomentation down off of the chest. Be sure to warn your client that the cold is coming, and encourage him or her to take a deep breath just as you lay on the cloth. Although the contrast will be dramatic, the client's chest will be very warm, and most clients find the cold refreshing.

10. Place another hot fomentation on the chest. Set the timer for 5 minutes (Fig. 5-10J).

11. Add more hot water to the footbath if needed so that the water remains at 105° to 110°F (Fig. 5-10K). Scoop some of the cooler water out, then remove the client's feet for a moment while you add more hot water and stir. Replace the client's feet.

12. By now, the client is usually becoming getting quite warm; provide water to drink as needed, and place a washcloth wrung out in ice water on the forehead (Fig. 5-10L).

13. When the timer rings, repeat steps 9 to 12.

14. After 5 more minutes, remove the fomentation on the chest and rub the chest with ice water as in step 9 (Fig. 5-10M). Dry the chest thoroughly.

15. Immediately have the client sit up. Remove the fomentation on the table and rub the entire back briefly with ice water (Fig. 5-10N). Dry the back. Do not let the client become chilled.

16. Take the client's feet out of the hot water, pour ice water (left from the cold application to the chest) over them, and dry them off (Fig. 5-10O).

17. Make sure the client is dry.

18. The towel under the client will be damp, and it should be removed and the client covered with a dry sheet. The massage session may begin.

CHAPTER SUMMARY

In this chapter you have learned about a variety of treatments that heat only one part of the body without immersion in liquid water and their effects and benefits. During massage sessions, therapeutic heat can help relieve musculoskeletal pain and promote mental relaxation and increased local circulation, as well as helping to warm and soften stiff muscles before exercise and stretching. Your therapy "toolbox" has just begun to expand, however; each of the chapters ahead discusses more new treatments, and you will learn even more about how to fine-tune them for yourself and for your clients. Soon you will be able to combine treatments, if desired, for particular clients.

REVIEW QUESTIONS

Short Answer

1. What is the primary hazard of heat applications?

2. Name five conditions for which local heat is contraindicated.

3. Name three conditions for which local heat may be indicated.

4. Discuss the difference between the heat provided by a hot water bottle or dry heating pad versus that of a silica gel pack or fomentation.

5. Describe the effect of local heat on myofascial trigger points.

Multiple Choice

6. Local application of heat
   a. Relaxes connective tissue
   b. Improves healing
   c. Causes local vasodilation
   d. Relieves pain
   e. All of the above

7. Which of these treatments has a heating effect?
   a. Local salt glow
   b. Cold footbath
   c. Tepid footbath
   d. Cold compress
   e. Castor oil pack

8. Local application of heat is indicated for all but one:
   a. Chronic arthritis
   b. Increased circulation
   c. Acute sprain
   d. Prior to exercise

9. The combination treatment is indicated for all but one of these conditions:
   a. soreness in the chest muscles from prolonged coughing
   b. deep tension in the chest muscles
   c. kidney failure
   d. arthritic back pain
   e. muscle spasm

10. The desired effects of a mustard plaster include all but one:
    a. provide soothing heat
    b. prepare muscles for massage
    c. increase local circulation
    d. cause a blister
    e. relieve arthritis or muscular pain

True/False

____11. Moist heat has the same effect as dry heat.

____12. A hot pack application prior to massage aids in muscle relaxation.

____13. Mustard plasters must be carefully monitored because they can burn the skin.

____14. Castor oil packs are used to soften adhesions.

____15. The combination treatment, when administered correctly, causes a drop in core temperature.

REFERENCES

1. Belanger A. *Evidence-Based Guide to Therapeutic Physical Agents*. Baltimore: Lippincott Williams & Wilkins, 2002.
2. Boyle W, Saine A. *Lectures in Naturopathic Hydrotherapy*. Sandy, OR: Eclectic Medical, 1988.
3. Doub L. *Hydrotherapy*. Fresno, CA: Author, 1971.
4. Kober A. et al. Local active warming: An effective treatment for pain, anxiety and nausea caused by renal colic. *J Urol* 2003;170:741–744.
5. Simons D, Travell J. *Myofascial Pain and Dysfunction: The Trigger Point Manual*, vol 1, 2nd ed. Baltimore: Lippincott Williams & Wilkins, 1999, pp 133, 170.
6. Thrash A. Thrash C. *Home Remedies: Hydrotherapy, Charcoal, and Other Simple Treatments*. Seale, AL: Thrash, 1981, p 75.

RECOMMENDED RESOURCES

Sister Kenny. 1946. Movie starring Rosalind Russell.
Ice Therapy. 1993. Video by massage therapist Harold Packman.

COLD PACKS, COMPRESSES, AND ICE MASSAGE: LOCAL COLD APPLICATIONS

6

What actually happens when you apply cold to an area? The cold constricts the local blood vessels, which results in a decrease of bleeding of an injury and swelling. This holds true for both internal bleeding such as bruises and open wounds. Cold immediately decreases the painful spasm of an injured muscle. It provides a numbing effect on nerves just below the skin thereby reducing the pain. Taking into consideration all of the aspects of cold therapy as stated above; you are now helping to provide an environment where the body helps to rebuild and repair damaged tissue.

—Harold Packman, Ice Therapy: Understanding Its Application

Chapter Objectives

After completing this chapter, the student will be able to:
- Describe the effects of local cold applications.
- Explain the contraindications to local cold applications.
- Name and describe local cold applications.
- Explain the four stages of ice massage.
- Perform local cold treatments using the procedure included with each treatment.

In this chapter, you will be introduced to some common local cold applications that will continue to expand your therapy "toolbox" (Fig. 6-1). Like the local heat applications covered in Chapter 5, local cold applications are effective, inexpensive, and in most cases quite portable. They require little preparation, can be easily incorporated into your massage sessions, and have different effects from those of local heat treatments. The benefits of cold applications have been recognized throughout history. Because of these effects, modern medicine uses ice in numerous ways (Box 6-1).

How can applying local cold treatments improve a massage session? Here are some examples: Before work with a muscle that is in spasm, cold gel packs, ice packs, ice bags, **ice massage** (applying an ice cube or ice cup over an area with a rotating motion) or **iced compresses** (frozen wet cloths) can relieve the spasm. **Ice stroking** (stroking the length of a muscle with ice to temporarily release muscle tension and suppress pain)

can temporarily deactivate trigger points so you can stretch taut muscles to their full length. Ice massage can prevent posttreatment soreness of a muscle that has been treated with deep transverse friction. Before massaging someone with arthritis pain, cold applications may relieve the client's pain better than heat. Before massage near an injured muscle, cold applications can help reduce tissue swelling and pain. Finally, cold applications such as a flat plastic water bottle filled with chilled water or an ice water compress can cool an overheated client. Cold applications penetrate deep into tissues more easily than hot ones do; when blood vessels are dilated under a hot application, cooler blood from the rest of the body flows in constantly, but a cold application causes vasoconstriction, so little fresh warm blood can flow in to rewarm the cold area. Thus, after a 20-minute ice pack application, a muscle may take an hour or more to reach normal temperature again.

Many cold applications can be combined with hot ones. For example, when a heat treatment is needed for

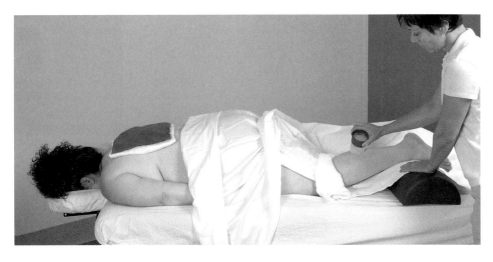

FIGURE 6-1 ■ Client with cold gel pack on upper back, ice pack on hamstring muscles, and ice massage being performed on the gastrocnemius.

clients who are likely to become overheated, adding an application of cold somewhere else on the body will help keep them comfortable. Hot and cold applications can also be combined to form contrast treatments which stimulate local circulation and relieve pain. After you learn how to use local cold treatments, you can both design an in-office massage session using them and perform many of these treatments in settings other than your office. You can also give your clients simple treatments that they can perform at home.

BOX 6-1 | *Point of Interest*

THE FIVE PRIMARY EFFECTS OF ICE APPLICATIONS

Ice has a wide range of uses in modern medicine because of its five main effects:

1. Ice reduces sensation by slowing down the messages from local sensory nerve fibers to the brain. The numbing effect of ice is widely used in medicine to reduce discomfort of musculoskeletal injuries, such as bruises, muscle strains, hematomas, and fractures; to reduce pain after orthopedic surgery; to numb skin which is going to be injected with anesthetic or stung by bees in bee sting therapy; and to numb the tongue to decrease the unpleasant taste of certain bad-tasting medications.
2. Ice reduces inflammation. This anti-inflammatory effect is widely used in medicine to reduce swelling after musculoskeletal injuries, such as bruises, sprains, strains, and torn muscles; to reduce swelling after orthopedic surgery; to decrease the itching caused by some types of cancer; to decrease the itching caused by some medications used for cancer; and to decrease the itching and oozing of mild poison ivy.
3. Ice reduces local blood flow by reflex vasoconstriction. In one study, the effect of an ice wrap applied to one knee was compared to a room temperature wrap applied to the opposite knee. Researchers found that the ice wrap caused a 38% decrease in arterial blood flow, a 26% decrease in soft tissue blood flow, and a 19% reduction in blood flow to the bone itself.(1) As little as 5 minutes of icing a knee can decrease blood flow to both soft tissue and bone in the knee.(2) The reason ice applications are generally limited to 15 to 30 minutes is because the tissues under the ice may become so ischemic that they are injured: frostbite and nerve palsy have resulted from longer applications. The blood

flow–reducing effect of ice is used in medicine for these purposes:

- To decrease blood flow into tissues after musculoskeletal trauma
- To decrease blood flow to the brain during a migraine headache
- To decrease blood flow into the joints of hemophiliacs during a bleeding episode
- To decrease the metabolism of local tissues, as shown in Figure 3-11
- To decrease blood flow to the nose during a nosebleed
- To decrease blood flow to the skin to slow the absorption of medications given by injection
- To decrease blood flow to the scalp during administration of some chemotherapeutic drugs that cause hair loss, with ice applied to the skull
- To decrease blood flow to an erupting herpes blister to arrest its development and shorten its healing time

4. Ice decreases muscle spasm. This effect is used in medicine to decrease muscle spasm in specific muscles, to deactivate trigger points and release muscle tension long enough for individual muscles to be gently but thoroughly stretched, and to increase range of motion before stretching.
5. Ice reduces body temperature. This effect is used in medicine to reduce core temperature in patients with heatstroke, heat exhaustion, and high fevers.

References
1. Ho SS et al. The effects of ice on blood flow and bone metabolism in knees. *Am J Sports Med* 1994;22:537.
2. Ho SS et al. Comparison of various icing times in decreasing bone metabolism in the knee. *Am J Sports Med* 1990;18:376.

INDICATIONS, CONTRAINDICATIONS, AND CAUTIONS FOR LOCAL COLD APPLICATIONS

Below are the primary indications, contraindications, and cautions for local cold treatments. Unless otherwise indicated, these apply to all treatments in this chapter.

INDICATIONS FOR ICE APPLICATIONS

1. Muscle strains for the first 24 to 48 hours
2. Contusions for the first 24 to 48 hours
3. Joint sprains for the first 24 hours
4. Vigorous exercise that might lead to delayed-onset muscle soreness
5. Acute low back pain
6. Chronic low back pain
7. Rheumatoid arthritis if beneficial for the client (heat may work better for some)
8. Osteoarthritis if beneficial for the client (heat may work better for some)
9. Bursitis if beneficial for the client (heat may work better for some)
10. Chronically stiff or spastic muscles due to damage to the brain or spinal cord
11. Temporary stimulation of muscle contraction in muscle weakness brought on by conditions such as stroke, spinal cord injury, or muscular dystrophy (see Chapter 14)
12. Stimulation of local circulation (when used as part of a contrast treatment)
13. To reduce blood flow in congested areas by creating a derivative effect (fluid-shifting). For example, when cold is applied on the back of the neck, it causes local vasoconstriction and may be helpful in treating a migraine headache.
14. Overheated client

CONTRAINDICATIONS TO ICE APPLICATIONS

1. Cold client. If it is important that a client who is cold have an ice treatment, first warm him or her by putting such materials as hot packs, blankets, hot water bottles, and/or warmed linens proximal to the iced area. A heating pad to the abdomen will raise core temperature and cause reflex vasodilation in the hands and feet.
2. Aversion to cold
3. Sensitivity to cold. This is common in clients with fibromyalgia.
4. Headache upon contact with cold
5. Inability to provide feedback about tissue temperature (impaired sensation) in the area to be

treated. Numbness can be caused by spinal cord injury, diabetic neuropathy, other medical conditions, or the use of some medications, which may cause the person to be unable to feel the pain of a too-cold application. Never put a cold application on a numb area.
6. Poor circulation. Because cold will further decrease blood flow, do not use over areas where circulation is already poor.
7. Raynaud's syndrome
8. Previously frostbitten areas should not have local cold gel packs or ice applications.
9. Peripheral vascular disease, including diabetes, Buerger's disease, and arteriosclerosis of the lower extremities
10. If an analgesic cream has been applied to the skin, do not cover that area with a cold application.
11. Wounds that are not completely healed
12. Malignancy in the area to be treated
13. Heart disease: do not apply cold over the heart, as this can cause a reflex constriction of the coronary arteries.
14. Implanted devices, such as cardiac pacemakers, stomach bands, and infusion pumps that are in the area to be treated
15. Marked hypertension. (Ice applications anywhere on the body normally cause a brief rise in blood pressure, so they are contraindicated for persons with marked hypertension.)
16. Lymphedema: avoid exposure to extreme cold for long periods. For example, avoid using cold gel packs, ice packs, and flat plastic water bottles filled with chilled water. However, cold compresses, iced compresses, and ice massage are safe to use.

CAUTIONS FOR ICE APPLICATIONS

1. Cold client. If it is important that cold clients have an ice treatment, warm them first by using such applications as hot footbaths, hot packs, blankets, hot water bottles, and/or warmed linens.
2. Elders, that is, clients who are over 60 years old, may not be able to keep warm during cold treatments; be careful not to chill them.
3. Children, especially preschool-age children, have difficulty describing their bodily sensations and may not be able to tell you if cold is causing pain, so use local cold with caution.
4. Use caution when applying cold over superficial nerves. Do not exceed recommended times, and do not tie cold applications over superficial nerves.
5. Clients may have decreased muscle strength and slowed reflexes for 30 minutes after ice treatment and may be prone to injury if they exercise right away.

6. Always check tissues periodically for cold damage. If an area has been cooled too much, there will be blotchiness, redness, or a welt underneath the cold application.

SILICA GEL COLD PACKS

There are many types of commercial cold gel packs, marketed under such names as Flex-Gel and Elasto-Gel, that are filled with a combination of water and various additives to form a gel which remains flexible even when it is frozen. They typically have a cover made of washable vinyl.

Cold gel packs are popular because they are an effective source of cold, they cool tissues faster than ice, and they require almost no preparation. All that is necessary is to place them in a freezer for 2 hours before you use them. Small freezers are inexpensive and take up little space in an office (Fig. 6-2). When they are ready for use, cold gel packs are very cold—about 25°F—and remain so for 15 to 20 minutes.

The advantage of a cold gel pack, that it can become very cold, can also be a disadvantage: while it is wonderful to have such an efficient source of cold, gel packs can also cause tissue damage. In one study, after 20 minutes on a patient's skin, the skin temperature under the cold gel pack had decreased from 93° to 32°F. If applied for 20 minutes, cold gel packs can reduce intramuscular temperature as much as 5–10°F. Tissues must not be chilled too much or they will be damaged.

Gel packs are most efficient at cooling large, flat surfaces, such as the thigh or the back, because it is difficult to wrap them around joints and other irregularly

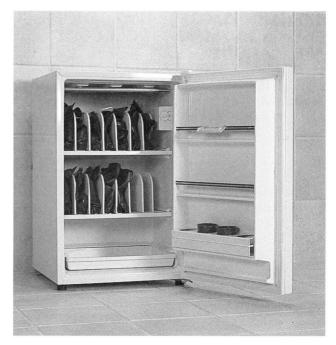

FIGURE 6-2 ■ Small freezer for storing cold gel packs and ice cups. (Photo courtesy of Whitehall Company. www.whitehallmfg.com/media.)

shaped surfaces (Fig. 6-3). Never let a client lie on a cold gel pack. Never tie a cold gel pack to any part of the body: this can compress the tissues underneath and cut off circulation.

The step-by-step procedure that follows shows how to use a cold gel pack on the upper back. However, gel packs can be adapted to treat almost any area of the body. They can also be combined with hot applications to create contrast treatments.

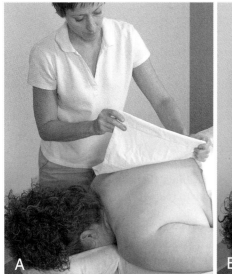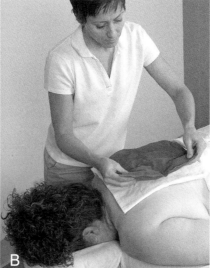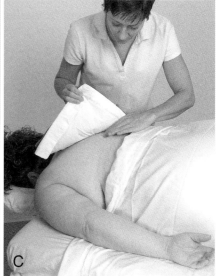

FIGURE 6-3 ■ Large gel pack on the back. **A.** With the client in prone position, place the cloth on the upper back. **B.** Place the cold gel pack on top of the cloth. **C.** Remove every few minutes to inspect the skin, then replace it.

Cold Gel Pack to Reduce Pain

Background

Leila was a healthy 38-year-old woman with a history of constant low-level pain in the lower back. At age 13 she had developed scoliosis and then wore a brace for 4 years. At age 17 she had surgery to fuse her spine at T4 to L3 level. Leila healed well from her surgery and had no complications. She had minimal pain prior to surgery but had lower back pain following surgery. Her **physiatrist** (doctor specializing in rehabilitation) recommended a program of regular aerobic exercise, periodic physical therapy to help her increase her strength and flexibility, and regular massage therapy. Leila managed her pain quite well on the program her doctor recommended, but she still had lower back pain late in the day. However, as she was not able to take any medication for it, her pain sometimes kept her from falling asleep.

Treatment

After having a cold gel pack applied to her back during a massage session, Leila realized that it helped numb her back and could be an option to help reduce her pain at bedtime. She purchased a large gel pack, kept it in the freezer, and began to use it every night before bed. She found that once the pack had been on her back for 20 minutes, the area became quite numb and she could then remove it and fall asleep easily.

Discussion Questions

1. Explain how the cold gel pack relieved Leila's pain.
2. What other local cold treatments could be added to Leila's massage sessions?

Temperature: 25 to 32°F

Time Needed: 20 minutes. To prevent cold damage, do not exceed this time.

Equipment Needed: Cold gel pack, thin cloth or towel to put between the gel pack and the client's skin. If the cloth is wet, it will conduct cold faster than if it is dry.

Effect: Primarily thermal

Cleanup: Launder cloth covering; clean the surface of the gel pack with soap and water if it comes in contact with the client's skin

Procedure

1. Check with the client to make sure there are no contraindications to the use of local cold.
2. Explain the use of local cold to the client and get consent.
3. Dampen a thin cloth.
4. With the client prone, place the cloth on the upper back (Fig. 6-3A).
5. Place the cold gel pack on top of the cloth (Fig. 6-3B).
6. Remove every few minutes to inspect the skin (Fig. 6-3C), then replace it.

Remove after a maximum of 20 minutes.

ICE PACKS AND ICE BAGS

Ice packs and ice bags are a popular method of treating many local musculoskeletal conditions. They are widely used in doctors' offices, hospitals, athletic facilities, physical therapy clinics, and massage therapy offices. They not only cool effectively, they are simple to prepare: ice packs can be easily made by with only a towel and ice cubes or crushed ice, and ice bags need only be filled with crushed or cube ice. If ice packs are applied to the client's skin for 20 minutes, they can reduce intramuscular temperature as much as 5–10°F.

Packs and bags of ice can be applied to almost any area of the body except over the eyes, and are especially suited for large, dense muscles that need real cold to chill them. Smaller areas without much insulation, such as the back of the hand, will not need to be iced for as long to become very cold.

ICE PACK

Ice packs made with towels can be large or small, depending upon the size of the towel. Here we show a small ice pack which can be used on the back of the neck, the front of the knee joint, or other small area. Never lie on an ice pack.

Temperature: Very cold (32°F)

Time Needed: 20 minutes. To prevent cold damage, do not exceed this time.

Equipment Needed: One damp towel and one dry towel, crushed ice or ice cubes

Effect: Primarily thermal

Cleanup: Launder towel.

Procedure
1. Check with the client to make sure there are no contraindications to the use of local cold.
2. Explain the use of local cold to the client and get his or her consent.
3. To make a small towel ice pack, dampen a small face towel, then lay it on a flat surface. Place about 4 cups of ice cubes on one end of the towel (Fig. 6-4A). Fold it over to make an ice pack which will fit easily on a small area (Fig. 6-4B).
4. Place the ice pack on the client's skin (Fig. 6-4C).
5. Cover the ice pack with a dry towel of the same size (Fig. 6-4D).
6. Remove every few minutes to check for cold damage, then replace.
7. Remove after a maximum of 20 minutes.

ICE BAG

Ice bags are simple, found in drugstores, many grocery stores, and massage therapy suppliers. They come in various sizes.

Temperature: Very cold (32°F)

Time Needed: 20 minutes. To prevent cold damage, do not exceed this time.

Equipment Needed: Ready-made ice bag or plastic resealable bag to make ice bag, crushed ice cubes to fill the bag, a thin cloth to be placed between the ice bag and the client's skin (optional). (Fig. 6-5 shows various types of ice bags.)

Effect: Primarily thermal

Cleanup: Launder cloth coverings and any other linens used. Clean the surface of the ice bag with soap and water if it comes in contact with the client's skin. Dispose of resealable plastic bag if used.

Procedure
1. Check with the client to make sure there are no contraindications to the use of local cold.
2. Explain the use of local cold to the client and get his or her consent.
3. Fill the bag with crushed ice or ice cubes. Remove as much air as possible from the bag before you seal it.
4. Place a thin cloth on the client's skin (Fig. 6-6A).
5. Place the ice bag on the client's skin (Fig. 6-6B).
6. Remove every few minutes to check for frostbite, then replace.

Remove after a maximum of 20 minutes.

FLAT PLASTIC WATER BOTTLE

Chapter 5 explains the use of a flat plastic water bottle filled with hot water. When it is filled with cold water at the appropriate temperature, a flat plastic water bottle can also be effectively used for several cold applications. When laid flat on a massage table before a session begins, it cools the table. On a hot day, by cooling the entire torso and abdomen or the entire back, it can keep the client's entire body cool and can also cool and stimulate

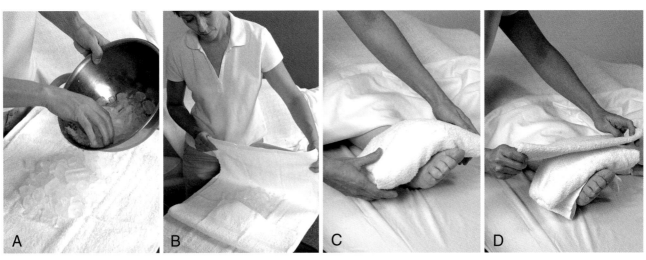

FIGURE 6-4 ■ Homemade ice packs. **A.** Placing ice cubes on a towel. **B.** Folding the ice inside the towel to form an ice pack. **C.** Placing ice pack on client's skin. **D.** Placing dry towel on top of ice pack.

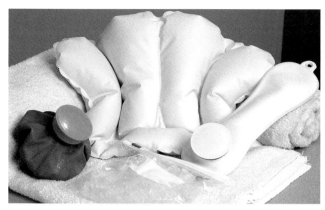

FIGURE 6-5 ■ Ready-made ice bags come in various sizes.

local areas before they are massaged. It will stay cool for approximately 30 minutes, depending upon the temperature of the water it is filled with and the client's core temperature. Obviously, a very warm person who lies on any cold object will warm it faster than someone who is not so hot.

An advantage of this particular hydrotherapy treatment is that it is inexpensive and fairly low tech: all the therapist needs is the bottle and cold water. Unlike gel cold packs or ice packs, it is also safe to lie on, as it begins to warm up as soon as the client lies on it. Flat plastic water bottles filled with cold water also can be combined with various heat applications—including another bottle filled with hot water—to create contrast treatments. If filled with very cold water and placed in a ice chest along with a bag of ice, they can stay cold for hours. When the water bottle is placed on the top half of the massage table, the front or back of the entire torso can be cooled while the client lies on it. Although the legs can also be

cooled with a flat water bottle, the upper body is the most effective place to apply it.

The following procedure shows the most convenient place to apply the water bottle, on the massage table underneath a cloth, where it can cool the client's entire back.

Temperature: Cold (water is 55°F)

Time Needed: 5 to 30 minutes. The client's tissue will begin to cool after about 5 minutes.

Equipment Needed: Water thermometer, water bottle, and a thin cloth to cover or wrap the filled water bottle (a pillowcase is ideal)

Effect: Primarily thermal

Cleanup: Launder cloth; empty the water bottle and lay it flat with the lid off, so the last drops of water will evaporate; then fold and store it.

Procedure

1. Check with the client to make sure there are no contraindications to the use of local cold.
2. Explain the use of local cold to the client and get his or her consent.
3. Use a thermometer to ensure the water is 55°F (Fig. 6-7A). Fill bottle about one-third full of cold water that has been chilled in the refrigerator or room temperature water that has been mixed with crushed ice to chill it and strained to remove any pieces of ice (Fig. 6-7B). About 6 cups of water will be needed for a large 18 × 24 inch bottle.
4. Carry the open bottle carefully to the massage table. Lay it flat on the table. Use your hand to expel the air bubbles, and check to make sure the top is snapped on securely so it does not leak (Fig. 6-7C).
5. Cover it with a cloth or pillowcase or place it inside a pillowcase (Fig. 6-7D).
6. As the client lies supine on the cloth that is covering the cold water bottle, say, "Be sure to let me know if this ever feels like it is too cold."

Although the chance of cold injury is minimal, be sure to ask your client for feedback. The bottle will be intensely cold when it is first lain upon but will begin to warm up almost immediately.

ICE MASSAGE

Ice massage is a method of cooling tissue using an ice cube or a chunk of ice applied to the skin. The ice is moved over and around the area to be cooled with a gentle rotary motion but no pressure. Ice massage may be performed on any part of the body, from large dense muscles, such as the quadriceps, to small areas, such as

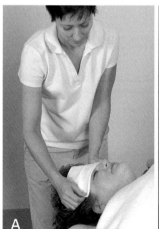
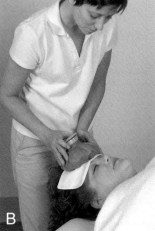

FIGURE 6-6 ■ Applying an ice bag. **A.** Placing cloth on client's skin. **B.** Placing ice bag on client's skin.

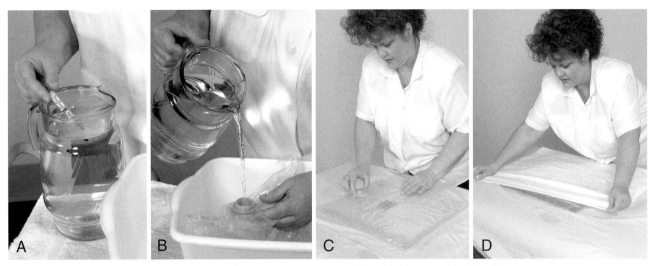

FIGURE 6-7 ■ Flat plastic water bottle. **A.** Check the water temperature. **B.** Fill bottle about one-third full with cold water. **C.** Carry the open bottle carefully to the massage table, lay it flat on the table, use your hand to expel the air bubbles, and check to make sure the top is snapped on securely so it does not leak. **D.** Cover it with a cloth or pillowcase or place it inside a pillowcase.

the back of the hand. After an injury such as a blow which leaves a bruise, a muscle strain, or a joint sprain, ice massage, like other cold applications, can decrease local swelling and inflammation and relieve spasm and pain. It may be used after deep transverse friction to reduce posttreatment soreness. Ice massage is also an excellent home treatment you can teach your clients. For example, someone who wakes up with an acutely stiff neck or other muscle spasm can perform ice massage on the area.

Some practitioners prefer ice massage over ice packs or bags, and each has its advantages and disadvantages. Ice massage not only reduces tissue temperature as well as ice packs and ice bags do; it does so much faster. One study comparing the cooling effect of ice massage to that of ice bags found that ice massage cooled the gastrocnemius muscle as much as 10 minutes faster than an ice bag. Therefore, using ice massage during a massage session means you will not have to wait as long for the area to cool. However, the advantage of rapid cooling must be weighed against the fact that ice massage is more intensely cold, and some clients find the sensation much too intense. For these clients, a cold application that chills the area more slowly will be tolerated better. In this case, you might prefer to apply an ice pack or ice bag while performing massage on another part of the body. You might also choose ice massage because herbs, essential oils, or other chemical substances can be applied to an area this way if you add them to the water before making ice cups. As the ice melts, the dissolved chemical will come into direct contact with the skin. Another consideration when choosing which cold application to use is that time will be taken away from manual massage while you are performing ice massage.

To begin, you will need a chunk of ice made by freezing water in a paper cup or a plastic cup that is designed especially for ice massage (Fig. 6-8A).

As you perform ice massage, keep in mind that the thicker the area you wish to cool, the more time will be

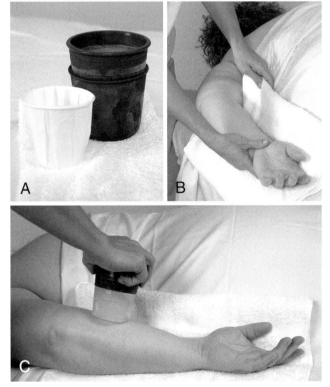

FIGURE 6-8 ■ Ice massage. **A.** Ice cups, made from paper cups or commercial ice massage cups. **B.** Drape towels around the area to be iced. **C.** Hold the cup of ice in one hand and gently rub it in a circular motion. Shown: ice massage on the forearm.

required for the cold to penetrate. Tissues that are near the body surface and have little subcutaneous fat to insulate them, such as the front of the knee, will require relatively little time, and tissues that are deeper or covered by more subcutaneous fat, such as the gluteal muscles, will require more time. The tissues of a small, thin person who takes cold easily will need to be treated differently from those of a larger person with well-developed muscles or a great deal of subcutaneous fat. For this reason, the stages of ice massage listed below give you a better guide to the amount of time a client will require than a set number of minutes. Never exceed 15 minutes of ice massage.

Generally, the client will feel four sensations:

1. A sensation of cold
2. Burning or pricking
3. Aching
4. Numbness; take the ice away as soon as this happens.

It is important to explain the benefits of ice massage to clients before you begin, since they may want you to stop performing it when the area begins burning or aching. When the aching stage is reached, tell them that this is beneficial because their tissue is just about to become numb. Once past the aching stage, clients will be happy with the relief that they receive.

Here we show a step-by-step procedure for performing ice massage on the flexor muscles of the forearm, but ice massage can also be performed on many other parts of the body, including the entire back, all four limbs, and the neck. A simple variation of ice massage for the arch of the foot follows the basic procedure.

Temperature: Very cold (32°F)

Time Needed: 5 to 15 minutes, depending upon the thickness of the tissue and individual tolerance

Equipment Needed: Ice in paper cup or in specially designed plastic cup for ice massage, medium-size to large towel

Effect: Primarily thermal

Cleanup: Dispose of ice, launder towel, and sanitize plastic cup.

Procedure
1. Check with the client to make sure there are no contraindications to the use of local cold.
2. Explain the use of local cold to the client and get his or her consent.
3. Explain the four stages of ice massage to the client. It is important that he or she realizes that the ice massage must last to the point of numbness.
4. Drape towels around the area to be iced so melting ice will not drip onto other parts of the body (Fig. 6-8B).

5. Hold the cup of ice in one hand and gently rub it in a circular motion over the area you are treating and a few inches above and below the area as well (Fig. 6-8C). Here we show ice massage on the forearm.
6. Continue until the area is numb.
7. Remove ice and dry the area.

Variation: Ice massage for the arch of the foot, to be used for inflammation, tightness of arch muscles, and arch muscle strain

1. Fill a 20-oz plastic soft drink bottle with water and freeze it.
2. Have the client roll the affected foot over the bottle for 10 to 15 minutes. Rather than leaning the entire body weight on the bottle, the pressure should be no more than will gently stretch the muscles, tendons, and fascia.
3. Begin massage.

ICE STROKING (INTERMITTENT COLD WITH STRETCH)

During treatment of active trigger points with massage techniques, ice stroking can temporarily release muscle tension and suppress pain. This will assist the therapist in stretching tight muscles to their full length without aggravating them. Normally, trying to stretch a tight muscle beyond its limited range of motion causes pain, an involuntary tightening of the muscle, and soreness afterward. However, ice stroking can release or deactivate trigger points in individual muscles long enough for them to be gently, thoroughly, and painlessly stretched during a massage session. Three sweeps with ice, each lasting 2 to 3 seconds, are made over the length of the muscle, and then it is gently stretched to its full length. Ice is wrapped in thin plastic so that the skin remains dry. When ice is stroked over the muscle to be stretched, it causes a sudden drop in skin temperature, which is a strong tactile stimulation, and keeping the ice moving sends a continuous barrage of nerve impulses to the spinal cord. This stimulus inhibits the normal reflex tightening of the muscle that would otherwise occur with stretching.

Ice stroking can be incorporated into most massage sessions. Do not use ice stroking in acute injuries with inflamed tissue, such as sprains or whiplash injuries. For more information on this technique, see *Myofascial Pain and Dysfunction*, by Janet Travell and David Simons.

The procedure that follows shows you a step-by-step procedure for using ice stroking during trigger point treatment of the triceps muscle. This technique can be used for all muscles with active trigger points.

CASE HISTORY 6-2

Ice Massage for Muscle Spasm

Background

Suzanne Smith was a 28-year-old nurse who had received massage in the past for relaxation. Suzanne was generally very healthy but had mild whiplash due to a sledding accident and was taking prescribed muscle relaxants and anti-inflammatory and pain medications. She was receiving physical therapy for neck and upper back pain and frontal headaches but had never received massage therapy. She requested massage because she had a very uncomfortable feeling in her right mid scapular region. She said it felt as though the area "needed to be popped." Suzanne had never had this feeling (likely a muscle spasm stemming from her injury) until a few days ago. She then asked her father to "pop her back" in the mid scapular region. He did so, using a great deal of force, and she immediately had a severe headache which lasted for 4 hours. Now that she knew "popping the area" was not helpful, she hoped that massage could help relieve the sensation.

Treatment

The massage therapist, after taking Suzanne's history, consulted with her physical therapist, who approved of ice massage and hands-on massage for Suzanne's entire back. The massage therapist began the session with 15 minutes of Swedish massage of the back to assess Suzanne's muscles and to relax the most superficial layers. Among other tight muscles, she identified active trigger points in the right rhomboid major and right lower trapezius muscles. At the end of the 15 minutes, Suzanne said her back felt more relaxed, but the uncomfortable sensation remained. The massage therapist then performed ice massage over the midthoracic region, concentrating on the right side. After 10 minutes of ice massage, Suzanne said the uncomfortable sensation was gone, and the massage therapist showed her how to perform self-massage of the mid scapular muscles by lying supine and using a tennis ball. At the end of this time, Suzanne stood up and found that that not only was the uncomfortable sensation still gone, but her back muscles felt comfortable and relaxed. The therapist gave her instructions on how to use an ice pack or bag to chill her midthoracic muscles before using the tennis ball for self-massage, should the uncomfortable feeling recur.

Discussion Questions

1. Why did ice massage relieve Suzanne's uncomfortable sensation?
2. What other hydrotherapy treatment that you have learned could be used in this situation?

Temperature: 32°F

Time Needed: 1 minute or less

Equipment Needed: Ice cup or ice cube, thin plastic bag to wrap ice

Effect: Primarily thermal

Cleanup: Dispose of ice and plastic bag; sanitize plastic cup if used.

Procedure

1. Check with the client to make sure there are no contraindications to the use of local cold.
2. Explain the use of local cold to the client and get his or her consent.
3. Treat trigger points with massage techniques.
4. Place the ice in a thin plastic bag (Fig. 6-9A).
5. Gently stretch the muscle to the greatest extent possible without overstretching.
6. Maintaining the muscle stretch, stroke the entire length of the muscle three times with the ice, moving at about 4 inches per second (Fig. 6-9B).
7. Gently stretch the muscle to the greatest extent possible without overstretching (Fig. 6-9C).
8. If the muscle still does not fully lengthen without pain, try applying direct pressure to the trigger point, then gently stretching the muscle again, or have the client contract the antagonist muscle for 30 seconds and relax completely as you gently stretch the muscle again.
9. Repeat steps 4 to 6 until the muscle is pain free when completely stretched.
10. Gently return muscle to a comfortable position (Fig. 6-9D) and massage the area further if desired.
11. Apply a heating pad or moist hot pack to the muscle for 5 minutes or more (Fig. 6-9E) to reduce any posttreatment soreness.

COMPRESSES

Compresses are cloths that are soaked in water or another substance, wrung out, and applied to various parts of the body. Compresses can be hot, warm, cold, or

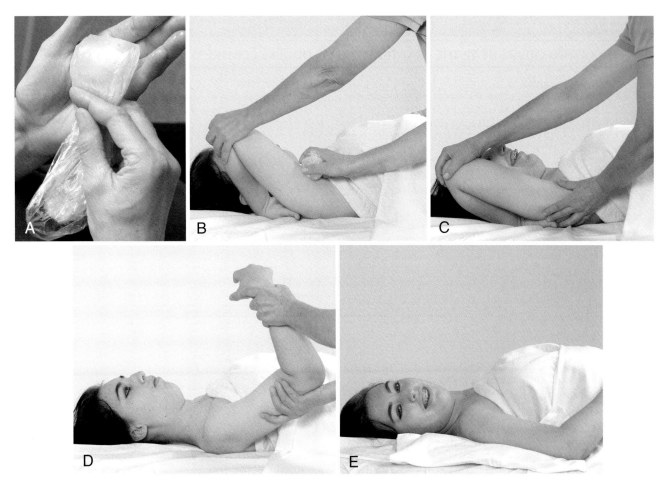

FIGURE 6-9 ■ Ice stroking. **A.** Place the ice in a thin plastic bag. **B.** Gently stretch the muscle to the greatest extent possible without overstretching. Maintaining the muscle stretch, stroke the entire length of the muscle three times with the ice. **C.** Gently stretch the muscle to the greatest extent possible without overstretching. **D.** Gently return muscle to a comfortable position. **E.** Apply a heating pad or moist hot pack to the muscle.

iced. They are used to apply heat or cold over the skin or to apply any of a variety of chemical solutions to the skin. This section discusses two cold compresses, one made with cold tap water and one frozen. (Box 6-2 has information on a special type of cold compress which is particularly appropriate for a home treatment.)

Cold compresses are a milder form of the intense cold of cold gel packs and ice. Cold compresses may be more appropriate over delicate areas, such as the eyes or for an especially sensitive person. Cloth molds to body curves well and has a slight weight, and so it may feel better to some clients. Historically, many chemical solutions have been added to cold compresses for special purposes, such as anti-inflammatory herbs, rubefacient herbs, Epsom salts over bruises and sprains, and antiseptic herbs or essential oils over wounds, to name just a few. (Although these chemical solutions are not covered here, additional information may be found in books on herbs and essential oils.) Cold compresses have also been combined with various hot applications to create contrast treatments. For example, a client's foot can be treated with a paraffin dip

followed by a cold compress or a client's back can be treated with a hot silica gel pack followed by a cold compress.

You can easily make cold compresses to suit the individual client. A tiny cold compress to cover the eyes may be made by soaking a washcloth in cold water and then wringing it out. Small or medium-size cold compresses may be made with a few layers of cloth or with small towels. Large cold compresses that can cover the entire back can be made with a bath towel.

COLD COMPRESS

Cold compresses of various sizes may be used to apply cold to any place where applications of ice are not suitable, such as over the eyes; to keep the forehead cool during whole-body heating treatments; to gently cool an overheated client; as part of a mild contrast treatment along with hot compresses; to relieve itchy skin; and to treat clients who cannot tolerate applications of intense cold.

BOX 6-2 | *Point of Interest*

USING COLD TO CREATE HEAT: THE HEAT-TRAPPING OR DOUBLE COMPRESS

A heat-trapping compress is an ingenious application of cold which ultimately becomes a mild moist heat treatment. It was widely used in the days of the water cure and is still an effective and safe home treatment. It begins with applying a cold compress—a cotton cloth dipped in cold water—to one part of the body, then covering that cold compress with dry cloth. The area under the two layers of cloth is cooled initially, but then the body creates a burst of heat in that area through reflex vasodilation, and because body heat cannot escape, the area begins to warm up. The heat-trapping or double compress must be worn for at least several hours—overnight is ideal—so it is a good treatment for clients to use at home but not practical for use during a massage session.

Heat-trapping compresses are used to warm and relax muscles and relieve musculoskeletal pain, and they have a derivative effect, since blood flow is increased once the compress becomes warm. They can be used on any part of the body and have no contraindications except skin rashes or other conditions that are irritated by moisture.

Elke Fraser, LMT, a massage therapist for 45 years, swears by the heat-trapping compress as a way to relieve hand and arm pain after a day of massage. At night she wraps her hands and forearms with cold, damp cloths, followed by dry cloths, and sleeps with them on. In the morning, the heat trapped by the compress has dried the wet cloth, and her symptoms are greatly decreased (personal communication, Corvallis, Oregon, September 5, 2005). Heat-trapping compresses are effective for many musculoskeletal conditions, such as backache, arthritis, and joint injuries. They can be wrapped around the chest for sore or tight chest muscles; around the abdomen and lower back for backache; around joints such as the wrist, elbow, knee, or ankle for joint pain; even around the throat to relieve muscle tension and strain. They also improve local circulation, and so they can be used for derivation. Using cold wet socks covered by dry socks is a classic treatment for sinus congestion.

If more than one-fifth of the body is covered by a cold compress, the core temperature will begin to fall, so it is important to monitor whether the client is warm or cold at all times. The skin should be monitored occasionally, but because the cold compress is much warmer than applications of ice, there is very little danger of cold damage to the skin. This is how to make a cold compress for the front of the lower leg:

Temperature: Cold (40–50°F)

Time Needed: 10 to 20 minutes unless used as part of a contrast treatment. For a contrast treatment, leave on for 1 minute.

Equipment Needed: Water thermometer, container for water, a towel of suitable size to use for the compress, and another towel to be placed under the client where the compress will be used

Effect: Primarily thermal

Cleanup: Launder used linens.

Procedure
1. Check with the client to make sure there are no contraindications to the use of local cold.
2. Explain the use of local cold to the client and get his or her consent.
3. Add crushed ice or ice cubes to a container of water until it is 40–50°F (Fig. 6-10A).
4. Soak a towel of the appropriate size in the water, then wring it out (Fig. 6-10B).
5. Apply to the client's shin (Fig. 6-10C).

The towel will begin to warm up after a few minutes on the client's skin; reapply if desired.

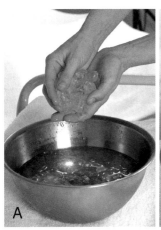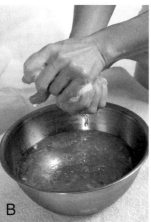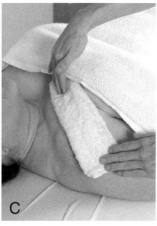

FIGURE 6-10 ■ Cold compress. **A.** Add crushed ice or ice cubes to a container of water until it is 40° to 50°F. **B.** Soak a towel of the appropriate size in the water and wring it out. **C.** Apply to the client.

ICED COMPRESS

An iced compress consists of a wet towel (various sizes) placed in a resealable plastic bag and then frozen; when removed from the freezer and placed on the client's body, it can remain cold for as long as 20 minutes. Colder than the cold compress but less cold than cold gel packs or ice, iced compresses are ideal for clients who would benefit from a local cold treatment but cannot tolerate the intensity of cold gel packs or ice. Iced compresses are safe for clients to lie on, unlike cold gel packs or ice, as they will begin to warm up as soon as they come into contact with the client's body. Iced compresses are safe on any part of the body, and placed on an area at the beginning of a massage session, they begin to warm up after a few minutes but can remain on an area for 20 minutes. An iced compress for the hands can be made by wetting and freezing a pair of wool gloves; they can be taken from the freezer and worn on hands which are tired from repetitive physical work.

Iced compresses are also easy and convenient to make up ahead of time. All you have to do once the client arrives is to pull them from the freezer. Place the compress on the body at the beginning of a massage and leave it on until you massage the area. Iced compresses are an excellent home treatment which can be recommended to clients.

To make an iced compress, wring out a hand towel in cold water, fold it in half lengthwise and then in half again, and put it into a resealable plastic bag. Lay it flat in the freezer. Chill for at least 2 hours. When ready to use, remove the iced compress from the bag and lay it directly on the body. It will be stiff at first but will soon warm up enough to conform to the part of the body. Here is how to use an iced compress on the lateral shoulder muscles.

Temperature: Very cold (32°F for a short time; then the compress will begin to warm up)

Time Needed: 20 minutes

Equipment Needed: Hand towel, resealable plastic bag, freezer

Effect: Primarily thermal

Cleanup: Dispose of plastic bag and launder the used towel.

Procedure

1. Check with the client to make sure there are no contraindications to the use of local cold.
2. Explain the use of local cold to the client and get his or her consent.
3. Soak a towel of the appropriate size in cold water, then wring it out (Fig. 6-11A). It should be wet but not dripping.
4. Fold towel in half lengthwise and in half again (Fig. 6-11B).
5. Place in plastic bag, seal it, and put it in the freezer (Fig. 6-11 C).
6. When ready to use an iced compress, first check with the client to make sure there are no contraindications to the use of local cold.
7. Explain the use of local cold to the client and get his or her consent.
8. Remove iced compress from bag and apply it to the client's shoulder (Fig. 6-11D).
9. The towel will begin to warm up after a few minutes on the client's skin and become more flexible. Wrap it more closely around the area as it softens.

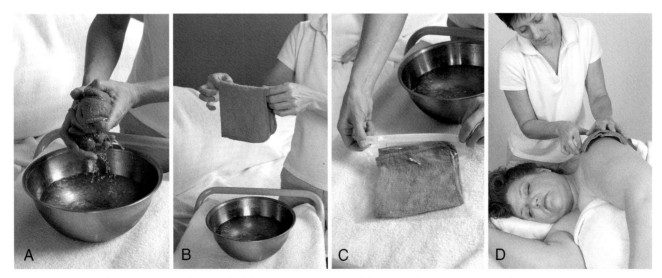

FIGURE 6-11 ■ Iced compress. **A.** Soak a towel of the appropriate size in cold water and wring it out. **B.** Fold towel in half lengthwise and in half again. **C.** Place in plastic bag, seal, and put in freezer. **D.** Remove from bag and apply iced compress to the client's shoulder.

CONTRAST COMPRESSES: ANOTHER COMBINATION TREATMENT

A **contrast compress treatment** consists of hot compresses alternated with cold ones. As noted in Chapter 3, contrast treatments can be used over many areas of the body to dramatically increase circulation. During a massage, contrast compresses are a simple way to prepare an area for massage by increasing blood flow, stimulating the skin and muscles underneath the compress, and relieving musculoskeletal pain. As with any hot or cold compress used by itself, chemical additives, such as herbs, essential oils, and salts, can be easily added to the compress water.

A procedure for performing a contrast treatment over the eyes is used here as one example of an alternating hot and cold application of compresses. In this case, the goal is to dramatically increase circulation around the eyes to relieve eyestrain and muscle tension, and to prepare the client's tissue for massage around the eyes. A similar treatment could be done to any part of the body to enhance its circulation and relax it before beginning massage. Here are two more examples: contrast compresses over the knee can be especially effective to stimulate healing after surgery, and contrast compresses over the lower back can increase blood flow to the lower back muscles and relieve pain. When would contrast compresses be preferred to contrast treatments using other types of heat and cold? When a slightly less intense treatment is preferred (not as hot and not as cold as some other applications), when a small irregularly shaped area needs treatment, or when the massage therapist has only hot and cold water and cloths available.

Temperature: Hot (102°–110°F) alternated with cold (32°–55°F)

Time Needed: 10 minutes

Equipment Needed: Water thermometer, containers of hot and cold water, three washcloths, one towel to place under the head to keep the sheets on the massage table dry

Effect: Primarily thermal

Cleanup: Clean and sanitize containers; launder washcloths and towel.

Procedure
1. Check with the client to make sure there are no contraindications to the use of local heat or cold.
2. Explain the use of local heat and cold to the client and get his or her consent.
3. With client supine, place towel under client's head.
4. Soak one washcloth in hot water and wring it out (Fig. 6-12A).
5. Fold in half lengthwise and lay over the client's eyes (Fig. 6-12B).
6. Check with the client to make sure it is not too hot.
7. After 2 minutes, soak the other washcloth in cold water and wring it out, fold it in half lengthwise, and lay it over the client's eyes (Fig. 6-12C).
8. After the cold compress has been on for 30 seconds, remove it.
9. Repeat steps 4 through 8.
10. Repeat steps 4 through 8 again for a total of three rounds.
11. Gently dry the area around the eyes with the last washcloth (Fig. 6-12D).

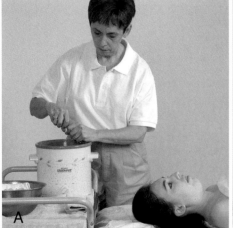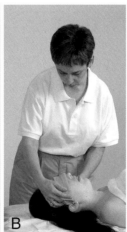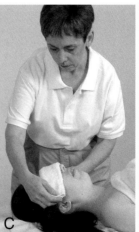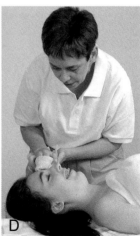

FIGURE 6-12 ■ Contrast compresses. **A.** Soak one washcloth in hot water and wring it out. **B.** Fold the hot washcloth in half lengthwise and apply over the client's eyes. **C.** Soak the other washcloth in cold water and wring it out. Fold it in half lengthwise and apply it over the client's eyes. **D.** At the end of three rounds of hot followed by cold, gently dry off the area around the eyes.

CHAPTER SUMMARY

In this chapter you have learned about a variety of treatments that cool just one part of the body without immersion in liquid water and about their effects and benefits. During massage sessions, therapeutic cold can help relieve acute inflammation, muscle spasm, and musculoskeletal pain as well as keep clients from being overheated, deactivate trigger points, and help increase local circulation when used in a contrast treatment. Your therapy "toolbox" has just gotten larger with these cold treatments. In each of the chapters ahead, you will learn more new treatments and learn even more about how to fine tune them for your massage practice.

REVIEW QUESTIONS

Multiple Choice

1. After application, how long do cold gel packs retain their cold?
   a. 5 minutes
   b. 15 to 20 minutes
   c. 30 to 45 minutes
   d. 60 minutes

2. Local application of cold is most often used
   a. To reduce swelling and pain
   b. In chronic conditions
   c. To prevent hypothermia
   d. To torment your clients

3. Local application of cold is contraindicated for patients with
   a. Inability to provide feedback about tissue temperature
   b. Chilled body
   c. Raynaud's syndrome
   d. Aversion to cold
   e. All of the above

4. In patients with acute muscle strain or contusion, cold is the best choice for
   a. The first 48 hours
   b. The first 12 hours
   c. The first 8 hours
   d. The first week

5. Which application is used to deactivate trigger points, allowing stretching a muscle to its full length?
   a. Cold flat water bottle
   b. Cold gel pack
   c. Contrast compress
   d. Ice stroking
   e. Iced compress

True/False

_____ 6. An iced compress can be used when pain is caused by acute swelling.

_____ 7. A cold water–filled water bottle gel pack cools tissues more than any other cold application.

_____ 8. The primary hazard of cold applications is cold-induced tissue damage.

_____ 9. Local cold applications can have effects on local tissue temperature, blood flow, edema, nerve function, muscle strength, and muscle tone.

_____ 10. Ice massage may be chosen over other local cold applications because it creates a mild relaxing sensation.

REFERENCES

1. Belanger A. *Evidence-Based Guide to Therapeutic Physical Agents*. Baltimore: Lippincott Williams & Wilkins, 2002.
2. Ho SS et al. The effects of ice on blood flow and bone metabolism in knees. *Am J Sports Med* 1994; 22:537.
3. Ho SS et al. Comparison of various icing times in decreasing bone metabolism in the knee. *Am J Sports Med* 1990;18:376.
4. MacAuley DC. Ice therapy: How good is the evidence? *Int J Sports Med* 2001;22:379.
5. Michlovitz S. *Thermal Agents in Rehabilitation*. Philadelphia: FA Davis, 1996.
6. Packman H. *Ice Massage: The Ultimate Cryotherapeutic Alternative*. Victoria, BC: Trafford Publishing, 2007.
7. Taber C et al. Measurement of reactive vasodilation during cold gel pack application to nontraumatized ankles. *Phys Ther* 1992;72:294.
8. Thrash A, Thrash C. *Home Remedies: Hydrotherapy, Charcoal, and Other Simple Treatments*. Seale, AL: Thrash, 1981.
9. Travell J, Simons D. *Myofascial Pain and Dysfunction: The Trigger Point Manual*. 2nd ed. vol 1. Baltimore: Williams & Wilkins, 1999.
10. Zemke J et al. Intramuscular temperature response in the human leg to two forms of cryotherapy: Ice massage and ice bag. *J Orthop Sports Phys Ther* 1998;27:301.

IMMERSION BATHS

7

Mollie [Mary McMillan, nurse, physical therapist, author of Massage and Therapeutic Exercise, *and founder of the American Physical Therapy Association] was arrested in Manila and put into a prison camp in 1942. Mollie made her bed on an inverted wooden filing cabinet to avoid sleeping on the ground, and she shared four toilets and three showers with 469 other women. But with her indomitable spirit, she still managed to set up a physical therapy clinic for the prisoners, performing miracles with her clever hands, hot water, a few pails and towels. As one admirer would later recall, "Aching backs and arthritis from sleeping on cold cement, pulled muscles, painful feet, infected bedbugs bites and rashes— all manner of aches and pains were brought in. And every day people went away feeling better."*

—Wendy Murphy, Healing the Generations: A History of Physical Therapy and the American Physical Therapy Association

Chapter Objectives

After completing this chapter, the student will be able to:

- Describe the effects of various local and whole-body baths.
- Explain the contraindications to various local and whole-body baths.
- Name and describe local baths of different temperatures, including foot, hand, leg, arm, and half-body baths.
- Describe a variety of applications for local baths.
- Name and describe full body baths, including hot, warm, neutral, cold, and contrast whole-body baths.
- Name and describe various full-body baths using warm water and bath additives.
- Describe a variety of applications for full-body baths.
- Give local and whole-body baths using the procedure included with each treatment.

A bath is defined as "the immersion of the body or some of its parts in liquid." As noted in Chapter 1, baths are one of the most ancient and popular of all medical treatments throughout the world because they are convenient and effective and may be used for a variety of therapeutic purposes over many body regions. For the massage therapist, they can complement hands-on techniques. Depending upon the type of bath, they can relax muscles and prepare them for massage, stimulate the circulation in many ways, relieve muscular fatigue and pain, relieve joint pain, raise or lower core temperature,

induce a general relaxation response, and even stimulate muscle contractions for a short time. An easy way to administer therapeutic substances, such as herbs, salts, clays, essential oils, vinegar, baking soda, oatmeal, muds, seaweeds, and other chemicals is to dissolve them in water and immerse the body part or the entire body in it. When liquid completely surrounds a body part or the entire body (Fig. 7-1), the heat or cold it contains is transferred to the entire area better than with hydrotherapy applications such as moist heat packs or cold packs that are merely laid on the area. This makes water baths a more practical choice for some situations. This chapter

127

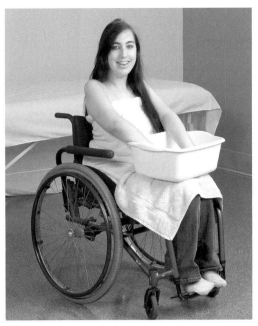

FIGURE 7-1 ■ Hand bath.

discusses commonly used partial-body baths and whole-body baths. (To learn more about some less commonly used baths, see Box 7-1.) We begin our discussion with the wide variety of partial-body baths.

PARTIAL-BODY BATHS

For the massage therapist, baths which immerse only one part of the body are a particularly convenient hydrotherapy treatment. They are inexpensive, require only basic equipment, and may be used for a variety of clients and situations. They are also simple, safe home treatments for your clients. Partial-body baths may use hot, warm, neutral, or cold water, or hot water alternated with cold water. Partial baths can be taken in all sorts of containers, from large bowls and plastic tubs to stainless steel whirlpool baths. The partial baths and the various types of additives given here are only a small sampling of the most common ones that have been used in the past.

When would you use a partial-body bath rather than another local hydrotherapy application? Here are some factors to consider when making your choice:

1. Water has a soothing feel on the skin that is enjoyed by most people and, hence, is more enjoyable than many treatments that are laid on top of the skin, such as ice packs. In addition, tissue that is too sensitive to have any weight on it can be better treated with liquid water.
2. When you do not have time to prepare a more elaborate treatment, such as a fomentation, partial-body baths are fast. Just get the water to the correct temperature and you are ready to go. However, any

---

BOX 7-1 | *Point of Interest*

CLASSIC BUT NOT COMMONLY USED BATHS

The baths discussed here have been used not only for a thermal effect but also to apply a wide variety of chemicals, including herbal preparations, salts, essential plant oils, clays, seaweeds, and even muds.

SCALP BATHS

Scalp baths can be performed by leaning over a container of water and immersing the scalp in it or with the receiver supine, head hanging over the head of the table and resting in a bowl of water. This little-used bath can be used to warm or cool the scalp or apply chemical preparations to it. Hot or warm scalp baths can be used to relieve some types of head pain and to encourage healing of injuries to the cranial bones or scalp. Cold scalp baths can decrease circulation to the scalp to help relieve tension or migraine headaches. Contrast baths can increase circulation to the scalp. In Chinese medicine, stroke patients are sometimes given scalp baths with hot ginger tea to relieve head pain. Epsom salt scalp baths have been used to relieve swelling of the scalp after head injury.

EYE BATHS

Eye baths, using bowls of water or glass eye cups, are used to warm or cool the eyes and the muscles around them or to apply chemical preparations to them. Warm eye baths can be used to soothe muscle tension and eyestrain. Cold eye baths relieve tired, itching eyes. Contrast baths stimulate circulation in the muscles around the eyes. Someone with eye irritation from dust or allergies may find relief by bathing the eyes in cool water.

SINUS BATHS

Sinus baths rinse the nasal passages, using bulb syringes, neti pots, or special tips on irrigating devices (Water Piks). They are used to ease sinus congestion, improve local circulation, and to apply chemical preparations such as salt water or herb teas. Water may be hot, warm, or cool.

THROAT BATHS

Throat baths, or gargling, are used to warm or cool the throat or to apply chemical preparations such as salt water or herb teas. Warm throat baths can be used to relieve tension in the throat muscles or soothe the throat irritation which occurs after too much singing or public speaking or after having a cold, and contrast baths can increase local circulation.

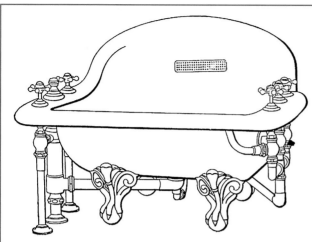

Porcelain sitz bath manufactured in 1905 by Standard Sanitary Manufacturing Company of Pittsburgh, Pennsylvania.

SITZ BATHS

Sitz baths are immersion of the pelvic region, covering about the same area as a pair of shorts. They are given in specially designed chair-shaped bathtubs to warm or cool the muscles of the pelvic and lower back areas and to apply chemical preparations such as salts, essential oils, and herbal preparations. The pelvic area is large and difficult to cover with other thermal applications, such as moist heat packs or ice packs, and hence, water baths to the pelvic area may be the most efficient way to treat it in some situations. Hot sitz baths have been used to relieve sciatica, lower back pain, dysmenorrhea, spastic constipation, kidney stone pain, and poor local circulation; to raise core temperature; and to create a fluid-shifting (derivative) effect. Warm sitz baths can also warm the entire body, soothe the perineum after labor and delivery, and speed healing of perineal stitches. Short, cold sitz baths can be used to increase muscle tone in the smooth muscles of the uterus, bladder, and colon; to relieve atonic constipation; and to stimulate circulation in the abdominal muscles and organs. Long, cold sitz baths can be used to treat local muscle problems, such as pulled muscles in the groin area, and to cool the entire body. Contrast sitz baths can be used to increase circulation to the muscles of the pelvis and lower back, to prevent menstrual cramps, and to relieve chronic pelvic pain.

ARM AND LEG WHIRLPOOLS

Arm and leg whirlpools, made of stainless steel and marketed under such names as HI-Boy and Low-Boy, are most commonly used in physical therapy settings. They are used to relieve joint stiffness and muscle spasm in an arm or leg, to make therapeutic exercise easier, and to relieve pain. Local whirlpools are often warm. They may be used for posttraumatic pain;, cleansing of wounds; swelling in the hands and feet; acute orthopedic trauma at the onset; acute edema; acute muscle spasm; scar tissue contractures from burns, wounds, or adhesions; or as a preparation for massage to leave tissues supple, warm, and relaxed. Athletic trainers sometimes use whirlpools to treat athletic injuries with hot, cold, or contrast temperatures. A typical whirlpool has at least six jets, some with low pressure to make water swirl and some with high pressure for vigorous hydromassage. Unlike hot tubs, because they are constructed of stainless steel, they can be sterilized after use.

HUBBARD TANK

The Hubbard tank is a very large steel whirlpool with a turbine at one end, invented in the 1920s by American engineer Carl Hubbard. With a 425-gallon capacity, the tank is similar to a shallow swimming pool, and the entire body can be immersed to allow motion and exercise. Because the person in a Hubbard tank is actively exercising, the water temperature is cooler than in a standard whole-body whirlpool, generally between 90° and 104°F, unless an artificial fever is being induced.

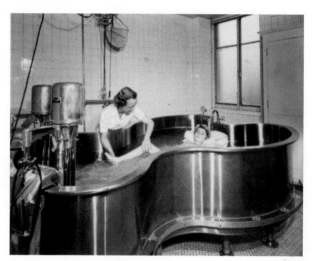

Physical therapist working with polio patient in Hubbard tank, 1949.

As can be seen in the 1949 photograph above, the unique figure-8 or butterfly shape of the tank allows a therapist to get close enough to work with the patient during the treatment but still stay dry. And because it is stainless steel, it can be sterilized after each use, making it suitable for people with open wounds and burns that would be in danger of infection if they were exercising in a swimming pool.

tub used for water baths must be cleaned, disinfected, and dried between each use.

3. When you do not have elaborate hydrotherapy equipment, a clean container, running water, and a towel are all you need. However, if running water is far from the room in which massage is performed, it may be too difficult to carry a heavy container of water there.

4. When you wish to heat or cool an entire area, surrounding it with hot or cold liquid is the most effective way to do that. In one study, the gastrocnemius muscle was much colder after a cold immersion bath than after an ice pack applied to it for the same amount of time. Following a 20-minute leg bath at 50°F, it took a full 3 hours for the muscle to return to its normal temperature, whereas following a 20-minute ice pack application, it took an hour and a half for the muscle to warm back up to its normal temperature.(1)

5. When you wish to apply a chemical preparation that must be dissolved in water to the skin, such as

Epsom salt, adding it to a local bath is an easy way to do that.

6. During a local bath, massage and stretching may still take place. Ischemic compression of trigger points will be more effective if the area is immersed in warm water, and tight muscles can be stretched while they are in a hot bath.(2)

A NOTE ON SANITATION

Any tub that you use for a water bath, whether partial or whole body, must be cleaned, disinfected, and dried between each use. This is important to prevent transmission of pathogens from one client to another. (Athlete's foot fungus and *Streptococcus* bacteria are examples of pathogens which can be transmitted by water.) Begin by cleaning the tub with a cleanser, then disinfect it by spraying or wiping it with a disinfectant solution.

Disinfectant solutions range from highly toxic disinfectants intended for cleanup of blood or body fluids to alcohol or citrus essential oils that are less toxic. You may need to consider what works best for your facility. For example, chlorine bleach is a common and effective disinfectant, but it is considered too strong smelling for many offices. It is recommended that you investigate the different kinds and pick a product that is suitable for your facility. When purchasing a whole-body hydrotherapy tub, check with the manufacturer for recommended disinfectants.

FOOTBATHS

A footbath, made by filling a tub large enough to hold the client's feet (Fig. 7-2), is easy to integrate into a massage session. It can have a variety of effects, depending upon the duration of the bath; the temperature of the water; whether there are any chemical additives, such as Epsom

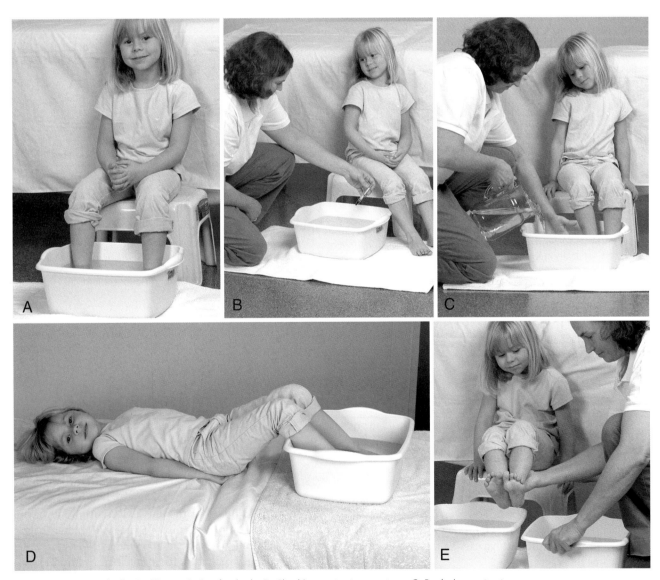

FIGURE 7-2 ■ Footbath. **A.** Client enjoying footbath. **B.** Checking water temperature. **C.** Replacing water to maintain desired temperature. **D.** Footbath with client reclining on massage table. **E.** Massage therapist moving client's feet from one tub of water to another during a contrast treatment.

salt, herbs, or essential oils in it; and whether it is combined with other hydrotherapy treatments.

Hot Footbath

A hot footbath is an easy-to-perform treatment that many clients find relaxing and nurturing. A client with chronically cold feet will especially enjoy this treatment before a massage, and someone who is going to receive a cold treatment may feel better about receiving it if a hot footbath is given first. If prolonged, footbaths can not only warm the feet but raise the core temperature significantly and encourage sweating. Hot footbaths are an excellent treatment for insomnia: numerous studies have found that when the feet are warmed before bed, a person goes to sleep much faster and often sleeps more deeply as well.(3–6) In a massage practice, a hot footbath before or after an evening massage would be an excellent way to help a client who struggles with insomnia. Or, when a client comes into your office feeling cold, a footbath can be given while the client is filling out forms or talking to you; it also can be done with the client lying on the massage table. A large rectangular container such as a plastic dishpan provides space for both feet without crowding them and has enough room for water to cover them up to the top of the ankles.

Temperature: Hot (102°–110°F)

Time Needed: 20 minutes

Equipment Needed: Water thermometer, container for water, 1.5 to 2 gallons of water, a large towel to go under the footbath and a small towel for drying the feet, cold water and cloth for cold compress (optional)

Effect: Primarily thermal

Cleanup: Clean, disinfect, and dry tub; launder towels.

Indications: Chilled person, preparation for cold treatment, cold feet, cramps in the feet and legs, menstrual cramps, arthritis pain, gout pain, derivation for migraine headache, insomnia (if given shortly before the client goes to bed), general relaxation. A hot footbath is an excellent, easy way to apply chemicals contained in herbs, salts, or essential oils.

Contraindications: Loss of sensation, lymphedema of lower extremity, peripheral vascular disease (which includes diabetes), Buerger's disease, arteriosclerosis of the lower extremities, lymphedema

Procedure
1. Check with client to make sure there are no contraindications to the hot footbath.
2. Explain the use of the hot footbath to the client and get consent.
3. Have the client seated in a chair next to the massage table. Place a towel on the floor under the client's feet.

---

4. Put the container of hot water on the towel, rest the client's feet in the container. Cover him or her with a blanket if body warming is desired (Fig. 7-2A).
5. Using a water thermometer, monitor the water temperature from time to time (Fig. 7-2B) and add more hot water if it is needed to keep the water at the desired temperature. Do not pour this water directly on the feet; have the client move the feet to the side of the container when you pour fresh water in (Fig. 7-2C).
6. If the client begins to sweat, add a cold compress to the forehead.
7. Massage of other parts of the body that can be done in a seated position may proceed at this time.
8. To end the foot soak, have the client lift the feet out of the water, move the container to one side, place the client's feet on the towel, then cover the feet with the towel.
9. Remove the container.
10. Dry the feet.
11. Have the client move onto the massage table without touching the bare floor with his or her feet.

Variations
1. Footbath with client lying down (Fig. 7-2D). A hot footbath can be easily given right on a massage table if a large towel is placed under the container of water to protect the sheets. The client reclines on the table and places the feet in the water. In this case, it is important that the container be heavy enough so it does not slide, then clients can rest their feet in the water and not have to use energy holding the legs up. A plastic milk crate can be used for this purpose: place the milk crate on the towel, place the footbath inside it, then have the client put his or her feet in the water. For hygienic purposes, any part of the milk crate that will touch the client's skin should be draped with a towel. To prevent the footbath from cooling off, a piece of wood may be cut to cover most of the top of the container with a half-circle cut out for the legs. Then the person's feet go in the water and the wooden lid is put on top of the container.
2. Sweating footbath. The client is seated in a chair, covered with a blanket, and given a cold compress to the head as soon as sweating begins. When the body is covered so that no heat escapes, the client's core temperature will rise higher than if the body is not covered.
3. Vasodilating footbath. Powdered mustard, ginger, or cayenne will cause vasodilation in the feet. To 2 gallons of water add 2 teaspoons of mustard powder, 1 teaspoon of powdered ginger, and $1/4$ teaspoon of cayenne pepper. Do not use with open skin or on clients with sensitive skin, as burning and stinging sensations may result.

Warm Footbath

Temperature: Warm (98°–102°F)

Time Needed: 15 to 20 minutes

Equipment Needed: Water thermometer, container for water, 1.5 to 2 gallons of water, a large towel to go under the footbath, a small towel for drying the feet

Effect: Primarily thermal

Cleanup: Clean, disinfect and dry tub; launder towels.

Indications: Mild warming of the body; cold feet; for someone who should not have a hot footbath, such as a diabetic; general relaxation

Contraindications: None

Procedure
Same as for hot footbath, but adjust water temperature to warm.

Variation
Epsom salt footbath. A footbath with Epsom salt can be used for soreness after vigorous exercise, painful bruises, or edema of pregnancy. Add 1 cup of Epsom salt per gallon of warm water. More information on the effects of Epsom salt is given later in this chapter.

Cool Footbath

Temperature: Cool (66°–98°F)

Time Needed: 15 to 20 minutes

Equipment Needed: Water thermometer, container for water, 1.5 to 2 gallons of water, a large towel to go under the footbath, a small towel for drying the feet

Effect: Primarily thermal

Cleanup: Clean, disinfect, and dry tub; launder towels

Indications: Mild cooling of the body, hot feet, general relaxation

Contraindications: None

Procedure
Same as for hot footbath, but adjust the water temperature to cool.

Cold Footbath

Short, cold footbaths are stimulating to the local circulation, refreshing, and invigorating, while long, cold footbaths are depressing to the local circulation. Short, cold footbaths also cause a reflex contraction of the blood vessels of brain, pelvic organs, bladder, liver, and gastrointestinal tract and thus were once used by hydrotherapists to treat uterine, bladder, or kidney bleeding. Any prolonged footbath with a water temperature of less than 98°F will cool the body to some extent, and the colder the water, the greater the heat loss. Some of these effects are due to the reaction of the nervous system to cold, including reflex effects such as changes in the size of local blood vessels. However, much of the effect of a cold immersion is strictly an effect of tissues becoming colder. In one study, men with spinal cord injuries exercised until their core temperature was elevated, then took cold footbaths. This lowered their core temperature by 4°F. Spinal cord injuries cause damage to the nervous system, and these men's brains could not receive sensory information that would normally cause their central nervous system reactions to the cold. It was clear, then, that the change in their core temperatures was from cooling of tissues. Chilled blood in the feet, carried back to the heart and pumped from there out to the whole body, lowered core temperature.(7)

Temperature: Cold (55°–65°F); 55°F water may be difficult to tolerate for long. Crushed or cube ice may be used to achieve lower temperatures.

Time Needed: 2 to 20 minutes, depending on tolerance.

Equipment Needed: Water thermometer, container for water, large towel to go under the footbath, small towel to dry the feet

Effect: Primarily thermal

Cleanup: Clean, disinfect, and dry tub; launder towels.

Indications: Stimulation of the entire body when used for 2 minutes or less; cooling of the entire body, especially when used for longer than 2 minutes; ankle sprains (2–10 minutes; water must be over the top of the ankles); for learning to tolerate colder temperatures; as part of a contrast treatment; for stimulation of the muscle tone of the extensor muscles of the toes and ankles. (See the section on muscle weakness in Chapter 14.)

Contraindications: Chilled client, Raynaud's syndrome, high blood pressure. Prolonged cold footbaths are contraindicated for clients with lymphedema.

Procedure
Same as for hot footbath, but use cold water. Immerse feet for 2 minutes or longer, depending upon the purpose of the footbath and the person's tolerance. Clients who have difficulty tolerating cold water may be more comfortable if the footbath water is gradually cooled by adding ice cubes or crushed ice after 1 to 2 minutes. Anytime the footbath water warms up too much, take some of the warmer water out and replace it with colder water or ice.

Variation
Ice-cold footbath to stimulate muscle tone of extensors of the toes and ankles. This footbath and exercise routine can be used to help build muscle strength for clients with muscle weakness from stroke, muscular dystrophy, spinal cord injury, postpolio syndrome, and

A Cooling Footbath for Hot, Burning Feet

Background

Rachel was a 45-year-old schoolteacher who exercised regularly, practiced yoga, and was in excellent health. She received massage therapy regularly to help her deal with a high level of stress. One hot summer day she arrived for her regular appointment and told the therapist that she had been on her feet for 3 hours that morning. Her feet were swollen, she said, because of the combination of prolonged standing on them and the summer heat, which always caused her to retain water. Upon questioning, she also told the therapist that she had had this problem for many years and that her family doctor told her not to worry about it. However, as she lay down on the massage table, her discomfort was evident: she did not want anything covering her feet, complained that they were burning, and moved her legs restlessly.

Treatment

The therapist placed a towel at the foot of the table and a plastic tub with 75°F (cool but not cold) water on top of it. Rachel placed her feet in the water, exclaimed that the water was cold for just a moment, and then sighed with relief as her feet began to adjust to the colder temperature. The therapist began her massage routine at Rachel's head while Rachel kept her knees bent and her feet in the footbath. After 2 minutes she said that her feet felt better but were still somewhat hot. The therapist added a cup of ice cubes and 2 drops of oil of peppermint to the water, then continued the massage for another 5 minutes, when Rachel indicated that her feet felt "nice and cool" and that she was tired of holding up her legs. The tub was removed, and Rachel's wet feet were left to dry in the air. She quickly became more relaxed and commented on the wonderful sensation of the breeze blowing over her feet.

Discussion Questions

1. Explain why the therapist chose the cool footbath for this situation.
2. Give examples of other hydrotherapy treatments you have learned that would also help Rachel's feet feel better.

---

some types of cerebral palsy. Muscle tone will be stimulated for about 20 minutes after completing the cold footbath. For more on this topic, see section on muscle weakness in Chapter 14.

1. Explain the use of the ice water bath to the client and get his or her consent.
2. Because the sensation of very cold water can be quite startling, it is important to explain the rationale for this treatment.
3. Add equal parts of ice and water to a large container.
4. Place a towel under the ice water bath.
5. Warn the client that the water will be very cold.
6. With the client seated, immerse the feet in the ice water for 3 seconds.
7. Remove the feet from the cold water for 30 seconds while the client exercises the extensors of the toes and ankles.
8. Repeat steps 6 and 7 five more times, for a total of six cold water dips.
9. Dry the foot well.

The client's extensor muscles will be able to contract more strongly for about 20 minutes after the completion of this footbath.

Contrast Footbath

A contrast footbath is actually a sequence of hot footbaths alternated with cold footbaths. By causing blood vessel dilation in the hot footbath and then blood vessel constriction in the cold footbath, the combination results in significant fluctuations in arterial blood flow during the treatment, about double the arterial blood flow of someone sitting quietly and not moving the feet at all. The muscles that change the diameter of the arterial walls will contract more strongly if this treatment is performed regularly, so contrast footbaths encourage good circulation in the feet. As with the hot footbath, as the circulation in the feet increases, circulatory congestion in other areas, such as the pelvic or abdominal organs, is reduced.

Although contrast footbaths can increase circulation, they do not warm deeper tissues. Therefore, although they can increase circulation in sprained ankles, they do not induce edema, as a hot treatment would by itself. Contrast footbaths are also useful for passive swelling of the ankles. Because increased circulation is known to promote healing, foot ulcers, varicose ulcers, and other poorly healing wounds have been treated with contrast foot and leg baths by physicians at Wildwood Hospital and other Adventist medical facilities for generations.

(However, massage therapists should not treat these conditions unless directly under doctor's supervision.) The muscles of the arterial walls, which dilate with heat and constrict with cold, generally become fatigued after three or four rounds. Therefore, if the treatment is to continue, the temperature contrasts must be greater—the hot water hotter and the cold water colder. To increase the circulatory effect of a contrast footbath even further, have the client contract (make active movements of) the muscles of the feet and ankles while the feet are immersed.

Temperature: Hot footbath at 110° to 115°F, cold footbath at 50°F

Time Needed: About 10 minutes

Equipment Needed: Water thermometer, two containers for water, two large towels to go under footbaths, one small towel to dry the feet

Effect: Primarily thermal

Cleanup: Clean, disinfect, and dry tub; launder towels.

Indications: Poor circulation in feet; tendonitis in feet; tarsal tunnel syndrome; derivation for migraine headache; ankle sprains (water must cover the ankles). Perhaps as many as 10 rounds of hot and cold may be necessary to decrease swelling and pain as much as possible in an acute ankle sprain. In this case, more attention will have to be paid to maintaining water temperature, since the hot bath will begin to cool down and the cold bath will begin to warm up. For more information, see the section on ankle sprains in Chapter 13.

Contraindications: Same as for both the hot and the cold footbath

Procedure
1. Check with client to make sure there are no contraindications to the contrast footbath.
2. Explain the use of the contrast footbath to the client and get his or her consent.
3. Set up everything just as you would for a hot footbath except prepare one container of hot water and one container of cold water. Keep a towel under each container, so that even when you switch from one to the other, neither one will be resting directly on the floor.
4. Begin with the hot footbath, soaking the client's feet for 2 minutes.
5. Replace hot footbath with the cold, soaking the client's feet for 30 seconds.
6. Repeat steps 2 and 3 for a total of three rounds.
7. Dry the client's feet.

HAND BATHS

A hand bath, made by filling a tub large enough to accommodate both hands (Fig. 7-3) is easy to integrate into a massage session and can have a variety of effects depending upon the duration of the bath, the temperature of the water, any chemical additives such as Epsom salt, herbs, or essential oils, and whether it is combined with other hydrotherapy treatments. Figure 7-4 shows a combination arm and leg bath, which can be used to perform two partial baths at once. It might be used to treat someone with a migraine headache by having both legs and arms immersed in hot water.

Hot Hand Bath

A hot hand bath is another easy-to-perform treatment that can warm the hands, prepare them for massage, relieve hand pain, and if prolonged, warm the entire body. Hand baths are a simple, excellent way to apply chemical treatments such as herbs, salts, or essential oils. With a hot hand bath, dilation of the blood vessels also means that less blood flows into congested areas in other parts of the

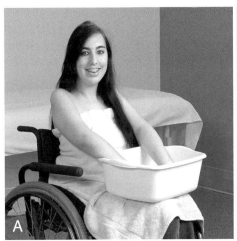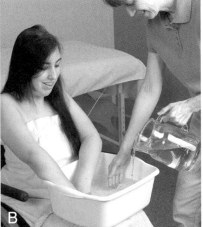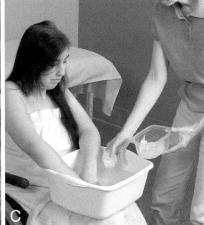

FIGURE 7-3 ■ Hand bath. **A.** Client enjoying hand bath. **B.** Replacing water to maintain desired temperature. **C.** Adding ice cubes to maintain the cold hand bath temperature at 55° to 65°F.

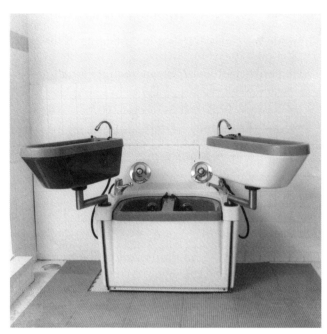

FIGURE 7-4 ■ Combination arm and leg bath. (Courtesy of HEAT Spakur Therapy Development Inc. Calistoga, California.)

body. One migraine sufferer discovered this effect on her own while she was washing dishes in hot water:

> For years I have suffered from recurring migraine headaches. . . . [One day] I was struck by another migraine. I was determined to keep functioning—feeding my daughter, doing the laundry and washing the dirty dishes. I ran hot, hot water to rinse off my dishes, and, while rinsing, I felt my headache ebb. I could feel the blood draining out of my head like the tide washing away from the shore. It dawned on me that I was practicing my own biofeedback, by immersing my bare hands in the hot water. The blood vessels in my hands were dilating to allow blood to rush to the area and carry away the heat. That took the pressure out of my head. The dishes were clean and my headache was gone.(4)

Temperature: Hot (110°F)

Time Needed: 15 to 20 minutes

Equipment Needed: Water thermometer, a container for water such as a large bowl or plastic dishpan, 1 gallon of water, one large towel to go under the hand bath, one small towel for drying the hands

Effect: Primarily thermal

Cleanup: Clean, disinfect, and dry tub; launder towels.

Indications: Cold hands, arthritis pain, muscle cramps when the hand muscles have been overused, preparation for stretching of muscles and fascia (stretching of hand muscles can be performed in the hot water), migraine headache (for 20 minutes at the beginning of

a headache; finish with brief cold water pour), as part of a contrast treatment

Contraindications: Loss of sensation in the hands, lymphedema of the upper extremity

Procedure

1. Check with client to make sure there are no contraindications to the hot hand bath.
2. Explain the use of the hot hand bath to the client and get his or her consent.
3. Place the large towel on a table.
4. Fill a large bowl or plastic tub with hot water. Place it on the large towel.
5. Have the client sit in a chair in front of the hand bath.
6. Have client immerse the hands for 15 to 20 minutes. Massage may be performed on other parts of the body during this time if desired. The container of water can be placed in the client's lap on a towel if desired (Fig. 7-3A).
7. As the water cools, take some out and replace it with hotter water to maintain the temperature at 110°F. Do not pour hot water directly onto the hands (Fig. 7-3B).
8. Have the client take his or her hands out of the hand bath and dry them.

Variation

Epsom salt hand bath. A hand bath with Epsom salt can be used for soreness after vigorous exercise, painful bruises, or for edema of pregnancy. Should a client with bruises also have open abrasions, an Epsom salt hand bath is safe. Add 1 cup of Epsom salt per gallon of warm water. For more information on Epsom salt and its effects, see the section on Epsom salt bath in this chapter.

Cold Hand Bath

Short, cold hand baths are stimulating to the local circulation and feel refreshing and invigorating, while long, cold hand baths are very cooling but depressing to the local circulation. Both are easy to perform and especially welcome to clients who are overheated but would find a cold footbath intolerable. They can cause a reflex contraction of the blood vessels of the nasal mucosa and thus were once used by hydrotherapists to treat nosebleeds. Clients who have difficulty tolerating cold water may be more comfortable if the hand bath water is gradually cooled by adding ice cubes or crushed ice after 1 to 2 minutes of immersion.

Temperature: Cold (55–65°F); 55°F water may be difficult to tolerate for long. Crushed or cube ice may be used to achieve the lower temperatures.

Time Needed: 15 to 20 minutes

Equipment Needed: Water thermometer, container for water, approximately 1 gallon of water, one large towel to go under the hand bath, one small towel to dry the hands

Effect: Primarily thermal

Cleanup: Clean, disinfect, and dry tub; launder towels.

Indications: Arthritis pain in finger joints, writer's cramp, poor circulation in the hands (use twice daily), strain of the hand muscles (use twice daily), cooling of the entire body if prolonged, as part of a contrast treatment

Contraindications: Chilled client, Raynaud's syndrome, high blood pressure; prolonged cold hand baths are contraindicated for clients with lymphedema.

Procedure

1. Check with client to make sure there are no contraindications to the cold hand bath.
2. Explain the use of the cold hand bath to the client and get his or her consent.
3. Place the large towel on a table.
4. Fill a large bowl or plastic tub with cold water and ice. Place it on the large towel.
5. Have the client sit in a chair in front of the hand bath.
6. Have client immerse the hands for 15 to 20 minutes. Massage may be performed on other parts of the body during this time if desired. The container of water can be placed in the client's lap on a towel if desired.
7. As the water warms, take some out and replace it with ice cubes to maintain the temperature at 55° to 65°F (Fig. 7-4C).
8. Have the client take his or her hands out of the hand bath and dry them.

Variation

Cold hand bath to stimulate muscle tone of extensors of the fingers and wrists. This hand bath and exercise routine can be used to help build muscle strength for clients with muscle weakness from stroke, muscular dystrophy, spinal cord injury, postpolio syndrome, and some types of cerebral palsy. Muscle tone will be stimulated for about 20 minutes after the cold hand bath. For more on this topic, see section on muscle weakness in Chapter 14.

Procedure

1. Explain the use of the ice water bath to the client and get his or her consent. Because the sensation of very cold water can be quite startling, it is important to explain the rationale for this treatment.
2. Add equal parts of ice and water to the tub.
3. Place a towel under the ice water bath.
4. Warn the client that the water will be very cold.
5. With the client seated, immerse the hands in the ice water for 3 seconds.

6. Remove the feet from the cold water for 30 seconds while the client exercises the extensors of the toes and ankles.
7. Repeat steps 1 and 2 five more times for a total of six cold water dips.
8. Dry the hands well.

The client may now perform exercises for extensor muscles as prescribed by the physical therapist. The extensor muscles will be stimulated and flexors inhibited for about 20 minutes.

Contrast Hand Bath

As seen in Figure 7-5, in this treatment the hands alternate between hot and cold water. A contrast treatment for the hands can be created from almost any heat treatment by dipping the hands in very cold water afterwards. For example, the hands could be dipped in paraffin or wrapped in hot fomentations instead of dipped in hot water. Contrast hand baths can dramatically increase the circulation, and when performed regularly, they are a general tonic for the hands and wrists. They are effective for anyone doing heavy work with the hands, such as massage therapy. In fact, this treatment can be done immediately after a massage session to relieve muscle fatigue and increase local circulation. To increase the circulatory effect of a contrast hand bath even further, have the client contract (make active movements of) the muscles of the hands and wrists while they are immersed.

Temperature: Hot (110°F) followed by cold (55°F)

Time Needed: 10 minutes

Equipment Needed: Water thermometer, two containers for water, towel to dry hands

Effect: Primarily thermal

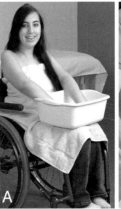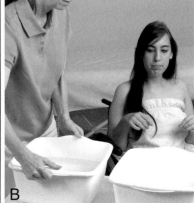

FIGURE 7-5 ■ Contrast hand bath. **A.** Immersing the hands in hot water. **B.** Changing from tub of hot water to cold.

Cleanup: Clean, disinfect, and dry tub; launder towels.

Indications: Muscular fatigue in the hands and wrists, muscular pain in the hands and wrists, poor circulation in the hands and wrists, repetitive stress in the hands and wrists, wrist sprains, healed fractures after the cast is removed, when prescribed by a doctor to promote healing of infections.

Contraindications: Same as for hot and cold hand baths

Procedure

1. Immerse the hands in hot water for 2 minutes.
2. Immerse the hands in cold water for 1 minute.
3. Repeat steps 1 and 2 twice, for a total of three rounds.

ARM BATHS

An arm bath, including both the hands and arms, is also easy to integrate into a massage session and can have a variety of effects depending upon the duration of the bath; the temperature of the water; any chemical additives such as Epsom salt, herbs, or essential oils; and whether it is combined with other hydrotherapy treatments. Giving the client an arm bath requires a somewhat larger container than for a hand bath, such as a rectangular plastic flower box (Fig. 7-6), an extra-large plastic dishpan, a baby bathtub, or even a 5-gallon plastic bucket.

Hot Arm Bath

A hot arm bath can warm the hands and arms, prepare them for massage, relieve hand pain, and if prolonged, warm the entire body. After 20 minutes in a 111°F whirlpool, the temperature in the muscles of the arm rises as much as 4°F.(8) This is a significant finding, because when the temperature in any limb increases by 4°F, twice as much blood flows into it. With a hot arm bath, there are even more blood vessels to dilate than with a hand

bath, and if blood flow to the arms doubles, there is less blood available to flow into congested areas in other parts of the body.

Temperature: Hot (110°F)

Time Needed: 15 to 20 minutes

Effect: Primarily thermal

Equipment Needed: Water thermometer, a container for water such as a large bowl or plastic dishpan, 1 to 1.5 gallons of water, one large towel to go under the arm bath, one small towel for drying the hands and arms

Cleanup: Clean, disinfect, and dry tub; launder towels.

Indications: Arthritis pain; muscle cramps after overuse of arm and hand muscle, such as carpentry, massage or writing; preparation for stretching of arm muscles and fascia; derivation for migraine headache (use for 20 minutes at the beginning of a headache and finish with a brief cold water pour)

Contraindications: Lymphedema of the arm, loss of sensation

Procedure

1. Check with client to make sure there are no contraindications to the hot arm bath.
2. Explain the use of the hot arm bath to the client and get his or her consent.
3. Place the large towel on a table.
4. Fill a large bowl or plastic tub with hot water. Place it on the large towel.
5. Have the client sit in a chair in front of the arm bath.
6. Have client immerse one or both arms as far as possible for 15 to 20 minutes. Massage may be performed on other parts of the body during this time if desired. The container of water can be placed in the client's lap on a towel if desired (Fig. 7-6A).
7. As the water cools, take some out and replace it with hotter water to maintain the temperature at 110°F. Do not pour hot water directly onto the arms (Fig. 7-6B).
8. Have the client take the arms out of the bath and dry them.

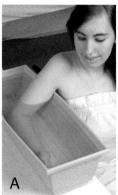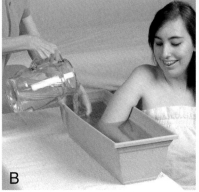

A   B

FIGURE 7-6 ■ Arm bath. **A.** Immersing one arm. **B.** Replacing water to maintain desired temperature.

Cold Arm Bath

To perform a cold arm bath, first read the section on cold hand baths and follow the step-by-step directions given there. To treat the arms, simply use a larger container and enough water to fill the container. Otherwise, all directions apply.

All indications and contraindications are the same, but in this case they apply to the muscles and joints of the arms as well as the hands. Because more of the body is cooled when the entire arm is immersed rather than just the hand, a cold arm bath may cool the entire body to a greater extent.

Contrast Arm Bath

In a contrast arm bath, the hands and arms are immersed to the elbows first in hot water and then in cold water for the purpose of increasing local circulation. A contrast treatment for the arms can be created by applying almost any warming application, then following that with a cold water immersion. For example, the arms could be painted with paraffin, soaked in hot water, or wrapped in hot fomentations, then plunged into cold water, and all three would have a similar effect. To increase the circulatory effect of a contrast arm bath even further, have the client contract (make active movements of) the muscles of the elbows and wrists while they are immersed.

Temperature: Hot (110°F) alternated with cold (55°F)

Time Needed: 10 minutes

Equipment Needed: Water thermometer; two containers for water such as large bowls or plastic dishpans or plastic buckets, each holding 1 to 1.5 gallons of water; one large towel to go under each arm bath; one small towel for drying the arms and hands

Effect: Primarily thermal

Cleanup: Clean, disinfect, and dry tub; launder towels.

Indications: Relieves muscular fatigue in the arms, and eases muscular pain. It is indicated for wrist and elbow sprains, healed fractures after the cast has been removed, and when prescribed by a doctor to promote healing of infections. It can also be a general tonic for the circulation in the arms for the massage practitioner.

Contraindications: Same as for both the hot arm bath and the cold arm bath

Procedure

Same as for contrast hand bath, but immerse the entire arm or arms in the water.

HALF BATH

As shown in Figure 7-7, a hot half bath is one in which the client sits waist-deep in hot water so that the upper body is entirely out of the water. This bath can be used when body warming is needed but the client cannot tolerate a full hot bath; when it is desirable to encourage blood flow to the lower body, as in migraine headache; to allow substances such as herbs or essential oils to be absorbed through the skin; or when a leg bath is desired and no leg-sized tub is available. The tub is filled half-full with 104°F water. The client will be exposing the lower half of the body to the water, so from the waist down he or she must be undressed or wearing shorts or a bathing suit. The top of the body should still be warm so the client can either wear a shirt or be covered with a small blanket or towel. As soon as sweating begins, place a cold compress or ice bag on the head. At the end of the bath, give the client a brief cold pour from the waist down only and finish with a rest of 20 minutes or more.

Temperature: Hot (104°F)

Time Needed: 15 minutes

Equipment Needed: Water thermometer; two large bath towels, one for the floor and one to go behind the client's head; a bowl of cold water and washcloth for cold compress (optional); a shirt or small towel to cover the upper body if needed

Effect: Primarily thermal

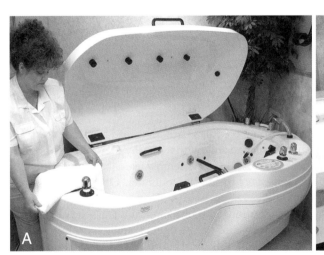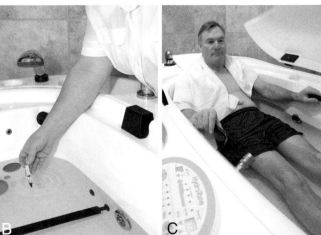

FIGURE 7-7 ■ Half bath. **A.** Placing towels. **B.** Filling tub and checking water temperature. **C.** Client resting in half bath.

CASE HISTORY 7-2

Hot Half Bath for Migraine Headache

Background

Christina was a 53-year-old massage therapist in excellent health. Christina very occasionally had a type of headache called an occipital or basilar artery migraine. After her first migraine, her optometrist explained to her that an occipital migraine is caused by a constriction of the basilar artery; this causes the person to see vivid flashes of light or bright zigzag patterns, which slowly spread and move from the person's central vision to the peripheral vision. Occipital migraine may or may not cause pain, and Christina had no pain with her migraines. She had had these migraines only five times before and had not been able to relate them to any particular event. One day, after typing at her computer for an hour, Christina started to see flashing lights again. They appeared as bright moving zigzag patterns across her entire field of vision, and she found them extremely disorienting.

Self-Treatment

Christina had read about using hot water to relieve migraine headaches and decided to try a hot half-bath. After seeing the flashing lights for 10 minutes, she ran about 6 inches of 110°F water into her bathtub. Leaving her shirt on, she got into the water, which covered her feet and legs. She took her watch into the tub with her, the better to observe the effects. After a time, she noticed the flashing lights started to diminish, and consulting her watch, she realized she had been in the water for 4 minutes. Another 2 minutes later the flashing lights were completely gone. Greatly relieved, Christina stayed in the water for another 5 minutes (a total of 11 minutes in the water) and then got out tentatively, afraid that the migraine would recur at any moment. However, she dressed and continued her day with no further problem: the flashing lights did not recur and she felt entirely normal.

Discussion Questions

1. Explain why hot water to the legs and feet affected this migraine headache.
2. What other hydrotherapy treatment could be used for the same purpose as the hot half-bath?

Cleanup: Clean, disinfect, and dry tub; launder towels.

Indications: Arthritis of the lower extremities, acute or chronic low back pain, sciatica, migraine headache, chilled client: before a cold treatment

Contraindications: Diabetes, lymphedema in legs, loss of sensation, peripheral vascular disease (arteriosclerosis of the lower extremities or Buerger's disease)

Procedure

1. Check with client to make sure there are no contraindications to the hot half bath.
2. Explain the use of the hot half bath to the client and get consent.
3. Place towels on floor in front of tub and behind where client's head will be.
4. Fill tub to waist level, checking temperature with water thermometer.
5. Have the client enter the tub, wearing a dry shirt or sheet to keep the upper body warm if desired.
6. After 15 minutes, have the client leave the tub, dry off vigorously, and lie down for rest or massage.

Variations

Warm half bath. This bath is suitable for clients who would benefit from a half bath but have diabetes, because they can safely take a bath if the water is 102°F or less. Simply follow the directions for the hot half bath but use water that is 98° to 102°F.

LEG BATHS

Leg baths, made by filling a bathtub with enough water to cover both legs, can help treat many musculoskeletal aches and pains in the legs. They can also be used to change the temperature of the leg muscles and to apply salts, herbs, essential oils, or other substances to the skin. They will affect the general circulation if they are significantly hot or cold. Leg baths are also an excellent home treatment for clients. A leg bath may be given in a standard bathtub or a stainless steel whirlpool specifically designed for this purpose. If only the lower legs are to be treated, use two deep buckets, one for each leg.

Hot Leg Bath

Temperature: Hot (102°–110°F)

Time Needed: 20 minutes

Equipment Needed: Water thermometer, bath towel, shirt or small towel to cover the upper body if needed

Effect: Primarily thermal

Cleanup: Clean, disinfect, and dry tub; launder towels.

Indications: Tightness in the leg muscles; stiffness and poor circulation in the leg muscles after the removal of a leg or ankle cast; muscle soreness after vigorous exercise; arthritis pain in legs or feet; pain in an amputation stump, including phantom pain; scar tissue contractures on the legs from adhesions, wounds, or burns that are to be treated with massage. A hot leg bath can soften tissues before massage. A long hot leg bath will also warm the entire body.

Contraindications: Diabetes, lymphedema in legs, loss of sensation, peripheral vascular disease (arteriosclerosis of the lower extremities or Buerger's disease)

Procedure

1. Check with client to make sure there are no contraindications to the hot leg bath.
2. Explain the use of the hot leg bath to the client and get his or her consent.
3. Place towels on floor in front of tub and behind where client's head will be.
4. Fill tub to a level that covers the legs (usually about 8 inches deep), checking temperature with water thermometer.
5. Have the client enter the tub, wearing a dry shirt or sheet to keep the upper body warm if desired.
6. After 20 minutes, help the client to leave the tub and dry off vigorously, and then he or she can lie down for a rest or massage.

Variations

1. Warm leg bath (98°–102°F). This bath is safe for clients who would benefit from a leg bath but have diabetes or lymphedema of the legs. Bath water must be 102°F or less.
2. An Epsom salt leg bath can be used for painful bruises or soreness after vigorous exercise. Add 2 cups of Epsom salt to a leg bath. More information on Epsom salt is given later in this chapter.
3. Lower leg bath. Use two large buckets and immerse the lower legs up to the knee.

Cold Leg Bath

Cold leg baths are not for everyone, as many people find exposure of such a large portion of the body to cold very unpleasant. However, they are useful to prevent muscle soreness after vigorous exercise and much used by college and professional runners. A classic study of the effects of cold leg baths on leg muscles also found that cold baths greatly increased their strength. Subjects were given 54°F leg baths for 30 minutes. Each subject was tested for leg strength 11 times during the 30 minutes and every 20 minutes for 3 hours after the treatment while he rested. Subjects' leg muscles showed increased strength during the cold bath and afterward for up to 6 hours. The researchers concluded that this increased strength was due to increased blood flow to the deep leg muscles, caused by restriction of peripheral blood flow during the treatment.(9)

Temperature: Cold, 50° to 60°F for a strong reaction, up to 70°F if the client cannot tolerate a very cold bath

Time Needed: 5 to 20 minutes

Equipment Needed: Water thermometer, bath towel, shirt or small towel to cover the upper body if needed

Effect: Primarily thermal

Cleanup: Clean, disinfect, and dry tub; launder towels.

Indications: To prevent muscle soreness after vigorous leg exercise (15–20 minutes), to stimulate circulation in legs (2–5 minutes), to cool an overheated client (5–15 minutes)

Contraindications: Marked hypertension; Raynaud's syndrome; if prolonged, cold leg baths are contraindicated for lymphedema.

Procedure

Follow the procedure for the hot leg bath but use cold water.

Variation

Lower leg bath. Use two large buckets and immerse the lower legs up to the knee.

Contrast Leg Baths

Contrast leg baths can have a powerful influence on blood flow to the legs. For example, one study conducted in 2005 examined arterial blood flow in the lower legs during hot, cold, and contrast treatments. The contrast treatment consisted of 4 minutes of immersion in hot water (104°F) alternated with 1 minute of cold (55°F). There were significant fluctuations in arterial blood flow throughout the 20-minute treatment. There was an increase in arterial blood flow in the first hot water bath and then a decrease in blood flow when the bath was changed from hot to cold and the muscles of the artery contracted. This was followed by another increase in blood flow each time the water bath was changed back to hot and another decrease when the water was changed to cold again. The increase in arterial blood flow was greatest on the first change back from a cold bath to a hot one and became less with each successive hot bath. This suggests that the muscles of the artery wall became progressively more fatigued. Experimenters also found that contrast baths caused a greater increase in local circulation than a simple hot bath, and the arterial blood flow at the end of the contrast bath sequence was double that of subjects who were simply sitting quietly (10). To increase the circulatory effect of a contrast leg bath even further, have the client contract (make active movements of) the muscles of the lower legs, feet, and ankles during immersion.

The following directions for the contrast leg bath rest on the assumption that the therapist has two tubs, one for hot and one for cold, but this treatment may also be done with a bathtub for the hot water followed by a cold leg shower.

Temperature: Hot (102°–110°F) alternated with cold (55°–70°F)

Time Needed: 10 minutes

Equipment Needed: Two bathtubs, water thermometer, bath towel, shirt or small towel to cover the upper body if needed

Effect: Primarily thermal

Cleanup: Clean, disinfect, and dry tub; launder towels.

Indications: Muscular fatigue in legs, poor circulation in legs, joint sprains, passive swelling in legs, stiffness and poor circulation in the leg muscles after a cast has been removed, when prescribed by a doctor to promote healing of infection

Contraindications: Same as for hot and cold leg baths

Procedure
1. Follow the procedure for a hot leg bath; then, while the client is in the hot leg bath, fill the other bathtub with cold water.
2. After 2 minutes, help the client to leave the tub of hot water and move into the tub of cold water.
3. After 30 seconds, help the client to leave the tub of hot water and move into the tub of cold water.
4. Repeat steps 3 and 4 for a total of three rounds.
5. Dry the lower body vigorously and lie down for a rest or massage; or exercise until the legs are warm first.

Variation
Lower leg bath. Use two buckets and immerse the lower legs up to the knee.

PARAFFIN BATH

A paraffin "bath" is the immersion of a body part, usually the hands or feet, in a tank of melted paraffin (Fig. 7-8). In the United States, paraffin formulated for baths also contains mineral oil, which makes it easy to peel off the skin and leaves the skin soft. Dipping a body part into paraffin a number of times produces a coat of wax that not only warms the tissue underneath but traps heat at the skin's surface so it cannot radiate off. Instead, heat goes into the joint. A paraffin bath can significantly increase the temperature of both the skin it coats and the muscles and joint capsules underneath (Box 7-2).

When might a massage therapist choose melted paraffin to treat a client? The deep heating of a painful or stiff body part makes it an excellent treatment for relieving joint stiffness in conditions such as arthritis, poorly healed sprains, nonacute bursitis, and fractures after the client's cast has been removed. When used before massage, the deep heat of the bath also softens tissues and makes them more pliable, which is especially helpful when treating scar tissue. For example, by using a combination of paraffin baths followed by stretching, patients with burn scars can gain significant increases in their joint range of motion.(8) Another time you might choose to use melted paraffin is for a client who does not have joint problems or pain but would like a novel or a pampering treatment.

However, sometimes paraffin is not the right hydrotherapy treatment. Some disadvantages of using paraffin: Melted paraffin is easy to spill, difficult to clean up when spilled, and more expensive than water. A paraffin bath must be plugged in 3 hours before it is used. And finally, only the hands and the feet can be easily immersed in a paraffin bath. Deciding when to use paraffin will depend upon your practice, your clients, and the type of facility where you practice massage.

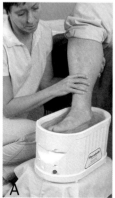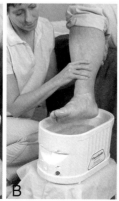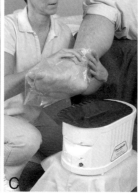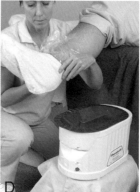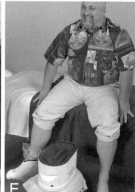

FIGURE 7-8 ■ Paraffin footbath. **A.** Dipping client's foot in paraffin bath. **B.** Paraffin-coated foot drying. **C.** Wrapping the foot in plastic bag. **D.** Placing bootie on client's foot. **E.** Client resting with one foot drying.

BOX 7-2 *Point of Interest*

HISTORY OF THE PARAFFIN BATH

According to English physical therapist Olive Millard, who practiced in Europe from 1913 to 1940, the melted paraffin bath was first introduced into the practice of physical medicine in 1917. W. L. Ingle, of the English firm of Messrs. Ingle, Ltd., Tanners and Curriers, heard that a Frenchman was employing melted paraffin wax in the treatment of rheumatism. Ingle also noticed that a number of his workers were immersing their hands and feet in a vat of wax that was used for preparing animal skins at his plant in Churwell, Yorkshire. So many found benefit from using paraffin, probably for arthritic pain, that Ingle presented a paraffin bath to Colonel Littlewood, the commanding medical officer of the Second Northern General Hospital, to treat wounded soldiers.(1)

Paraffin baths were enthusiastically adopted for physical therapy and quickly became very common. They were used throughout Europe and North America by physical therapists,

athletic trainers, and massage therapists. At Warm Springs (Georgia) Rehabilitation Institute, a state-of-the-art facility founded in 1927, paraffin was one of the treatments used for musculoskeletal problems. For example, a patient with clubfeet might be treated with serial casting, which is used to gradually straighten out twisted limbs. To begin, the feet were reshaped as much as possible toward a normal position and then put in a cast for a week or two. Every few weeks each foot would be taken out of its cast and dipped in hot paraffin to make the tissue more pliable; then massaged, stretched, and reshaped more toward a normal position; and finally put into another cast. Melted paraffin was also used to treat arthritis pain and soften scar tissue prior to stretching.

Reference
1. Millard O. *Under My Thumb.* London: Christopher Johnson, 1952.

The procedure below, which describes a paraffin bath for the feet, is also suitable for the hands.

Temperature: Hot (123°–126°F)

Time Needed: 15 minutes

Equipment Needed: Paraffin bath containing 3 pounds of paraffin, small plastic bags, booties or oversized socks to slip on the feet. These supplies are often included when a paraffin bath is purchased.

Effect: Primarily thermal

Cleanup: Throw away plastic bags and used paraffin; launder towel and booties or socks.

Indications: Poorly healed sprains, nonacute bursitis, fractures after cast removal, joint contractures, of scar tissue, muscle strains, muscle spasm, gout, joint stiffness, pain of osteoarthritis and rheumatoid arthritis. Clients with arthritis can benefit from having a paraffin bath at home and using it daily.

Contraindications: Peripheral vascular disease, including diabetes, Buerger's disease, and arteriosclerosis of the lower extremities; lymphedema; skin that is open or contains cuts or sores; loss of sensation (lack of feeling); sensitivity to heat, especially in those with thin skin, such as the elderly and small children

Procedure
1. Check with client to make sure there are no contraindications to the paraffin bath.
2. Explain the use of the paraffin bath to the client and get his or her consent.
3. Have the client seated in a chair next to the massage table. Place a towel on the floor under the client's feet.
4. Put the container of hot water on the towel, rest the client's feet in the container, and briefly soak the feet. (If running water is not available, spray the feet with a sanitizer.) This step feels good to the client and keeps the paraffin bath clean.
5. Quickly dip the first foot in paraffin and remove it.
6. Wait about 3 seconds for the wax to harden slightly (the wax will just start to lose its shine), then dip the foot again.
7. Repeat steps 5 and 6 five times for a total of six dips and encase the foot in a plastic bag or cellophane wrap and then in an oversized sock, cloth bootie, or electric bootie.
8. Repeat steps 5 to 7 with the other foot.
9. Leave the paraffin on for about 10 minutes, then remove the sock or bootie, the bag or cellophane, and the paraffin from one foot.
10. Massage that foot.
11. Repeat steps 9 and 10 with the other foot.

Variations
1. Paraffin dip on massage table. The client may disrobe, wrap in a sheet, and sit on the side of the table while you bring the paraffin bath there. Once the feet are wrapped, it is easy for the client to lie down while you begin massage.
2. Contrast treatment. Paraffin foot dips can be used to create a contrast treatment by dipping the feet in cold water for 30 seconds after removing the paraffin. Perform three rounds of hot paraffin dips followed by cold water.

CONTINUOUS BATHS: INGENIOUS TREATMENTS FOR ANCIENT PROBLEMS

The continuous bath treatment was developed by a Viennese doctor in 1861. Patients remained in a tub of neutral temperature water (98°F) for extended periods, from a few hours to many days or weeks. They lay in a stretcher suspended inside the tub by clamps or hooks, which formed a hammock-type sling. The stretcher was covered with a blanket or mattress with a sheet on top, and rubber pillows were provided for the patient's head and feet. Once the patient was in the water, the top of the tub was covered with boards, which helped retain the heat and also provided a table for the patient (see Figure 1-13). Warm water ran in as cooler water ran out, so that not only did the bath stay at a constant temperature, but water constantly ran gently over the skin. Normally a waterproofing ointment was applied to the patient's skin at the beginning of the bath, since he or she stayed in the water for many hours at a time. Some patients would be removed periodically only long enough for the tub to be cleaned and more waterproofing ointment applied.

Continuous baths met some medical needs that today are treated by medications, but when they were developed, there were no effective medications for many of the problems they addressed. These included reflex spasms from spinal cord injuries, paralysis of the legs, and joint stiffness and pain from advanced arthritis. Because bacterial growth in infected areas was reduced while the person remained in the bath, until the advent of antibiotics the continuous bath was also a standard treatment for such conditions as nonhealing pressure sores,

gangrene, ulcers from radiation burns, fecal and urinary fistulas, and extensive burns.(1)

Floating in the bath also decreased pressure and pain on sores or wounds on the back part of the body, and reduced the number of painful dressing changes on badly infected wounds.(2) The continuous bath has also been useful for relieving the pain and stiffness of rheumatoid arthritis and the pain, spasm, burning sensation, and tremors of Parkinson's disease.(3) When hydrotherapy was popular in mental hospitals, continuous baths were used extensively to sedate agitated mental patients. Physical therapist Earl Qualls saw the continuous bath being used in California state mental hospitals as late as 1952, for both musculoskeletal pain and for a tranquilizing effect (E. Qualls, personal communication, July 5, 2005).

Continuous baths have fallen out of use because of their time-consuming nature, but research is needed to find out whether they could be useful when medication is not effective, such as when pressure sores do not heal even when treated with antibiotics, or when side effects of medication are very serious.

References

1. Baruch S. *An Epitome of Hydrotherapy for Physicians, Architects and Nurses.* New York: Saunders, 1920, p 95.
2. Jelinek R. Continuous bath treatment in surgical therapy. *J Int Coll Surg* 1953;20:156.
3. Thrash A, Thrash C. *Home Remedies: Hydrotherapy, Charcoal, and Other Simple Treatments.* Seale, AL: Thrash, 1981, p 120.

WHOLE-BODY BATHS

In this section, you will learn about a number of different bath treatments in which the entire body is immersed in water. A variety of bath treatments can be performed in any standard bathtub and with different effects depending upon the temperature of the water, the duration of the bath, and any additives in the water. From hot, warm, neutral, cold, or contrast whole-body baths to baths with additives, and from jetted tubs to Watsu pools, baths have different effects that complement massage treatments. If you work in a facility that has either a standard bathtub or a specialty bathtub, it is easy to add whole-body baths to your repertoire of hydrotherapy treatments; you may also give your clients instructions on how to take different types of baths at home. The continuous bath, an ingenious use of whole-body immersion to treat a variety of problems, is not used today because it is extremely time consuming. However, the wide variety of problems it was used to treat makes clear how varied the effects of whole-body baths can be (Box 7-3).

STANDARD BATHS

Many bath treatments can be performed in a single standard bathtub. The therapeutic effects can be varied by changing or alternating water temperatures.

Hot Bath

Almost everyone loves a full-body hot bath like the one pictured in Figure 7-9, especially those who are cold or have musculoskeletal pain. The combination of the warmth of the water, the soothing sensation of water on the skin, and the temporary release from the pull of gravity draws healthy and sick people alike to hot springs all over the world, to spas and health clubs that have hot tubs, and to home bathtubs. According to Patrick Horay and David Harp, authors of *Hot Water Therapy*, "There is something almost magical about hot water. It was probably in the environment of hot water that the primordial soup coalesced into the dance of spinning molecules known as life. All the conditions had to be just right—plus something extra. Something that calls life out of chaos; something that heals. Slipping into a warm bath, a part of you remembers and allows itself to be supported and buoyed up, warmed and nurtured to the core. It reminds you to let go of physical and mental tension, to give up all the striving and activity, to be just held by the penetrating warmth."(11)

Temperature: Hot (102°–104°F), depending upon the client's tolerance. Clients vary widely as to their ideal temperature, and what is an extremely hot bath to one

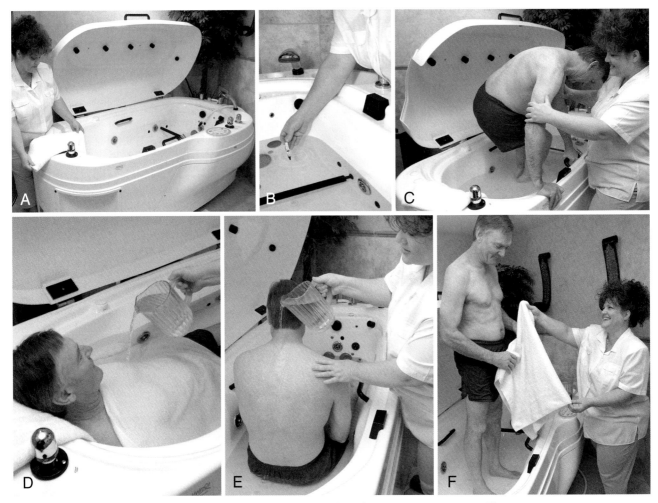

FIGURE 7-9 ■ Hot bath. **A.** Placing bath mat and towel. **B.** Filling tub and checking water temperature. **C.** Client entering the tub. **D.** Covering chest and shoulders with towel. **E.** Pouring cold water over the client. **F.** Giving client a towel after bath.

person will be almost a cold bath to another. If the water temperature is not comfortable, however, no clients will want to stay in for very long. For someone who is not accustomed to taking a hot bath, begin with no more than 15 minutes.

Equipment Needed: Water thermometer, tub, two bath towels, bath mat

Effect: Primarily thermal

Cleanup: Clean and sanitize tub; launder towels and bath mat.

Indications: Before massage, hot baths can soften connective tissue, relax muscles, enhance circulation, and encourage mental relaxation. The whole-body heating effect relieves many types of musculoskeletal pain, including pain from osteoarthritis, gout, dysmenorrhea, back pain, arthritis, neuralgia, muscle soreness, sprains, strains, bruises and contusions, and is known to help a person fall asleep faster and sleep more deeply.(5,6)

Contraindications: Systemic or chronic conditions, including cardiovascular problems, diabetes, hepatitis, lymphedema, multiple sclerosis, seizure disorders; loss of sensation; great obesity; pregnancy; inability to tolerate heat; ingestion of alcohol or drugs; recent meal (wait at least an hour after a meal). Very frequent hot baths are not recommended for clients with hypothyroid conditions.

Procedure
1. Check with client to make sure there are no contraindications to the full hot bath.
2. Explain the use of the full hot bath to the client and get his or her consent.
3. Place bath mat on the floor in front of the tub and a towel behind where client's head will rest.
4. Begin filling the tub and check the water temperature with a thermometer.
5. When the tub is half full, have the client get in the tub and sit down: assist as needed.
6. Have the client adjust the temperature to a tolerable level as the bath finishes filling.

---

7. Have the client remain in the tub for 15 minutes or longer, depending upon tolerance.
8. If the bathtub is too small for someone to be entirely immersed, cover the chest and shoulders with a large towel and pour water over it frequently. This way, the client's skin that is above the water will be warm and moist.
9. A brief cold shower or simply pouring cold water over the body will help reinvigorate someone who is feeling drained after a hot bath. However, many clients find this step unpleasant, so it is optional.
10. If lightheaded or dizzy, the client should sit in the tub while the water is draining out before getting out. This will bring down the core temperature slightly. The client should not try to get out of the tub until the lightheaded or dizzy feeling passes.
11. Hand the client a towel to dry off with before he or she gets out of the tub.

Variation

Brief cold bath, cold shower, or even a pouring of cold water over the client. When the cold water is in contact with the skin, it causes vasoconstriction of the blood vessels under the skin. This is difficult or unpleasant for many people but results in a prolonged feeling of warmth and invigoration. The cold exposure should be about 30 seconds but no longer than 2 minutes. Do not perform unless the client is quite warm.

Warm Bath

Warm baths are soothing and relaxing, but they are less challenging to the body: maintaining core temperature at 98.6°F is not as difficult in a warm bath as it is in a hot bath. The client's will still experience the bodily changes that come from adjusting to a temperature higher than 98.6°F, such as vasodilation of the skin and sweating, but these changes will be less extreme, as there is less heat to throw off. For this reason, warm baths are practical for many people for whom hot baths are contraindicated, such as people with diabetes or pregnancy. However, musculoskeletal pain will be less dramatically affected by a warm bath.

Temperature: Warm (99°–102°F). Clients vary widely as to what is the most comfortable temperature for them. If the water temperature is beyond the client's tolerance, he or she will not be able to stay in for very long. For someone who is not accustomed to taking a warm bath, begin with no more than 15 minutes.

Equipment Needed: Water thermometer, tub, two bath towels, bath mat

Effect: Primarily thermal

Cleanup: Clean and sanitize tub; launder towels and bath mat.

Indications: Before massage, to soften connective tissue, relax muscles, enhance circulation, and encourage mental relaxation; musculoskeletal pain, including the pain of osteoarthritis, gout, dysmenorrhea, back pain, arthritis, neuralgia, sprains, strains, bruises and contusions. Combats insomnia if given before bed.

Contraindications: Seizure disorders, due to the danger of a client having a seizure in the tub; loss of sensation; great obesity; inability to tolerate heat; ingestion of alcohol or drugs; recent meal (wait at least an hour after a meal)

Procedure
Follow the procedure for hot baths but use warm water.

Neutral Bath

The neutral bath places the client in an environment with as little thermal or mechanical stimulation as possible. (For more on its use with mentally disturbed people, see Box 1-2.) This lack of stimulation, along with the sensation of water surrounding one's body on all sides and a sense of buoyancy, is unusually soothing and calming. Heart rate drops, while skin blood flow, skin temperature and core temperature remain the same.(12) This calming effect can be further enhanced by eliminating all noise, extraneous conversation, bright lights, and other stimuli that would require a response on the part of the client. A massage after a neutral bath is a wonderful complement to a relaxing hydrotherapy treatment, but it should also be done in a quiet and calm manner. A neutral bath at bedtime is an excellent home treatment clients may use for insomnia.

Temperature: Neutral (94–98°F)

Time Needed: 20 minutes or more

Equipment Needed: Water thermometer, tub, two bath towels, bath mat

Effect: Primarily mechanical (lack of sensory stimulation)

Cleanup: Clean and sanitize tub; launder towels and bath mat.

Indications: Insomnia, nervousness, anxiety, depression, and diseases of the heart and blood vessels with which more extreme hot and cold temperatures cannot be used, such as arteriosclerosis or diabetes; when performed under doctor's supervision, sometimes used to lower blood pressure in a hypertensive person

Contraindications: Hypotension (because it may lower the systolic blood pressure 20 points) unless prescribed by a doctor; severe cardiac weakness; eczema.

Procedure

1. Follow the procedure for hot baths, using neutral water. The temperature of the bath water must remain the same throughout the bath.
2. Keep the environment calm and quiet.
3. Have the client dry off gently so as not to stimulate the skin, and then he or she may lie down to rest or to receive a massage

Short, Cold Bath

A short (30 seconds to 2 minutes) cold plunge bath is a traditional hydrotherapy treatment which, when given regularly, stimulates the muscles of the arteries of the skin to contract more strongly. A short, cold bath has little or no cooling effect on the body, because the body is not chilled for long enough to lower the core temperature. The body's defense mechanisms are stimulated, however, to such a degree that if a person jumps in a short, cold bath and then immediately dries off and gets dressed, he or she will actually feel warmer than before the bath. A feeling of invigoration is common, as the body's functions are stimulated, and for this reason a cold bath is a classic ending to a sauna. Longer cold baths have been used in the past to reduce fevers, because they actually cool the body and bring the core temperature down, but they are not recommended for massage therapy unless a client has become overheated in a hot bath, sauna, or steam bath.

Temperature: Cold, generally below 65°F. (Cold tap water is usually 55° to 65°F.)

Time Needed: 30 seconds to 2 minutes

Equipment Needed: Water thermometer, tub, two bath towels, bath mat

Effect: Primarily thermal

Cleanup: Clean and sanitize tub; launder towels and bath mat.

Indications: Reversal of vasodilation of skin after a heat treatment; stimulation of blood flow to skin; invigoration; prevention of painful menstrual cramps (see Chapter 13)

Contraindications: Chilled client; extreme fatigue; kidney disease; cardiovascular disease. (The blood pressure will rise for a very short time and may be too much of a demand for a person with heart disease or arteriosclerosis.) When given very frequently, cold baths are contraindicated for clients with hyperthyroid conditions. (This is a disease in which the basal metabolic rate is too high, and a short, cold bath will further increase the metabolism.) Client with an aversion to cold.

Procedure
Follow the procedure for hot baths, using cold water and keeping the bath short, only 30 seconds to 2 minutes.

Contrast Bath

A contrast bath combines immersions in both hot and cold water. (see Fig. 5-13). By causing dilation and constriction of the blood vessels of the entire skin surface, it stimulates the circulatory system and leaves the client feeling both relaxed and invigorated. However, only the hardiest of clients can tolerate the temperature extremes of very hot alternated with very cold. Someone who would like to try a contrast bath but is not accustomed to such a circulatory system challenge would do better to try a warm bath alternated with a cool bath at first. If you do not have the two tubs that this treatment calls for, you can substitute a sauna or steam bath for the hot bath and use a cold shower for the cold bath. In Scandinavia, rolling in the snow is a traditional method of cooling the body after heat exposure; however, as discussed in the introduction to this chapter, immersion baths are truly the most efficient in warming and cooling the body. Be sure to explain the benefits of the contrast bath to your client, because the first immersion in the cold bath is often quite a strong sensation. The muscles of the blood vessels generally become fatigued after three changes. If the contrast bath is going to be prolonged after that, so that the blood vessels continue to respond, the hot bath must be even hotter and the cold bath even colder. To increase the circulatory effect of a contrast bath further, have the client exercise gently at the same time.

Temperature: Hot (102°–104°F) alternated with cold (65°F or less)

Time Needed: About 15 minutes

Equipment Needed: Water thermometer; two tubs, one filled with hot water and one with cold water; two bath towels; bath mat

Effect: Primarily thermal

Cleanup: Clean and sanitize tub; launder towels and bath mat.

Indications: When stimulation of blood flow to the skin or a feeling of invigoration is desired; when training the circulatory system to react faster to heat and cold in order to stay warmer in the winter (see Chapter 12); as a general tonic

Contraindications: Because it combines the effects of hot and cold baths, same as for both hot bath and short cold bath

Procedure
1. Check with client to make sure there are no contraindications to either hot or cold whole-body baths.
2. Explain the use of the contrast bath to the client and get his or her consent.

3. For each tub, place a bath mat on the floor in front of the tub and a towel behind where the client's head will rest.
4. Fill both tubs, one with hot water and the other with cold, and check the water temperature in both.
5. Have the client enter the hot bath and remain for 5 minutes so that his or her body is thoroughly warm.
6. Have the client move to the cold bath for 30 seconds to 1 minute.
7. Have the client move back to the hot bath and remain for 2 minutes for maximum skin vasodilation.
8. Have the client move to the cold bath for 30 seconds to 1 minute.
9. Repeat steps 7 and 8.
10. Hand the client a towel to dry off with as he or she gets out of the tub

BATHS WITH ADDITIVES

To vary or expand the therapeutic effects of a standard bath, consider adding chemicals to the water using one of the substances in this section. They are easy to find, inexpensive, contain no preservatives, and have beneficial effects on the skin, muscles, joints, or nervous system (Fig. 7-10). For all of the baths that follow, use warm, not hot water, because the goal of the treatment is not to heat or cool the client; instead it is to bring the substance that is dissolved in the water into contact with the client's skin. Warm water is helpful because it causes dilation of the blood vessels under the skin, which increases absorption of the chemical. A warm bath also provides a relaxing environment for the client. The water is pleasant, unlike very hot or cold water, which will prevent the client from staying in the bath long enough for absorption to occur.

Mineral water hot springs, mud baths, and seawater baths have all been used to treat musculoskeletal ailments for thousands of years. Natural mineral springs contain various mixtures of chemicals, such as potassium, magnesium, calcium, and sulfate; mud baths are used to stimulate circulation and metabolism and combat inflammation; and minerals found in seawater, including sodium chloride, are said to stimulate circulation of blood and lymph and speed elimination of toxins. Where these baths are available, massage therapy is almost always practiced as well. However, these treatments are not practical for the massage therapist except in a spa setting and for this reason are not discussed in detail here. For more information on these baths, refer to *Spa Bodywork* by Anne Williams.

Oatmeal Bath

Oatmeal has an anti-inflammatory effect that makes it suitable for a variety of skin irritations.(13) It contains essential fatty acids and other chemicals that can soothe and moisturize dry, itchy skin and can relieve many types of itching for as much as several hours. Powdered oatmeal is an ingredient in many commercial bath products, such as Aveeno, Episooth and Actibath, but oatmeal is easily added to a bath using simple uncooked rolled oats (Fig. 7-11).

Temperature: Warm (98°–102°F)

Time Needed: 15 to 20 minutes

Equipment Needed: Water thermometer, bath towel, bath mat, and one of the following:

1. One packet of commercial oatmeal preparation, such as Aveeno or Actibath. The oat preparation should be added to the bath as soon as it begins filling to make sure it dissolves fully.
2. One cup uncooked rolled oats that have been ground fine in a blender and mixed with three cups of cold water.
3. One cup of uncooked rolled oats in a muslin bag

Effect: Primarily chemical

Cleanup: Clean and sanitize tub; launder towels and bath mat.

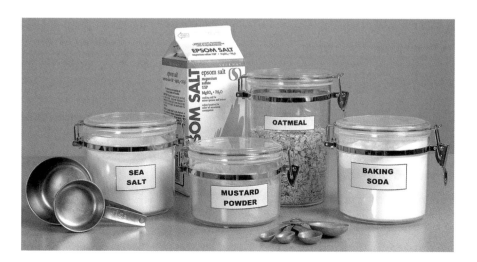

FIGURE 7-10 ■ Containers with bath additives.

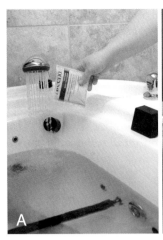
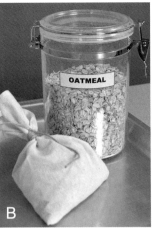
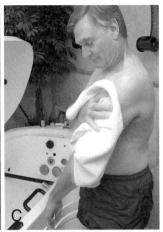

FIGURE 7-11 ■ Oatmeal bath. **A.** Adding oatmeal to bath water. **B.** Muslin bag containing oatmeal. **C.** Patting the skin dry.

Indications: Skin irritations such as poison oak, poison ivy, chickenpox, shingles, psoriasis, rashes, eczema, diaper rash, ichthyosis, sunburn

Contraindications: Same as for full warm bath

Procedure

Same as for a full warm bath, except directions are included for adding oatmeal to the bath.

1. Check with client to make sure there are no contraindications to a warm whole-body bath.
2. Explain the use of the bath to the client and get his or her consent.
3. Place a bath mat on the floor in front of the tub and a towel behind where the client's head will rest.
4. Begin filling the tub. Check the water temperature with a thermometer and then add the oatmeal preparation. If a muslin bag containing oatmeal is used, it should be put in the tub right away so that it becomes thoroughly saturated. During the bath, it should be squeezed occasionally to extract its beneficial properties.
5. Have the client enter the tub when it is half full. Assist as needed.
6. Have the client adjust the temperature to tolerance as the bath finishes filling.
7. Have the client remain in the tub for 15 minutes or longer, depending upon tolerance.

Hand the client a towel to dry off before he or she gets out of the tub. The skin should not be toweled vigorously. Instead the skin should be gently patted dry, so that some of the oat solution remains on the skin. Do not let the client become chilled during this process.

Baking Soda Bath

Sodium bicarbonate is widely used as an antacid. It is added to intravenous medication when a patient is in a state of acidosis; to many commercial preparations such as Alka-Seltzer to neutralize stomach acid; and to water

used to decontaminate the skin after some chemical exposures. Because it can neutralize toxins, normalize the skin's acid/base balance, and has mild anesthetic properties, baking soda is used to decrease many types of skin irritation. As a massage therapist, you can provide your clients with these beneficial effects by adding it to a bath treatment, or you can suggest that clients use a baking soda bath at home. For example, a client who has scheduled a massage but believes his or her skin might be too irritated to receive one could take a series of baking soda baths the day before the scheduled massage; this may improve the condition of his or her skin and make massage more comfortable.

Temperature: Warm (98°–102°F)

Time Needed: 15 to 20 minutes

Equipment Needed: Water thermometer, 1 cup of baking soda, bath towel, bath mat

Effect: Primarily chemical

Cleanup: Clean and sanitize tub; launder towels and bath mat

Indications: Skin irritations such as sunburn, heat rash, eczema, itching, hives, poison oak, poison ivy, and reactions from chemotherapy or radiation treatments for cancer

Contraindications: Same as for full warm bath

Procedure

Follow the procedure for the oatmeal bath, except add baking soda instead of oatmeal.

Epsom Salt Bath

Epsom salt is the common name for a mineral compound, magnesium sulfate heptahydrate, that was first prepared from the waters of the mineral spring in Epsom, England. That spring was discovered in the early 1600s, bubbling up through soil which contained the mineral epsomite. Its waters were found to be both relaxing and purgative. Enterprising businessmen soon began to prepare the crystalline form of Epsom salt by boiling down the mineral water, but it has been made synthetically since 1850.(14,15)

Today we are familiar with Epsom salt as a white or colorless crystal that is commonly found in grocery stores and pharmacies, where it can be purchased without a prescription. Since its discovery, hydrotherapists have used Epsom salt in partial and whole-body baths, body wraps, compresses, and constitutional treatments. Doctors have prescribed it for detoxification (magnesium is a necessary element in some enzymes responsible for detoxification), bruising, and drawing out of splinters. Because like other salts, it withdraws water from cells, Epsom salt is used as a fast-acting purgative in some types of poisoning, to draw water into the intestines thus reducing constipation, to withdraw toxins from the body, and to draw fluid from the brain in cases of cerebral edema. Because magnesium reduces striated muscle contractions, the muscle-relaxant action of magnesium is used to prevent convulsions in **preeclampsia** (hypertension or edema in a pregnant woman), to treat hyperreflexia in spinal cord injury, and to treat some cases of bronchospasm.(15,16) Dermatology Professor E. Proksch found that immersion of the skin of the forearm in a concentrated Dead Sea salt bath helped persons with atopic dermatitis (dry, rough, red skin) by moisturizing their skin and reducing inflammation and that this effect lasted for as long as 6 weeks after the end of the study. Probably the high magnesium content of the Dead Sea salts is responsible for these effects.(17)

As massage therapists, we can use Epsom salt in baths for its relaxing effect, to reduce soreness after massage or vigorous exercise, and to reduce inflammation caused by swelling and bruises.

Temperature: Warm (98°–102°F)

Time Needed: 15 to 20 minutes

Equipment Needed: Water thermometer, bath towel and bath mat, 2 cups Epsom salt for an adult or 1 cup Epsom salt for a child. Use double that amount when the bath is taken specifically for detoxification.

Effect: Primarily chemical

Cleanup: Clean and sanitize tub; launder towels and bath mat. Epsom salt is not corrosive to drainpipes.

Indications: Bruises, sprains in the subacute stage, soreness after exercise, nervous tension, arthritis pain, general tonic, detoxification

Contraindications: Same as for full warm bath

Procedure
Follow the procedure for the oatmeal bath, using Epsom salt instead. After the bath, Epsom salt should be thoroughly rinsed off with a brief shower or by pouring clean water over the client. Then apply a moisturizing lotion or oil to the skin: this is simple to do if the client is going to be receiving a massage.

Sea Salt Bath

Sea salt baths have traditionally been given as a general tonic and are also calming and relaxing. Use 1 to 3 cups of salt in a tonic bath, which may be taken daily. The water holds the heat better because of the salt. Salt baths have been used in the past for patients with severe burns, as a way of providing them with electrolytes. For burn patients 5 pounds of salt is added to 40 gallons of water, giving the same concentration of salt as ocean water. The tonic bath, however, uses less salt.

Time Needed: 15 to 20 minutes

Temperature: Warm (98°–102°F)

Equipment Needed: Water thermometer, 1 to 3 cups of sea salt, bath towel, bath mat

Effect: Primarily chemical

Cleanup: Clean and sanitize tub; launder towels and bath mat. Salt can be corrosive to drain pipes, so immediately after the bath, the pipes should be thoroughly flushed with tap water so that no salt water remains

Indications: General tonic, chronic sciatica, fractures after removal of the cast, dislocations, gout, arthritis

Contraindications: Same as for full warm bath

Procedure
Follow the procedure for the oatmeal bath, using sea salt instead. After the bath, the saltwater should be thoroughly rinsed off with a brief shower or by pouring clean water over the client. Then apply a moisturizing lotion or oil to the skin: this is simple to do if the client is going to be receiving a massage.

Powdered Mustard Bath

Powdered mustard, when mixed with water, has a warming and vasodilating effect. As discussed in Chapter 5, mustard can be extremely heating when used in a plaster or poultice. In a bath, however, the smaller amount is mildly warming, encourages sweating, relieves muscle soreness and fatigue, and is an excellent home treatment for insomnia.

Temperature: Warm (98°–102°F)

Time Needed: 15 to 20 minutes

Equipment Needed: Water thermometer, $1/3$ cup mustard powder for an adult, bath towel, bath mat

Effect: Primarily chemical

Cleanup: Clean and sanitize tub; launder towels and bath mat.

Indications: Muscle soreness or fatigue, insomnia

Contraindications: Same as for full warm bath

Procedure

Follow the procedure for the oatmeal bath, using mustard powder instead. As with oatmeal, mustard powder may be added directly to the water under the spigot. However, lumps may remain, so the mustard powder may also be combined with water in a bowl first. Stir until no lumps remain, then add the mixture to the bath water. Also, after the bath, mustard water should be thoroughly rinsed off with a brief shower or by pouring clean water over the client. Then apply a moisturizing lotion or oil to the skin: this is simple to do if the client is going to be receiving a massage.

Detoxification Bath

Detoxification baths that use salts and baking soda may be taken two to three times per week. This bath combines the detoxifying effects of three previous baths: baking soda neutralizes toxins; Epsom salt draws water and toxins and provides magnesium and sulfate needed for detoxification; sea salt draws water to and toxins; and the warm water promotes a moderate amount of sweating. Clients should replenish water and electrolytes afterward. See Chapter 12 for more information on detoxification.

Temperature: Warm (98°–104°F)

Time Needed: 15 to 20 minutes

Equipment Needed: Water thermometer; 1 cup sea salt, 1 cup Epsom salt, and 1 1/2 cups baking soda to put in tub; bath towel; bath mat

Effect: Primarily chemical

Cleanup: Clean and sanitize tub; launder towels and bath mat. Flush pipes with tap water to wash away salt.

Indications: As a general tonic, after recent exposure to toxins, or as part of a detoxification program

Contraindications: Same as for full warm bath

Procedure

Follow the procedure for the oatmeal bath, using baking soda and both types of salt rather than oatmeal. To make sure they dissolve, add them directly under the spigot as soon as the tub begins filling. At the conclusion of the bath, the bath water should be thoroughly rinsed off with a brief shower or by pouring clean water over the client. Then apply a moisturizing lotion or oil to the skin: this is simple to do if the client is going to be receiving a massage.

SPECIALIZED BATHS

In addition to the standard bath treatments presented, a massage therapist who is working in an athletic club, spa, or similar setting can perform other treatments that require special equipment. Here we cover baths taken in tubs with jets, spa bathtubs, or whole-body stainless steel whirlpools, along with Watsu treatments in swimming pools.

Tubs With Jets: Jacuzzis, Hot Tubs, or Spas

The terms used to describe tubs with jets are somewhat confusing, and they may be called Jacuzzis (named after the first manufacturer of jetted tubs), hot tubs, or spas. All are small pools containing jets of water or air or both, big enough for more than one person to use at a time. Today, tubs with jets such as the one pictured in Figure 7-12 can be found in athletic clubs, health spas, and some private homes. The bath water is generally heated to about 104°F, which is comfortable for most people, but it can easily be adjusted to lower or higher temperatures. Some jetted tubs have tile walls and floors, while others are made of fiberglass or other synthetic materials. Unlike a standard bathtub, water is not drained out at the end of the bath, and instead the water is treated with chemicals to disinfect it. Jetted tubs also contain equipment that heats and recirculates the bath water. Safe use of jetted tubs is important: water temperature must be carefully monitored and covers put back on properly after use. Accidental drownings have occurred when tubs were left uncovered.

Temperature: Hot (102°–104°F)

Effect: Thermal and mechanical

Equipment Needed: Water thermometer, tub, bath towel, bath mat

Cleanup: Clean and sanitize tub; launder towels and bath mat. Periodic maintenance should be done according to manufacturer's directions.

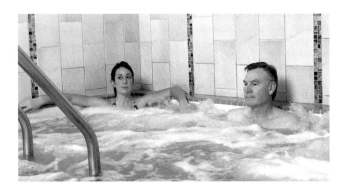

FIGURE 7-12 ■ Hot Tub.

CASE HISTORY 7-3

Client With Multiple Sclerosis

Background

Susan was a 51-year-old woman with no previous history of health problems who had just been diagnosed with **multiple sclerosis.** She had many of its typical symptoms, including extreme fatigue at times, muscle weakness, spasticity, and visual problems. However, susan had some of these symptoms for a full year before she was diagnosed.

Treatment

Even before she was diagnosed with multiple sclerosis, Susan had felt poorly for some time. She received hydrotherapy treatments and massage at a spa from Eva, a massage therapist, who tried a variety of treatment and massage combinations before finding the one that was the most relaxing and appropricite for Susan.

They began by using a soak in a jetted tub of hot water, followed by a massage. However, people with multiple sclerosis are advised to avoid sunbathing, hot showers, hot tubs, hot swimming pools, saunas, and even electric blankets because their symptoms worsen with elevations in body temperature of as little as 1°F. Just exercising on a warm day can raise their body temperature enough to exacerbate symptoms. For example Susan once had pain in her hands and feet, extreme fatigue, increased muscle spasms, and tunnel vision after a short hike on a hot day. She had not yet been diagnosed with multiple sclerosis, so her spa treatments began with a 15-minute stay in 102°F water. Soon, however, Susan realized that these soaks made her feel tired and weak, and then, trying different temperatures, she and Eva eventually found that soaking in a 97°F whirlpool for 10 minutes was relaxing and did not make her symptoms worse.

Again, guided by Susan's response, Eva and Susan also found another hydrotherapy treatment that helped meet Susan's needs. After taking the cooler soak, Eva gave Susan a salt glow using sea salt, oil of peppermint, and grapeseed oil. Eva had this combination available at the spa and felt comfortable using it because peppermint is such a common, widely used, and safe essential oil. Menthol, the main chemical in oil of peppermint, stimulates cold-sensitive receptors in the skin and gives a cooling effect.

After the cool soak, Susan's body would be frictioned, rinsed, and covered with plastic wrap, a sheet, and finally a blanket, and she would rest for 20 minutes. When uncovered, Susan was slightly warm and sweaty, but because of the peppermint oil she never felt hot, and she was very relaxed. She then took a brief shower, and finally received a Swedish massage from Eva. This combination of hydrotherapy and massage turned out to be relaxing and helpful for the emotional stress and spasticity that come with multiple sclerosis, but had unexpected benefits as well. If Susan was feeling a flare-up (temporary worsening of her symptoms) coming on, it would reduce her symptoms and shorten the length of time that she had them.

Discussion Questions

1. How did Eva, as a massage therapist, determine which treatments were effective for Susan?
2. What information relevant to hydrotherapy should be part of the medical history of someone with multiple sclerosis?

Indications: Same as for hot bath

Contraindications: Same as for hot bath, but clients with a rash or skin infection should not be in bath water that is agitated by jets, as this might spread the skin condition. While open wounds and pressure sores can be treated by a physical therapist in an individual stainless steel whirlpool that can be sterilized, jetted tubs are not suitable for this use.

Procedure
Same as for full hot bath

Spa Bathtub

Special European hydrotherapy tubs for one person may contain not only jets but specialized hoses so that a therapist can perform underwater massage. In this technique, the client lies in the warm tub while a stream of pressurized water is applied to various tissues. Underwater pressure massage may be used to promote general relaxation and to promote lymphatic drainage, but in Europe it is commonly used as a warm-down massage for athletes after hard training and for injuries such as subacute fractures, dislocations, sciatica, low back pain, joint contractures, scoliosis, and various types of paralysis.

Client With Encephalitis

Background

Kira was an 18-month-old girl who recently had a severe case of viral **encephalitis**. As a result, she was partially paralyzed on one side, with weakness in some muscles and spasticity in others. Her muscles were so contracted that she often woke in the night crying from pain. If the contractions continued, she would almost certainly develop permanent joint **contractures**.

Treatment

Jeff Bisdee, recreational therapist and Watsu practitioner, saw Kira three or four times a week for Watsu sessions. Kira floated in his arms as he manipulated and stretched her tight muscles. As can be seen in Figure 7-15, during the Watsu session Kira became profoundly relaxed, and she often fell asleep. After several sessions she began to sleep through the night. And because her muscles were not so contracted, she was no longer in danger of developing joint contractures.

Discussion Questions

1. What was the effect of Watsu on Kira's muscles?
2. What caused this effect?

These tubs are the same size as a standard one-person bathtub and can also be used for simple whole-body baths (Fig. 7-13). At this writing, they are very expensive, suitable only for high-end spas. For more information about these tubs, see *Spa Bodywork*, by Anne Williams.

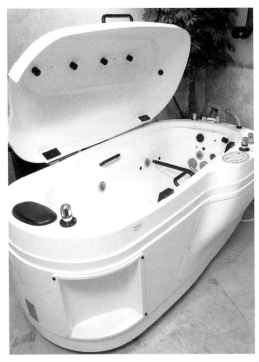

FIGURE 7-13 ■ Spa bathtub.

Stainless Steel Whole-Body Whirlpools

A whirlpool is a stainless steel bathtub containing one or more turbines which mix air with the water in the tub and can then direct jets of water to specific areas (Fig. 7-14). Pumps circulate warm or hot water, which is agitated and mixed with air; jets mounted in the body of the tub direct it against the affected area. Whirlpools are most often used in medical settings because they can be sterilized, making them suitable to treat patients with non-intact skin and problems, such as burns and pressure sores. The conditions most likely to be treated with a whirlpool are posttraumatic pain, swelling in the hands and feet, acute orthopedic trauma, acute edema, and acute muscle spasm. A 1998 study found that patients who took 15-minute whirlpool baths twice daily for the first 3 days after major abdominal surgery had significantly less postoperative pain and wound inflammation than controls. Researchers concluded that the decreased pain was due to the relaxing effect of the bath and improved movement of trapped anesthesia gases out of the intestines, and the wounds were less inflamed because of better cleansing of the incision itself.(18) Today, massage therapists are likely to encounter stainless steel whirlpools only if they work at a physical therapy clinic or athletic training facility.

Watsu

Watsu is a relatively new type of bodywork that takes place in a pool. It combines the effects of traditional Japanese shiatsu massage therapy with the buoyancy, pressure, and soothing sensation of warm water. As seen in

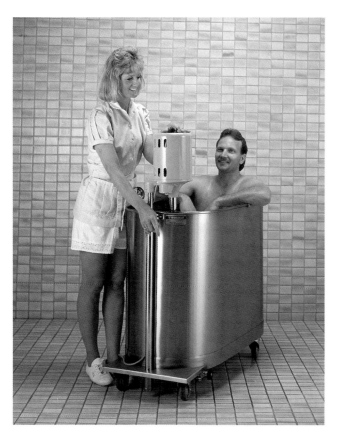

FIGURE 7-14 ■ Whole-body stainless steel whirlpool. (Photo courtesy of Whitehall Manufacturing Company, City of Industry, California.)

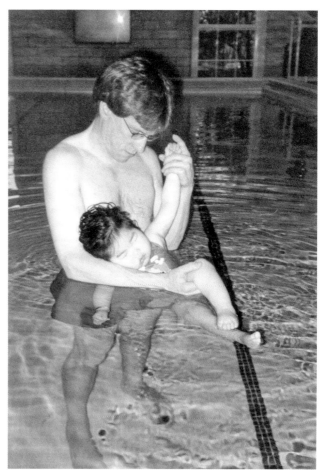

FIGURE 7-15 ■ Child receiving Watsu treatment. (Photo courtesy of Jeff Bisbee.)

Figure 7-15, the therapist stands chest deep in a swimming pool or specially made Watsu pool while the client floats in his or her arms. The therapist performs many of the techniques of shiatsu therapy, including pressure points, rocking movements, and gradual twists and stretches of different parts of the body. For best results, the water is kept at 93° to 98°F; because the receiver is barely moving and is not generating any extra body heat, this temperature means he or she will not become chilled. If the water drops below this temperature, the receiver's muscles will begin to contract and the person will not be able to relax.

Watsu is given to create deep states of relaxation, to free specific tight muscles, to increase range of motion, and to allow the spine to be moved in ways not possible on land. Neuromuscular disorders, stress-related disorders, and musculoskeletal pain may also be improved. Watsu may also bring up strong emotions elicited by the receivers being cradled in the therapist's arms. Training and certification are available for therapists who are interested in incorporating this treatment into their practice. For more information, visit the Web site www.watsuinstitute.com.

CHAPTER SUMMARY

In this chapter you have learned about a wide variety of baths that can be given for various parts of the body as well as for the entire body. Immersing one area or the entire body in hot, warm, neutral, cold, or alternating hot and cold water or in melted paraffin can have a wide variety of effects, and when therapeutic substances such as salts, oatmeal, or mustard powder are added to bath water, even more effects can be produced.

Now you can safely pick and choose water baths when they are suited to your clients' needs and your massage methods. The chapters ahead present more water treatments and you will learn even more about how to fine-tune them for you personally and for your clients.

REVIEW QUESTIONS

Short Answer

1. Name two baths that can be used to treat arthritis.

   _____

   _____

2. Name two baths that can be used for a migraine headache.

   _____

   _____

3. Explain how the additives in a detoxification bath work.

   _____

   _____

4. Give two examples of baths that can be used for insomnia.

   _____

   _____

5. Explain why baths are the most efficient way to heat or cool an area.

   _____

   _____

Fill in the Blank

6. Because they can be sterilized, stainless steel whirlpools are preferred for clients with _____ or _____ .

7. _____ baths are not used to increase local circulation in people with poor arterial circulation and diabetes.

8. A full-body contrast bath is a _____ treatment for clients who are sedentary or fragile.

9. Oatmeal baths are useful for clients with skin _____ .

10. One way to increase the effectiveness of a contrast bath is to have the client _____ .

REFERENCES

1. Zemke J et al. Intramuscular Temperature Response in the Human Leg to Two Forms of Cryotherapy: Ice Massage and Ice Bag. *J Orthop Sports Phys Ther* 1997;27:301.

2. Simons D, Travell J. *Travell and Simon's Myofascial Pain and Dysfunction: The Triggerpoint Manual*, vol 1, 2nd. ed. Baltimore: Lippincott Williams & Wilkins, 1999, pp 133, 170.

3. Karuchi K, Cajochen C, Werth E, Wirz-Justice A. Warm feet promote the rapid onset of sleep. *Nature* 1999; 401:36.

4. Ebben MR, Spielman AJ. The effects of distal limb warming on sleep latency. *Int J Behav Med* 2006; 13:221.

5. Raymann RJ, Swaab DF, Van Someren EJ. Cutaneous warming promotes sleep onset. *AM J Physiol Regul Integ Comp Physio* 2005;288:R1589. Epub 2005 Jan 27.

6. Sung, E, Tochihara Y. Effects of bathing and hot footbath on sleep in winter. *J Physiol Anthropol Appl Human Sci* 2000; 19:21.

7. Livingstone SD et al. Heat loss caused by cooling the feet. *Aviat Space Environ Med* 1995;66:232.

8. Belanger A. *Evidence-Based Guide to Therapeutic Physical Agents.* Baltimore: Lippincott Williams & Wilkins, 2002, pp 300, 369.

9. Thrash A, Thrash C. *Home Remedies: Hydrotherapy, Charcoal, and Other Simple Treatments.* Seale, AL: Thrash, 1981.

10. Fiscus KA. Changes in lower-leg blood flow during warm-, cold-, and contrast-water therapy. *Arch Phys Med Rehabil* 2005;86:1404.

11. Horay P, Harp D. *Hot Water Therapy.* Oakland, CA: New Harbinger, 1991.

12. Miwa C et al. Human cardiovascular responses to a 60 minute bath at 40°C. *Environ Med* 1994;38:77.

13. Vie K et al. Modulating effects of oatmeal extracts in the sodium lauryl sulfate skin irritancy model. *Skin Pharmacol Appl Skin Physiol* 2002;15:120.

14. Sakula A. Doctor Nehemiah Grew (1641–1712) and the Epsom salt. *Clio Med* 1984;19:1.

15. Childs PE. History of Epsom salt. *Chemistry in Action* 1993;40(summer):25.

16. Azaria E et al. Magnesium sulfate in obstetrics: current data. *J Gynecol Obstet Bio Reprod,* 2004;33:510.

17. Proksch E et al. Bathing in a magnesium-rich Dead Sea salt solution improves skin barrier function, enhances skin hydration, and reduces inflammation in atopic dry skin. *Int J Dermatol* 2005;44:151.

18. Meeker J. Whirlpool therapy on post operative pain and surgical wound healing: an exploration. *Patient Education and Counseling* 33(1998)39.

HOT AIR BATHS

I was without hope before I began detoxification. . . . until just a few weeks ago I was suffering. It is going to take hard work, but I believe I will be able to regain the ability to fly. The biggest obstacle, the one I saw no way to overcome, is now behind me. . . to say that my doctors have been amazed by the [sauna treatment] results is putting it mildly.

—*Helicopter pilot Sean Donahue, testimony before the New York City Council, February 2004*

Chapter Objectives

After completing this chapter, the student will be able to:

- Describe the effects of various hot air baths.
- Explain the contraindications to various hot air baths.
- Name and describe the various hot air baths.
- Describe a variety of applications for hot air baths.
- Give hot air baths using the procedure included with each treatment.

Hot air baths—stays in specially designed heated rooms filled with either dry air (saunas) or moisture-filled air (steam baths)—are another ancient and popular hydrotherapy treatment that may be used to advantage by massage therapists. After taking a sauna or steam bath of any kind, clients are comfortably warm and not likely to become chilled when receiving a massage. Their joint and muscle pain is reduced; their muscles are warm, relaxed, and pliable; and they feel mentally relaxed. Both dry and wet hot air baths are excellent for insomnia. After receiving a massage, a stay in a sauna or steam bath leaves clients even more relaxed, warmed to the core, and cleansed of all oil or lotions left on the skin from the massage. Saunas and steam baths may be combined with some of the other hydrotherapy treatments you have learned; for example, in Chapter 14 you will learn how to combine a sauna or steam bath with a local application of heat to treat an acute lower back spasm.

Some advantages to using hot air baths to warm clients:

- They require little labor. Unlike body wraps or other applications of moist heat that cover much of the body, hot air baths can be turned on with just a flip of a switch.
- They require little or no supervision. The client can be taking a sauna or steam bath either before or after a massage while the massage therapist is working with another client.
- They are preferred by some clients, who truly enjoy the sensation of sweating in hot air rather than sweating in a hot bath or body wrap.
- Hot air baths can also be used to administer therapeutic substances such as herbs and essential oils.

In the past, because they were more expensive and elaborate than many local hydrotherapy treatments, hot air baths were used almost exclusively by massage therapists who worked at athletic clubs or spas. Today, however, advances in technology are making them less expensive and more accessible to the massage therapist in private practice. This chapter discusses the uses and effects of hot air baths, including a classic local hot air bath, steam inhalation. We also discuss when the massage therapist will find hot air baths superior to other hydrotherapy treatments.

DRY HOT AIR BATH: THE SAUNA

A sauna is a cabinet, room, or other enclosure where room air can be heated to a high temperature. In the past, saunas have been constructed of materials as diverse as sod, stone, brick, metal, volcanic rock, wood, tent cloth, and heavy-duty plastic. They have been heated with energy sources as diverse as firewood, gas, electric light bulbs, electric heaters, and infrared heaters. **Turkish baths** are taken in large stone buildings. Today, however, most saunas are modeled after the classic Finnish sauna, which consists of a small room lined with wood and containing benches and a wood-burning, gas, electric, or infrared heater (Fig. 8-1). Soft aromatic woods such as cedar, redwood, or white spruce are used because they are porous—so they can readily absorb and eliminate moisture—and they stay cool to the touch.

Taking a sauna involves going into the heated room and remaining there for some minutes to absorb the heat through the hot dry air. Sauna temperatures can range from 145° to 200°F, with the average temperature being about 160°F. Sauna air is kept very dry, about 6% to 8% humidity, which is very different from the 100% humidity in a steam room. Intake and outlet vents that circulate hot air help to keep the humidity low. (Otherwise, the water released into the air by the bather's sweat would make the air less dry.) When the air is very dry, the human body can tolerate high temperatures because sweat evaporates almost immediately, and this produces an instant cooling effect. (In traditional Finnish saunas, dippers of water may occasionally be poured over stones lying on the stove. This produces steam, and a wave of heat and humidity rolls onto the bather. If the sauna is hot enough, however, this steam disappears into the air almost immediately.)

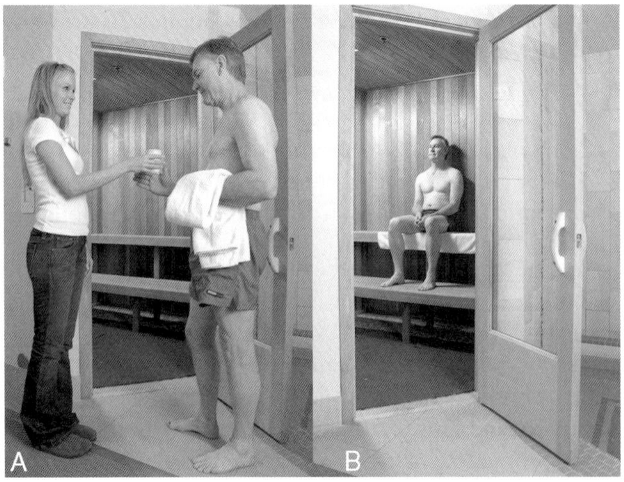

FIGURE 8-1 ■ Sauna. **A.** Therapist offering water to the client as he enters the sauna. **B.** Client seated in sauna.

Because it raises the client's core temperature, taking a sauna has the same physiological effects as other whole-body heat treatments, such as heating body wraps, steam baths, and full-body hot baths. As core temperature rises, the client experiences peripheral vasodilation, increased sweating, increased oxygen consumption, and relaxation of skeletal muscles. At the same time his or her heart beats faster and pumps out more blood with each beat. One study found that cardiac output of sauna takers increased by 60% to 70%, about as much as during a brisk walk, with blood being shifted from the internal organs to the skin. 50% to 70% of all blood pumped by the heart flowed to skin blood vessels.(1)

Levels of noradrenaline double after 10 minutes in a sauna and remain elevated after a cold plunge and a 15-minute rest. Heat to the entire body causes a brief rise in blood pressure, which is then followed by a fall in blood pressure as a result of vasodilation. Blood pressure remains lower for at least an hour after a sauna. In one study, the systolic blood pressure of hypertensive subjects was lowered about 35 mm Hg.(2) If the sauna is very hot, the blood pressure will stay high longer, and the heart rate will be even higher than in a moderate sauna. Just how high the client's body temperature will rise depends upon how hot the sauna is, how dry the sauna is, the client's sweating capacity, and how long he or she remains in the sauna. The core temperature may rise high enough that the healthy sauna bather goes directly from the sauna and takes a cold shower, jumps into a cold plunge, or rolls in the snow with no ill effects from the sudden change of 100°F or more. At the South Pole, where temperatures can be extremely cold, the "300°F club" has been formed by hardy souls who are able to run with only their boots on from a 200°F sauna to the pole itself, where the outside temperature is minus 100°F! At any other time, exposure to such extreme cold could be deadly, but the extreme heat of their sauna heats the body's tissues so well that they are not damaged during the short cold exposure.

Many wholistically oriented doctors recommend intense body heating at the onset of a viral infection to abort the illness or greatly reduce its severity. The heat, like that of a natural fever, is believed to weaken or kill the infectious organism. A 1990 study found that individuals who regularly took saunas had significantly fewer colds than those who did not.(3)

During a sauna, the body's metabolic rate increases 12% to 40% and then falls to slightly lower than it was before the sauna, which is why very frequent saunas or other whole-body heating treatments are not recommended for someone with a hypothyroid condition, in which the metabolic rate is already too low. (An occasional sauna is fine, however.) Because saunas can cause profuse sweating, dehydration can occur if extra water is not taken in. Competitive wrestlers are notorious for using saunas to sweat out water in order to lose enough weight to compete in a lower weight class. By cutting back on water drinking and then going into a sauna while wearing many layers of clothes, then exercising in the heat, a wrestler can lose as much as 6 pounds (3 quarts) of water in several hours. However, this practice is dangerous, and occasionally a wrestler actually dies of dehydration. On the other hand, in diseases that cause fluid overload, such as certain kidney diseases, saunas have been used therapeutically to help the body lose water.(4) In any event, therapists should be sure to encourage their clients to drink water before, during, and after a sauna to prevent dehydration. Persons who sweat frequently, either by being in hot environments or by exercising regularly, tend to sweat more profusely, and regular saunas will encourage this as well. But if your client is not accustomed to intense heat, he or she should be especially careful not to stay in too long.

Saunas have been used for detoxification for centuries, because heat mobilizes toxic substances that are dissolved in fatty tissues so they go back into the bloodstream, where they may leave the body via sweat or travel to the liver to be detoxified. For more on saunas and detoxification, see Case History 8-1 and Chapter 12.

The following are some directions to give your client before entering the sauna:

- Do not eat for at least an hour before you go in the sauna.
- After vigorous exercise, wait a few minutes before you go in to let your body cool down.
- Drink a glass of water before entering the sauna and another glass or two more during and after the sauna.
- Stay in for 10 to 15 minutes, until you are perspiring freely, but do not stay too long. As with a very hot bath, when you have been in too long, you may get lightheaded or dizzy—people have been known to pass out! Leave the sauna immediately if you begin to feel that you are not tolerating the heat well.
- Finish your sauna experience with a shower as cold as you can tolerate it and drink a final glass of water.

Air Temperature: Hot (145°–200°F) with 6% to 8% humidity

Time Needed: 10 to 15 minutes in the sauna plus a few minutes for a cool shower after the sauna (client may do more than one cycle)

Equipment Needed: Air thermometer, two bath towels, drinking water

Effect: Primarily thermal

Cleanup: Launder used towels. The sauna should be cleaned and sanitized periodically according to manufacturer's recommendations.

Indications: General relaxation, warming of tissue prior to massage, stimulation of circulation, muscle spasms in neck or back, arthritis pain, pain and joint stiffness in rheumatic disease, preparation for cold treatments, detoxification, onset of common cold or flu

Contraindications: Systemic or chronic conditions including cardiovascular problems, diabetes, hepatitis, lymphedema, multiple sclerosis, and seizure disorders. (These contraindications are the same as for any whole-body heating treatment.) Loss of sensation, great obesity, pregnancy, recent meal (wait at least an hour after eating), inability to tolerate heat, client who is under the influence of alcohol or drugs. (Deaths have occurred when alcohol and saunas were combined, usually because the intoxicated person lost consciousness in the sauna and then died of dehydration.)(5)

Sauna manufacturers usually install a sign on the doors stating that persons in poor health should consult their doctor before taking a sauna. Such a sign can serve as a visual reminder to the client and a reinforcement of the contraindications.

Cautions
1. Occasionally clients experience intense itching in a sauna, in which case they need only exit the sauna and the sensation will stop.
2. Very frequent saunas are not recommended for those with hypothyroid conditions.
3. Anyone who is at risk for lymphedema due to removal of lymph nodes should avoid prolonged (more than 15 minutes) or very hot saunas.

Procedure
1. Check with client to make sure there are no contraindications to the sauna.
2. Explain the use of the sauna to the client and get his or her consent.
3. Turn on the sauna. It may take 15 minutes for a completely cooled sauna to warm up. In an athletic club or spa, however, many saunas are left on all the time.
4. Have the client take a brief shower before entering the sauna.
5. Offer a glass of water before the client enters the sauna (Fig. 8-1A).
6. Have the client enter and stay seated for about 10 to 15 minutes (Fig. 8-1B) until he or she begins to perspire or feel too warm. Have the client exit the sauna immediately if he or she starts to feel dizzy, lightheaded, fatigued, or too hot, or when his or her heart is beating too fast. In other words, anytime the heat begins to be too extreme, it is time to get out of the sauna.

(continued)

CASE HISTORY 8-1

Rescue Worker Benefits From Sauna Treatments

Background

In 2001, 33-year-old Sean Donahue (real name used with permission) was a captain in the New York State National Guard. Sean, a Blackhawk helicopter pilot, was a healthy, highly conditioned athlete who worked as a computer consultant in lower Manhattan. On September 11, 2001, he was working just one block from the World Trade Center when he heard of the catastrophe. He hurried there, arriving just as the building's towers went down. He spent the rest of that day and the next performing search and rescue at the site, engulfed in deep smoke and airborne soot made up of such toxic substances as burning jet and diesel fuel, asbestos, benzene, dioxins, mercury, lead, manganese, polychlorinated biphenyls (PCBs), fiberglass, silicon, and sulfuric acid. He wore no special protective clothing except a simple dust mask some of the time. He began to have breathing difficulties on that first day but continued with the rescue work for 2 full days. He then returned to his work as a computer consultant. As he walked many blocks every day to his job, he continued to breathe in highly toxic materials from the cloud of tiny particles that had settled over lower Manhattan. Even the air inside his office was foul with soot.

On September 16, severe respiratory distress forced him to visit a local hospital, where he had to be intubated or he would have died. Sean gradually developed a variety of health problems, including shortness of breath, chronic cough (the most common health complaint of rescue personnel), sinus pain, severe stomach and chest pain, chronic nausea, vomiting, diarrhea, skin rashes, flashbacks, and inability to concentrate. Finally, in March 2003 (18 months after his initial exposure), Donahue had a physical and was found unfit to pilot an aircraft. By January 2004, he was taking 10 medications without any noticeable improvement and was considering taking whole-body steroids as a last resort. Concerned about side effects, however, he opted to begin the program offered by the New York City Rescue Workers Detoxification Project.

Treatment

Designed to help rescue workers (including police, fire, and medical personnel) excrete the toxins they absorbed, the detoxification program combined prolonged sweating in a sauna with nutritional supplements that support detoxification. For 33 days, Sean followed the same routine: vigorous exercise followed by a 140° to 180°F sauna bath for 2 to 5 hours, with frequent breaks to shower and rehydrate. (Detox personnel monitored all participants for heat exhaustion and dehydration.) At first, he felt no major difference. Although he never observed any highly colored sweat (many rescue workers have had purple, orange, gray, blue, or black sweat), he did notice that his sweat had a very strong odor. Then, after 8 or 9 days on the program, he noticed a dramatic improvement in how he felt. His symptoms slowly began to decrease, and although at the beginning of the detoxification he could not even walk up a flight of stairs, a few weeks later he could run 3 miles. His chronic cough disappeared, and he was able to discontinue his medications. (S. Donahue, personal communication, October 10, 2006.) Nothing else about Donahue's medical treatment changed during the detoxification program.

Today, Sean has not only returned to active duty, he has no health problems, takes no medications, runs miles every day, and is again approved to pilot aircraft. He has gone on to serve in combat zones in Afghanistan and Iraq and to assist in the recovery efforts in New Orleans after Hurricane Katrina.

References

1. Cecchini M, Root D, Rachunow J, Gelb P. Chemical exposures at the World Trade Center: Use of the Hubbard sauna detoxification regimen to improve the health status of New York City rescue workers exposed to toxicants. *Townsend Letter for Doctors and Patients*, 2006;April:58.
2. Donahue S. Testimony before New York City Council, found on Web site of New York City Rescue Workers Detoxification Project. www.nydetox.org/results3.htm. Accessed November 2006.
3. Root D. Downtown Medical: A detox program for World Trade Center responders. *Fire Engineering* 2003;June:12.

7. Have the client leave the sauna and take a tepid or cool shower. A rest can be taken in the cooler air outside the sauna for a few minutes if desired. The purpose of the shower is to cool down in between sauna sessions. If the client is not willing to take a cold shower or plunge, use the coolest water that he or she can tolerate.

8. At that point, if the client desires, he or she may go back to the sauna for another cycle of sweating and cooling. The perspiration and cooling may be repeated for a number of cycles, depending upon the bather's tolerance. However, 15 minutes is long enough to prepare the person for a massage session.

9. After the last stay in the sauna, have the client take a cool shower and dress in street clothes if the sauna was after a massage or in a bathrobe if he or she is now going to receive a massage. He or she should also drink a glass of water and rest for a few minutes.

WET HOT AIR BATHS: LOCAL AND WHOLE-BODY STEAM TREATMENTS

Like saunas, steam baths have such a strong appeal that they have been used in many different parts of the world and have been made of a variety of materials, including volcanic rock, wood, tile, and heavy-duty plastic. Water to make steam has been boiled with wood, gas, and electricity. In both partial-body and full-body treatments, hot, moist air coats and heats the skin.

LOCAL STEAM BATHS

Although local steam treatments are rarely used today except to treat the respiratory tract, they were common in the days of the water cure. For example, Sebastian Kneipp prescribed local steam to the feet for swollen or cold feet, eczema, or some foot diseases, and John Harvey Kellogg used a jet of steam to control local bleeding. (Very hot water can stop capillary ooze into tissues.) Medicinal herbs were sometimes added to the water that was boiled to make the steam.

One local steam bath that is still widely used is steam inhalation. An ancient remedy for nasal and chest congestion, inhaling small particles of hot water adds water to nasal mucus, liquifying it so that it drips out easily, and can have the same affect with congestion in the chest.(6) Steam inhalation moistens, soothes, and warms the respiratory tract, including the throat, and causes dilation of local blood vessels. Traditionally, many anti-inflammatory and antiseptic herbs have been added to the water that was boiled to make steam, and some essential oils have been used to open nasal passages and discourage bacterial

growth. For more on the use of steam for sinus problems, see *Sinus Survival* by Robert Ivker, MD. A traditional way to inhale steam is to boil water, pour it into a large heavy bowl, place the bowl on a tabletop, then sit over the bowl with a towel draped over the head so that the steam cannot escape. Steam is inhaled into through the nose and mouth, pulling hot, moist air into the nasal passages and bronchial tree. (Steaming the face with steam machines is common practice for aestheticians, who use it to warm and moisten the skin and open the pores before facials.)

Massage therapists do not treat the common cold; during a massage session, however, local steam treatments can ease "cradle congestion," a fullness in the sinuses and puffiness in the face that can occur when clients lie prone for an extended period. Clients with allergies or sinus headaches often find lying prone uncomfortable, and breathing steam can make them far more comfortable in this position. To add steam to the face during a massage, simply place a small steam vaporizer on a low table directly underneath the face cradle. When it is turned on, it emits a fine stream of steam that wafts up the inside of the cradle to the middle of the client's face. This may cause the client's nose to drip, so be sure to provide facial tissues.

Air Temperature: Hot (140°F) with 100% humidity

Time Needed: 10 to 15 minutes, while the client is receiving a massage in the prone position

Equipment Needed: Small steam unit, low table to place steam unit on, disposable tissues, two face towels (one to be placed underneath the small steam unit and one for the face cradle), wastebasket for used tissues

Effect: Primarily thermal

Cleanup: Have the client place used tissues in the wastebasket. The steam unit should be cleaned and sanitized periodically according to manufacturer's recommendations. Launder used face towels.

Indications: Sinus congestion and facial puffiness caused by lying prone on a massage table, sinus congestion from allergies or subacute stage of a cold, sinus headache

Contraindications: Congestive heart failure

Cautions: Some persons with asthma may be uncomfortable breathing hot moist air.

Procedure
1. Check with client to make sure there are no contraindications to the steam unit.
2. Explain the use of the steam unit to the client and get his or her consent.
3. Place a low table under the face cradle and cover it with a towel.

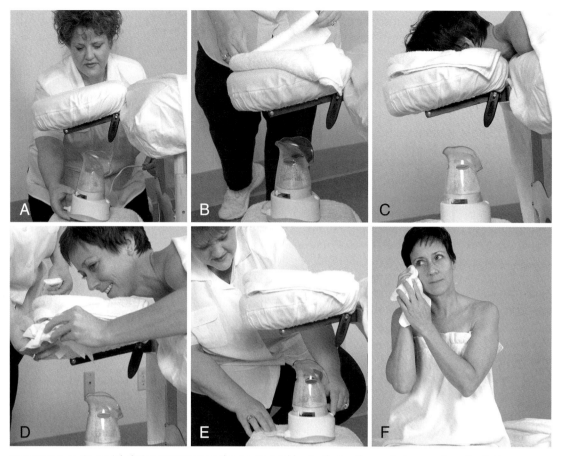

FIGURE 8-2 ■ Steam inhalation treatment on the massage table. **A.** Placing the small steam unit on the table underneath the face cradle. **B.** Placing the face towel over the face cradle. **C.** The client prone upon the table with face in the face cradle. **D.** Giving disposable tissues to the client. **E.** Turning on the steam unit. **F.** Client wiping her face with the face towel.

4. Place the small steam unit on the table under the face cradle (Fig. 8-2A).
5. Place the face towel over the face cradle (Fig. 8-2B).
6. Have the client lie prone upon the table with face in the face cradle (Fig. 8-2C).
7. Give disposable tissues to the client (Fig. 8-2D). Have a wastebasket available.
8. Turn on the steam unit (Fig. 8-2E).

At the conclusion of the treatment, have the client sit up and dry her face with the face towel (Fig. 8-2F).

WHOLE-BODY STEAM BATHS

A steam bath is a cabinet, room, or small structure which is designed to hold hot moist air and one or more bathers. Taking a steam bath involves going into the preheated enclosure and remaining there for some minutes, absorbing heat through the hot wet air. Unlike a liquid bath, in which the client is immersed in water, instead the client's skin becomes coated with hot water.

In the past, steam baths have been constructed of materials as diverse as blankets, animal skins, sheets of plastic, wood, and brick. Steam has been made using natural hot springs, firewood, gas, and electricity. Modern steam baths, whether rooms or small cabinets of different types, usually have electric steam generators outside of the bath. These generators make steam, which is injected into the enclosure.

The temperature in a steam bath ranges from 105° to 130°F, and the humidity is 100%. This is the real difference between the steam bath and the sauna, where temperatures are much hotter (145°–200°F) and the humidity is only 6% to 8%. The steam bath is at a lower temperature. Since steam bathers' skin is already wet, the normal cooling effect of sweat does not take place, and air as hot as that of the sauna would be much harder to tolerate.

Both the benefits and the dangers of any other whole-body heating treatment apply here. The contraindications to steam treatments are almost exactly the same as those for hot baths, saunas, and even heating body wraps.

Steam baths are excellent for relieving many kinds of musculoskeletal pain. Many long-time hydrotherapists believe that our muscles become more relaxed with steam than with any other type of heat, because moist heat penetrates deeper into the tissues and so heats them more effectively. The whole-body steam bath has an effect on the skeletal muscles similar to that of having moist hot packs applied all over the body. Louella Doub, a Seventh-Day Adventist nurse and chiropractor, used steam room treatments for more than 50 years to treat a wide variety of musculoskeletal and other types of ailments. She found that "perfect relaxation" of the muscles through the use of steam was a great aid to both massage and manipulative treatments.(7)

You may wonder why a massage therapist would choose to use a steam bath with a client rather than a sauna. In certain situations, steam baths may be preferable. Steam baths will bring the core temperature up more quickly than a sauna, since the cooling effect of sweating is not possible, and so they may be used if treatment time is at a premium. Another reason to pick a steam treatment over a sauna is when you feel moist heat is preferable to dry heat. You may want to use a steam treatment when herbal tea is used instead of water to administer herbs through the skin. Finally, some clients simply prefer the sensation of a steam bath over that of a sauna. Steam treatments may also be more practical for many massage therapists. Generally, they cost less than saunas and take up less space. With some types of steam treatments, such as a steam canopy, the client may be quickly washed with a warm wet towel, then dried with a dry towel and massage can proceed right away. Clients need to use a shower during and after a sauna, so both the expense and need for extra office space is substantially less with a steam canopy.

Head-Out Steam Baths

Steam canopies or cabinets, which treat the entire body except the head, are well suited for clients who enjoy steam heat but dislike breathing hot, moist air. Many versions of steam cabinets are being manufactured, from canopies that fit over a massage table to boxlike cabinets in which the client sits upright. Each one leaves the client's head out but steams the rest of the body. (Another head-out steam treatment can be performed with the hydrotherapy tub pictured in Figure 7-13. This tub contains a plate which can be fitted over the bottom of the tub. The client lies supine on the plate, the lid comes down and covers all but the head, and steam comes up through vents at the bottom of the tub.) A classic head-out steam bath that is seldom found anymore is a **Russian steam bath,** a tiled room with a circular hole in one wall. The client lies on a tiled bench inside the room, and the entire body is steamed except the head, which protrudes out of the hole.

Steam Canopy

A **steam canopy** suspended over a supine client is one way to give a steam bath for the entire body except the head (Fig. 8-3). The water-resistant canopy fabric is stretched over a wooden framework. During a session, the canopy is placed over the client, who is lying supine on a massage table, and covers the body from the feet to the head, leaving the head protruding from one end. At the foot of the table, a pot of simmering water produces steam, which rises into and fills the canopy within 2 minutes. (Herbal teas may also be used.) The client can be completely or partially undressed. To speed up heating or to retain heat longer, a thermal blanket may be laid over the canopy. The air temperature inside the canopy can rise as high as 130°F. Exposure to the hot, wet air, if prolonged, will have the same effects as any whole-body heat treatment as the client's core temperature rises above 98.6°F.

Because it is given directly on a massage table, a treatment with a steam canopy is perhaps the simplest

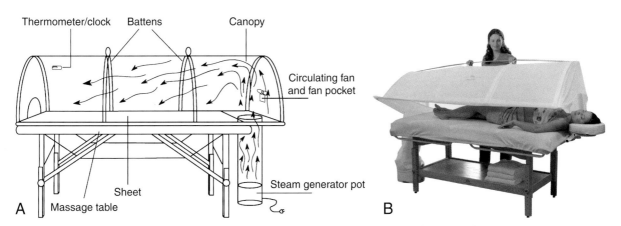

FIGURE 8-3 ■ Steam canopy. **A.** View inside steam canopy. **B.** Client receiving treatment. (Courtesy of Natural Health Technologies, Fairfield, Iowa.)

whole-body steam bath for before or after a massage, since the client does not have to leave the table. It may also be preferred by the massage therapist because it is far less expensive than most steam treatments and it uses little electricity and only a few cups of water.

Air Temperature: Hot (110–130°F with 100% humidity)

Time Needed: 15 to 20 minutes

Equipment Needed: Air thermometer, steam canopy, pot of water to make steam, sheets and one towel to cover the massage table, two additional towels to wash and dry client at the end of the steam bath

Effect: Primarily thermal

Cleanup: The inside of the canopy should be sprayed with a natural cleanser recommended by the manufacturer, then stood on end with a clean towel underneath it to air dry. It must be completely dry before the next use. Also launder used sheets and towels.

Indications: General relaxation; warming of tissue prior to massage; stimulation of circulation; muscle spasms in neck or back; musculoskeletal pain; pain of gout, osteoarthritis, rheumatoid arthritis, or sciatica; acute or chronic low back pain; sprains and fracture sites after a cast has been removed; preparation for cold treatments; onset of common cold or flu

Contraindications: Systemic or chronic conditions, including cardiovascular problems, diabetes if the steam bath is prolonged, hepatitis, lymphedema, multiple sclerosis, and seizure disorders. (These contraindications are the same as for any whole-body heat treatment.) Loss of sensation, great obesity, pregnancy, recent meal (wait at least an hour after eating), inability to tolerate heat, client under the influence of alcohol or drugs

Cautions
1. Very frequent steam baths are not recommended for persons with hypothyroid conditions.
2. Anyone who is at risk for lymphedema due to removal of lymph nodes should avoid prolonged (more than 15 minutes) or very hot steam baths.

Procedure
1. Check with client to make sure there are no contraindications to the steam canopy.
2. Explain the use of the steam canopy to the client and get his or her consent.
3. Cover the massage table with massage sheets and a large towel, and put the face cradle in place. Put water in the steam generator pot. Herbal tea may be used in place of water.
4. Offer water to the client just before he or she lies on the table.
5. Have the client lie on the towel-covered massage table, nude or wearing a bathing suit.

6. Place the steam canopy over the client with the head projecting through the open end.
7. Wrap a towel around the neck to keep steam from escaping and to ensure the client's skin does not touch the canopy.
8. Turn on the steam generator pot.
9. Have the client remain in the steam bath for 10 to 20 minutes.
10. Place a cold compress on the client's forehead when he or she begins to sweat.
11. Remove the canopy and quickly wash the client off with a warm wet towel, then dry the skin with a dry towel. Work quickly so that there is no chilling.
12. The towel underneath the client will be damp and should be removed. Have the client roll onto one side, bunch the towel up against his or her back, and then have the client roll onto the other side over the bunched-up sheet. Then you may easily gather it up and remove it (see Fig. 10-3, steps N–P). Or the client may stand up while you remove the towel, then lie back upon the table.
13. Cover the client with a dry sheet.
14. Offer water.
15. The massage session may now begin.

Variation
Steam canopy for a diabetic client. A short stay under a steam canopy—10 minutes or less—is acceptable for diabetics, as it will not significantly raise core temperature.

Steam Cabinet
A steam cabinet is a small box with a door. It contains a seat for the client, a hole for the head to protrude, and a port through which steam enters. (Fig. 8-4). The cabinet walls keeps steam from escaping so it surrounds the body except for the head.

Air Temperature: Hot (110°–130°F with 100% humidity)

Time Needed: 10 to 20 minutes

Equipment Needed: Steam cabinet; three towels to use on the seat, floor, and head opening of the cabinet; washcloth for cold compress; two additional towels to wash and dry client at the end of the steam bath; drinking water

Effect: Primarily thermal

Cleanup: Wipe down the walls of cabinet with a natural cleanser recommended by the manufacturer, then dry them. Launder washcloth and towels.

Indications: General relaxation; warming of tissue prior to massage; stimulation of circulation; muscle spasms

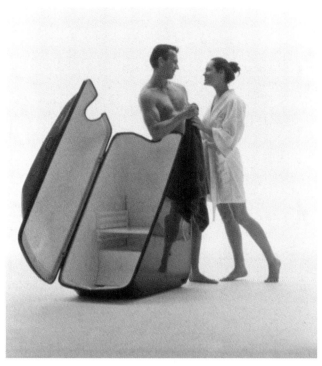

FIGURE 8-4 ■ Steam cabinet. (Courtesy of Steam Embrace, Inc., Oxnard, CA.)

in neck or back; musculoskeletal pain; pain of gout, osteoarthritis, rheumatoid arthritis, sciatica; acute or chronic low back pain; sprains and fracture sites after a cast has been removed; preparation for cold treatments; onset of common cold of flu

Contraindications: Systemic or chronic conditions, including cardiovascular problems, diabetes, hepatitis, lymphedema, multiple sclerosis, and seizure disorders (the same as for any whole-body heat treatment); loss of sensation; great obesity; pregnancy; recent meal (wait at least an hour after eating); inability to tolerate heat; client under the influence of alcohol or drugs

Cautions
1. Very frequent steam baths are not recommended for persons with hypothyroid conditions.
2. Anyone who is at risk for lymphedema due to removal of lymph nodes should avoid prolonged (more than 15 minutes) or very hot steam baths.

Procedure
1. Check with client to make sure there are no contraindications to the steam cabinet.
2. Explain the use of the steam cabinet to the client and get his or her consent.
3. Place water in the steam generator pot. Herbal teas may be used in place of water if desired, or essential oils may be added to the water.
4. Place towels on the seat itself, over the front of the seat so that steam will not burn the back of the legs, and on the floor where the client's feet will rest.
5. Offer water to the client just before he or she enters the cabinet.
6. Have the undressed or partially dressed client sit on the cabinet seat. Assist if needed.
7. Wrap a towel around the client's neck to keep steam from escaping and to ensure that the client's skin does not touch the sides or opening of the cabinet.
8. Have the client remain in the steam bath for 10 to 20 minutes.
9. Place a cold compress on the client's forehead when he or she begins to sweat.
10. After 10 to 20 minutes, assist the client out of the steam cabinet. Now wash the client with a warm wet towel, then dry the skin with a dry towel. Work quickly so that there is no chilling. A warm shower can be taken if one is available.
11. Have the client lie on the massage table and cover him or her with a dry sheet.
12. Offer water to the client.
13. The massage session may now begin.

Steam Room

Steam rooms are enclosed rooms with a port through which steam can enter. Unlike steam canopies or cabinets, steam surrounds the entire body and allows the client to breathe hot, humid air, as opposed to the steam cabinet, in which the person is breathing unheated room air. Thus, a steam room is better suited to someone who enjoys breathing warm moist air. Essential oils of eucalyptus or peppermint are sometimes added to steam rooms to help people with respiratory problems, such as the common cold or bronchitis, and these are, of course, not possible with head-out steam treatments.

The walls and benches of a traditional steam room are lined with ceramic tile (Fig. 8-5B). Newer steam rooms are being constructed in a variety of styles and of many different materials. For example, many newer steam baths are constructed of molded acrylic and include a built-in seat and a shower. Others, marketed as "steam capsules," have clear plastic walls with a plastic chair inside. Most have electric steam generators that make steam and inject it through a vent into the room. Many types have tiny ports for essential oils. Any bathroom may be turned into a steam room: simply turn on the shower full force with hot water and either sit in a bath chair in the shower stall or in a very small bathroom, sit on the toilet seat. Stay for about 15 minutes. (Many parents have been advised by their family doctor to use this treatment with small children who have respiratory problems.) Excess moisture in the bathroom may encourage mold, however.

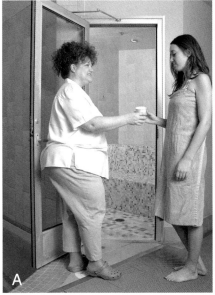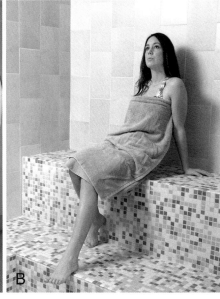

FIGURE 8-5 ■ Steam bath. **A.** Therapist offering water to the client as she enters the steam bath. **B.** Client seated in steam bath.

Below are some directions to give your clients before the steam room treatment:

■ Do not eat for at least an hour before you go in the steam bath.
■ Wait a few minutes after vigorous exercise before you go in to let your body cool down.
■ Drink a glass of water before the steam bath and a glass or two more during and after.
■ Be aware that wet tiled surfaces can be slippery. Take a towel into the steam room and sit on it. Then, when you are ready to get out of the steam room, move slowly.
■ Stay in for 10 to 20 minutes, until you are perspiring freely, but do not overdo it. As with a very hot bath, when you have been in too long, you may get light-headed or dizzy—people have been known to pass out!
■ Finish your steam bath with a cool or cold shower and another glass of water.

Air Temperature: Hot (105°–130°F with 100% humidity)

Time Needed: 10 to 20 minutes, depending upon the client's tolerance

Equipment Needed: Air thermometer, bath towel, steam room, drinking water

Effect: Primarily thermal

Cleanup: Must be cleaned periodically according to manufacturer's instructions. Public steam baths are usually cleaned with a cleanser recommended by the manufacturer, then sanitized at the end of each day. Also launder used linens.

Indications: General relaxation; warming of tissue prior to massage; stimulation of circulation; muscle spasms in neck or back; musculoskeletal pain, including pain of gout, osteoarthritis, rheumatoid arthritis, sciatica, acute or chronic low back pain; sprains and fracture sites after a cast has been removed; preparation for cold treatments; onset of common cold or flu

Contraindications: Systemic or chronic conditions, including cardiovascular problems, diabetes, hepatitis, lymphedema, multiple sclerosis, and seizure disorders (the same as for any whole-body heat treatment); loss of sensation; great obesity; pregnancy; recent meal (wait at least an hour after eating); inability to tolerate heat; client under the influence of alcohol or drugs

Cautions
1. Some persons with asthma may be uncomfortable breathing hot, moist air.
2. Very frequent steam baths are not recommended for those with hypothyroid conditions.
3. Anyone who is at risk for lymphedema due to removal of lymph nodes should avoid prolonged (more than 15 minutes) or very hot steam baths.

Procedure
1. Check with client to make sure there are no contraindications to the steam room bath.
2. Explain the use of the steam room bath to the client and get his or her consent.
3. Turn on the steam generator.
4. Have the client take a brief warm shower.
5. Offer the client water to drink just before entering the steam room bath (Fig. 8-5A).
6. Have the client enter the steam bath and remain for 10 to 20 minutes or as long as it is tolerable (Fig. 8-5B).

CHAPTER 8 ■ Hot Air Baths **165**

7. Have the client exit the steam bath and take a cool or cold shower to bring the body temperature down and give a feeling of invigoration.
8. The client may repeat the steam bath–shower cycle if desired.
9. Offer water to the client.
10. Have the client rest following the treatments, perhaps by lying down on the massage table if a massage session is planned.

CHAPTER SUMMARY

Hot air baths are an ancient and popular hydrotherapy treatment that massage therapists may use to advantage. You can use them to keep your clients comfortable, help them relax, and prepare their tissues for massage techniques. As you learn these hydrotherapy treatments in addition to those you have learned in earlier chapters and can begin to combine treatments, your ability to tailor sessions to many situations will continue to expand.

REVIEW QUESTIONS

Short Answer

1. What is the main difference between saunas and steam baths?

2. How does the body respond differently to each?

3. How is blood pressure affected by a sauna?

4. Explain the local effects of steam inhalation.

5. Why is congestive heart failure a contraindication to steam inhalation?

Multiple Choice

6. All but one of these uses steam:
   a. Canopy
   b. Russian bath
   c. Scotch hose
   d. Cabinet

7. All but one of the following can occur when a person is in a sauna too long:
   a. Profuse sweating
   b. Body cooling
   c. More concentrated blood
   d. Exhaustion

8. All but one is a chemical application:
   a. Medicinal herbs in local steam treatments
   b. Soft aromatic woods of sauna wall
   c. Essential oils of eucalyptus and peppermint in steam room
   d. Herbal teas in steam generator pot of steam canopy

9. Sweating can cause all but one:
   a. Dehydration
   b. Release of toxins
   c. Loss of fat
   d. Loss of electrolytes

10. All but one are contraindications to whole-body heat treatments:
    a. Pregnancy
    b. Muscle spasms in neck or back
    c. Cardiovascular problems
    d. Client under the influence of alcohol of drugs

REFERENCES

1. Husse E. Plasma catecholamines in Finnish sauna. *Ann Clin Res* 1977;9:301.
2. Hannuksela ML, Ellahham S. Benefits and risks of sauna bathing. *Am J Med* 2001;110:118.
3. Ernst E, Pecho E, Wirz P, Saradeth T. Regular sauna bathing and the incidence of common colds. *Ann Med* 1990;22:225.
4. Pyrih LA et al. Infrared sweat secretion stimulation as a means of homeostatic correction in patients with kidney dysfunction. *Fiziol Zh* 2003;49:25.
5. Press E. The health hazards of saunas and spas and how to minimize them. *Am J Publ Health* 1991;41:141.
6. Saketkhoo K, Januszkiewicz A, Sackner MA. Effects of drinking hot water, cold water, and chicken soup on nasal mucus velocity and nasal airflow resistance. *Chest* 1978; 74:408.
7. Doub L. *Hydrotherapy*. Fresno, CA: author, 1970, p 51.

RECOMMENDED RESOURCES

www.cyberbohemia.com/sweat. Web site by Mikkel Akkel, the author of *Sweat*, a book about his world travels to try different types of whole-body heat treatments. The site contains copious information on this topic.

SHOWERS

The healing time of practically any fracture can be shortened notably by the use of hydrotherapy as soon as the cast is removed. . . it eliminates the long periods of weakness, stiffness and partial disability that are commonly the sequel. . . . Sprays that may be given in the shower have a distinct value especially in the later stages of healing. They may be hot or cold or an alternation of both. They may be strong or soft, needle point or of a flooding type. They may be given with a hose by the operator, or they may be manipulated at the showerhead or regulated by the patient. The type suitable to the patient's condition and liking must be chosen.

—*Louella Doub, DC, RN, Hydrotherapy*

Chapter Objectives

After completing this chapter, the student will be able to:

■ Describe the effects of partial-body and whole-body showers.
■ Explain the cautions and contraindications to partial-body and whole-body showers.
■ Name and describe different partial-body and whole-body showers.
■ Perform partial-body and whole-body shower treatments using the procedure included with each treatment.

Showers—streams of water from a showerhead directed upon one or more parts of the body—are a common and very appealing water treatment. Shower treatments can be applied to the whole body, using one or more showerheads, or they can consist of just one stream of water directed at a particular part of the body. Showers can be useful for cleansing, stimulating the skin and the tissues underneath it, and for various hot, warm, cold, or contrast treatments. They may be used either before or after massage sessions, and as a home treatment for various musculoskeletal problems.

Although all showers have mechanical and thermal effects, they can be performed differently to produce specific effects. These depend upon how much of the body is treated, how hot or cold the water is, how hard the spray hits the body, and how long the shower lasts. For example, a short ice-cold high-pressure shower for the whole body will produce a very different effect from that of a long warm shower at mild pressure, and a hot shower for

the feet will produce a very different effect from that of a cold shower to the head. Multiple showerheads increase the effect of any shower, as not only is more water present to transfer heat or cold, but the added mechanical pressure stimulates the skin to a greater degree.

In a shower, the mechanical stimulation of the stream of water striking the skin stimulates receptors that are sensitive to pressure, resulting in both sedative and analgesic effects. Many people find this sensation pleasant and relaxing. (The mechanical effect of a shower can also be increased by adding friction. Beginning a shower with a salt glow, or scrubbing the skin with a loofah or brush, encourages the dilation of the blood vessels directly under the skin.) The thermal effects of showers are similar to those of baths, in which local and reflex effects take place as a result of the application of water at a specific temperature. Because the body part is not surrounded by water, however, the thermal effects are less intense. As with baths, the indications for shower treatments vary widely depending upon water temperature.

This chapter focuses on showers which are accessible to the massage therapist outside of a spa environment. It describes a variety of showers and explains how they can be used in your practice to benefit your clients and to complement your massage techniques. It also explains how in many cases the clients will benefit from using showers at home between sessions. For example, a client with an acute joint sprain or someone who has just had a cast removed can benefit from a partial-body shower over the area of concern as many as three times a day, which is practical only at home.

GENERAL CAUTIONS

Before beginning our discussion of shower treatments, it is important to note some general cautions and safety issues. Because wet tiled surfaces can be slippery, take care that clients do not slip getting into or out of a bathtub or shower or while standing in the shower. Always place a bath mat on the floor outside so that there are no puddles of water on the floor, and mop up any pools of water immediately. Be especially careful with anyone who is obese, walks with difficulty, or is unsteady on her feet for any reason. Grab bars outside the shower door are an important safety feature. Clients in wheelchairs can take showers, but they may require a transfer to a bath chair for the shower and then a transfer back to their wheelchairs.

Here are some other general precautions for shower treatment:

1. Never use these showers directly over implanted devices, such as cardiac pacemakers or Baclofen pumps, or over open skin, such as wounds or sores.
2. Never give a cold shower to a chilled client.
3. Water temperatures given in these showers should be followed as closely as possible but always within your client's tolerance. If water at the proper temperature for the treatment is intolerably hot or cold to the client, adjust it to a tolerable level. Explain that over time, tolerance to higher or lower temperatures will improve.
4. Water temperatures should be less extreme if a person has a diminished sensation. Although temperature ranges given here are safe, use milder temperatures at first to determine how the client will respond.

PARTIAL-BODY SHOWERS

Partial-body showers can be used much like many other local cold or hot treatments. For example, a prolonged very cold shower on a knee will cool it as much as an ice pack could, and contrast showers to the legs have an effect similar to that of alternating hot and cold leg baths or alternating hot and cold leg compresses. (For the partial-body showers described here, a standard fixed showerhead may be used, but it is far more effective to use a handheld shower that is connected by a hose to a shower stall or sink.) However, partial-body showers are also helpful when extra sensory stimulation is needed. Anytime a partial-body shower is used as a prelude to massage, the client will have a heightened awareness of the area before you begin. The extra sensory stimulation can also help in specific situations. A hot shower over a healed fracture when the cast has just been removed, or over an incision that has healed but is very sensitive, can help to desensitize an area, not only making it more comfortable but helping the client tolerate other types of tactile stimulation, such as massage. And a cold shower over an area where there has been a crush injury can make that area less sensitive to cold over time.

Water pressure affects how much the skin is stimulated by a partial-body shower. A fine low-pressure spray is unlikely to create a strong impression, and a spray with very high pressure may be too forceful for a hypersensitive area. Shower pressure should never be painful, and it must be adjusted to make a sensory impression without discomfort.

HEAD SHOWER

A shower to the scalp (Fig. 9-1) can be used to decrease the tightness of scalp tissue and to increase blood flow to the scalp. It can be taken sitting down in a bathtub,

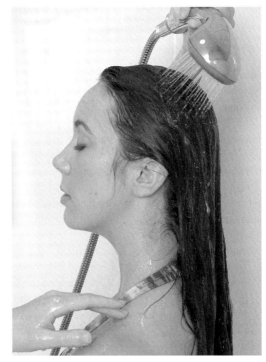

FIGURE 9-1 ■ Head shower.

standing up in a shower, or with the client's head over a sink. Here are directions for giving head showers in a shower stall as well as over a sink.

Temperature
- For hot head shower: 102° to 110°F
- For short, cold head shower: 55° to 70°F
- For long, cold head shower: 55° to 70°F
- For contrast head shower: 110°F alternated with 55°F

Time Needed
- For hot head shower: 2 minutes
- For short, cold head shower: 30 seconds to 2 minutes
- For long, cold head shower: 5 to 10 minutes
- For contrast head shower: 10 minutes: three rounds of 2 minutes of hot followed by 30 seconds of cold

Equipment Needed: Water thermometer, handheld shower, towel, bath mat, bathtub or shower stall

Effect: Thermal and mechanical

Cleanup: Clean and sanitize tiled area and tub or sink; launder used towel and bath mat.

Indications
- For hot head shower: nervous tension, tightness in scalp, poor circulation in scalp
- For short, cold head shower: mental fatigue, poor circulation in scalp, as part of a contrast treatment
- For long, cold head shower: overheated client, migraine headache, tension headache. The cold causes constriction of the blood vessels of the scalp much like an ice pack to the head.
- For contrast head shower: poor circulation in scalp, hematoma on scalp after 24 hours, migraine headache, any other condition in which increased circulation to the scalp is desired

Contraindications
- For hot head shower: migraine headache, acute bruise, or other injury on head
- For short, cold head shower: none
- For long, cold head shower: chilled client
- For contrast head shower: none

Procedure
1. Check with the client to make sure there are no contraindications to the head shower.
2. Explain the use of the head shower to the client and get his or her consent.
3. Place a bath mat in front of the bathtub or shower.
4. Have the client undress, or if preferred, put on a bathing suit or wrap a towel around the body.
5. Turn on the water in the shower, check the temperature with a thermometer, and adjust the flow as necessary to reach the desired temperature.
6. Spray the client's head for the desired amount of time. If the client prefers, demonstrate how to spray the head and allow the client to do it.
7. Turn off water.
8. Have the client towel off and dress quickly to avoid chilling.

Variation
Head shower using a sink.

Procedure
1. Check with the client to make sure there are no contraindications to the head shower.
2. Explain the use of the head shower to the client and get his or her consent.
3. Turn on the water in the sink, check the temperature with a thermometer, and adjust the flow as necessary to reach the desired temperature and pressure.
4. Place a towel around the client's neck to protect clothing.
5. Have the client stand in front of the sink, lean on the counter, and lower the head so the shower water will fall into the sink.
6. Spray the client's head for the appropriate time.
7. Thoroughly dry the client's head.

CHEST SHOWER

A shower to the chest (Fig. 9-2) can be used to warm or cool the chest muscles, change local blood flow, and stimulate the skin over the chest muscles. Hot showers relax muscles for easier breathing, and cold showers stimulate deeper breathing. In one study, not only did an ice-cold chest shower cause the subjects to gasp and breathe more quickly but sympathetic nervous system reflexes of the heart and blood vessels also caused an increase in the blood pressure and heart rate.[1]

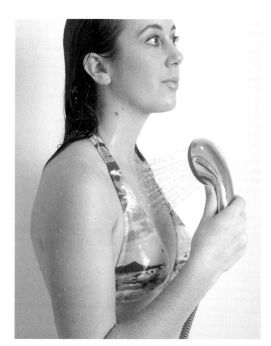

FIGURE 9-2 ■ Chest shower.

Temperature
- For hot chest shower: 102° to 115°F
- For short, cold chest shower: 55° to 70°F
- For long, cold chest shower: 55° to 70°F
- For contrast chest shower: 110°F alternated with 55°F

Time Needed
- For hot chest shower: 5 to 10 minutes
- For short, cold chest shower: 10 to 30 seconds
- For long, cold chest shower: 5 to 10 minutes
- For contrast chest shower: 10 minutes: three rounds of 2 minutes of hot followed by 30 seconds of cold

Equipment Needed: Water thermometer, handheld shower, towel, bath mat, bathtub or shower stall

Effect: Thermal and mechanical

Cleanup: Clean and sanitize tiled area and tub or sink; launder used towel and bath mat.

Indications:
- For hot chest shower: chest muscles that are sore and tight as a result of vigorous coughing, chest muscles that are aching or fatigued as a result of vigorous exercise, chronic tightness in chest muscles
- For short, cold chest shower: low energy, after heat treatment to chest, as part of a contrast treatment
- For long, cold chest shower: acute rib sprain, acute strain of chest muscles, subacute rib fracture (with doctor's permission)
- For contrast chest shower: poor circulation in chest muscles, subacute rib sprain, healed rib fracture, subacute chest muscle strain, chronic tightness in chest muscles

Contraindications
- For hot chest shower: acute injury to chest, such as a muscle strain; cardiac problems; cardiac pacemaker; chilled client
- For all cold or contrast chest showers: asthma, cardiac problems, cardiac pacemaker, chilled client

Procedure
1. Check with client to make sure there are no contraindications to the chest shower.
2. Explain the use of the chest shower to the client and get his or her consent.
3. Place a bath mat in front of the bathtub or shower.
4. Have the client undress, or if preferred, put on a bathing suit or wrap a towel around the body.
5. Turn on the water in the shower, check the temperature with a thermometer, and adjust the flow as necessary to reach the desired temperature.
6. Spray the client's chest for the desired amount of time. If the client prefers, demonstrate how to spray the chest and allow the client to do it. The sides of the chest should also be sprayed.
7. Turn off water.
8. Have the client towel off and dress quickly to avoid chilling.

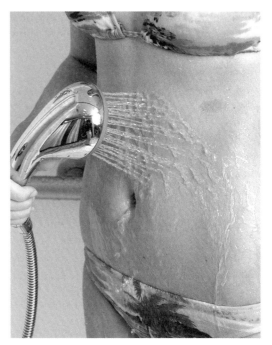

FIGURE 9-3 ■ Abdominal shower.

ABDOMINAL SHOWER

A shower to the abdomen (Fig. 9-3) can be used to warm or cool the abdominal muscles, change local blood flow, and stimulate the skin overlying the abdominal muscles. Hot showers relax abdominal muscles, and cold showers can stimulate them.

Temperature
- For hot abdominal shower: 102° to 115°F
- For short, cold abdominal shower: 55° to 70°F
- For contrast abdominal shower: 115°F alternated with 55°F

Time Needed
- For hot abdominal shower: 5 to 10 minutes
- For short, cold abdominal shower: 10 to 30 seconds
- For contrast abdominal shower: 10 minutes: three rounds of 2 minutes of hot followed by 30 seconds of cold

Equipment Needed: Water thermometer, handheld shower, towel, bath mat, bathtub or shower stall

Effect: Thermal and mechanical

Cleanup: Clean and sanitize tiled area and tub or sink; launder used towel and bath mat.

Indications
- For hot abdominal shower: chronic tension in abdominal muscles, menstrual pain, to soothe abdominal area at least 24 hours after delivery of a baby
- For short, cold abdominal shower: atonic constipation, general sluggishness

- For contrast abdominal shower: chronic tension in abdominal muscles, poor circulation to abdominal muscles

Contraindications
- For hot abdominal shower: acute injury, such as muscle strain; recent abdominal surgery unless with permission of the client's physician
- For short, cold abdominal shower: chilled client
- For contrast abdominal shower: acute injury, such as muscle strain; recent abdominal surgery unless with permission of the client's doctor; chilled client

Procedure
1. Check with client to make sure there are no contraindications to the abdominal shower.
2. Explain the use of the abdominal shower to the client and get his or her consent.
3. Place a bath mat in front of the bathtub or shower.
4. Have the client undress, or if preferred, put on a bathing suit or wrap a towel around the body. A shirt may be left on and pulled up to keep the shoulders and upper back warm.
5. Turn on the water in the shower, check the temperature with a thermometer, and adjust the flow as necessary to reach the desired temperature.
6. Spray the client's abdominal area for the desired amount of time. If the client prefers, demonstrate how to spray the abdominal area and allow the client to do it.
7. Turn off water.
8. Have the client towel off and dress quickly to avoid chilling.

ARM SHOWER

A shower to the arm (Fig. 9-4) can be used to warm or cool the arm muscles, change local blood flow, and stimulate the skin overlying the muscles. Hot showers relax the muscles and increase local blood flow to them, and cold showers can stimulate them. Although instructions are given for performing the arm shower in a bathtub or shower stall, it may also be possible to use a deep sink, depending upon the size of the client's arm and the part to be sprayed. Clients may also stand in a whole-body shower and direct the spray primarily on the arms, but this is not as effective.

Temperature
- For hot arm shower: 102° to 115°F
- For short, cold arm shower: 55° to 70°F
- For long, cold arm shower: 55° to 70°F
- For contrast arm shower: 110°F alternated with 55°F

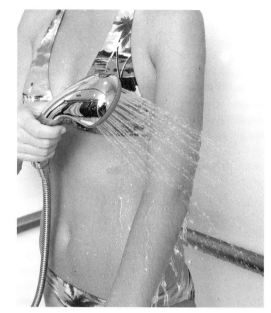

FIGURE 9-4 ■ Arm shower.

Time Needed
- For hot arm shower: 5 to 10 minutes
- For short, cold arm shower: 10 to 30 seconds
- For long, cold arm shower: 5 to 10 minutes
- For contrast arm shower: 10 minutes: three rounds of 2 minutes of hot followed by 30 seconds of cold

Equipment Needed: Water thermometer, handheld shower, towel, bath mat, bathtub or shower stall

Effect: Thermal and mechanical

Cleanup: Clean and sanitize tiled area or tub; launder used towel and bath mat.

Indications
- For hot arm shower: aching or fatigued arm muscles from vigorous exercise; derivation in migraine headache; preparation for stretching arm muscles; chronic tightness in arm muscles; musculoskeletal pain, such as arthritis pain
- For short, cold arm shower: aching or fatigued arm muscles from vigorous exercise; poor circulation in hands or arms; when exercises will be performed to strengthen a weak muscle, as in muscle weakness from stroke, muscular dystrophy, spinal cord injury, postpolio syndrome, and some types of cerebral palsy. (See section on cold footbaths, Chapter 7, for more information.)
- For long, cold arm shower: aching or fatigued arm muscles from vigorous exercise, poor circulation in hands or arms. Unlike a long, cold application to the chest, whose muscles are quite thin and can become very cold quickly, a long, cold shower to the dense muscles of the arms will stimulate circulation.

- For contrast arm shower: poor circulation in arms or hands, edema of hands caused by pregnancy, hematoma of arm muscle, arm muscle strain, healed fracture of arm bone after cast is removed, osteoarthritis pain, aching or fatigued arm muscles from vigorous exercise, derivation in migraine headache, chronic tightness in arm muscles

Contraindications

- To hot arm shower: lymphedema in arm, axillary lymph nodes removed, acute joint sprain, acute bruise
- To short, cold arm shower: Raynaud's syndrome
- To long, cold arm shower: Raynaud's syndrome, chilled client
- To contrast arm shower: lymphedema in arm, Raynaud's syndrome

Procedure

1. Check with client to make sure there are no contraindications to the arm shower.
2. Explain the use of the arm shower to the client and get his or her consent.
3. Place a bath mat in front of the bathtub or shower.
4. Have the client undress, or if preferred, put on a bathing suit or wrap a towel around the body.
5. Turn on the water in the shower, check the temperature with a thermometer, and adjust the flow as necessary to reach the desired temperature.
6. Spray the client's arm for the desired amount of time. If the client prefers, demonstrate and then allow the client to do it. The hands should be sprayed as well.
7. Turn off water.
8. Have the client towel off and dress quickly to avoid chilling.

Variation

Contrast forearm and hand shower using a sink.

This shower is especially helpful for clients who have repetitive stress injuries of the hands, such as carpal tunnel syndrome. It is an excellent self-treatment for anyone who performs heavy work with the hands and is especially suited for massage therapists to use on their own hands and forearms at the conclusion of a session. It is contraindicated for clients with lymphedema of the arm or Raynaud's syndrome.

Use hot water at 110° to 115°F and cold water at 40° to 70°F.

Procedure

1. Check with client to make sure there are no contraindications to the forearm and hand shower.
2. Explain the use of the forearm and hand shower to the client and get his or her consent.
3. Turn on the water in the sink, check the temperature with a thermometer, and adjust the flow as necessary to reach the desired temperature.
4. Have the client stand in front of the sink and put the forearms and hands under the stream of hot water for 2 minutes. Have the client move the arms so that the water stream continuously passes from the hands up to the elbows and back.
5. Turn the water to the maximum coldness that the client can tolerate, then have him or her move the forearms and hands under the stream of cold water for 30 seconds.
6. Repeat steps 4 and 5 for a total of three rounds of hot followed by cold.
7. Give the client a towel to dry the forearms and hands.

LEG SHOWER

A shower to the leg (Fig. 9-5) can be used to warm the leg or cool the leg muscles, change local blood flow, and stimulate the skin overlying the muscles. Hot showers relax the muscles and dilate their blood vessels, while cold showers can stimulate the muscles. Although instructions are given for the leg shower in a bathtub or shower stall, it may also be possible to use a deep sink if the feet alone are sprayed. Special leg tubs may be used for this purpose (see Appendix D). Clients may stand in a whole-body shower and direct the spray primarily on the legs, but this is less effective.

Temperature

- For hot leg shower: 102° to 115°F
- For short, cold leg shower: 55° to 70°F
- For long, cold leg shower: 55° to 70°F
- For contrast leg shower: 110°F alternated with 55°F

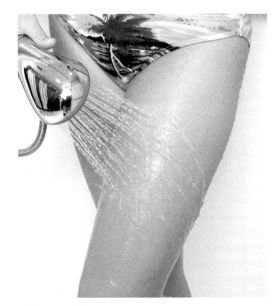

FIGURE 9-5 ■ Leg shower.

Time Needed

- For hot leg shower: 5 to 10 minutes
- For short, cold leg shower: 10 to 30 seconds
- For long, cold leg shower: 5 to 10 minutes
- For contrast leg shower: 10 minutes: three rounds of 2 minutes of hot followed by 30 seconds of cold

Equipment Needed: Water thermometer, handheld shower, towel, bath mat, bathtub or shower stall

Effect: Thermal and mechanical

Cleanup: Clean and sanitize tiled area or tub; launder used towel and bath mat.

Indications

- For hot leg shower: aching or fatigued leg muscles from vigorous exercise, derivation in migraine headache, preparation for stretching leg muscles, chronic tension in leg muscles, arthritis pain
- For short, cold leg shower: poor circulation in the legs, shown by chronically cold feet and poor healing of injuries; when exercises will be performed with a weak muscle, as in weakness from stroke, muscular dystrophy, some cases of spinal cord injury, postpolio syndrome, and some types of cerebral palsy. (See section on cold footbath, Chapter 7, for more information.)
- For long, cold leg shower: aching or fatigued leg muscles from vigorous exercise, to prevent delayed-onset muscle soreness after exercise
- For contrast leg shower: poor circulation in legs, edema of legs and feet caused by pregnancy, hematoma of leg muscle, leg muscle strain, healed fracture of leg bone after cast is removed, aching or fatigued leg muscles from vigorous exercise, derivation in migraine headache, chronic tension in leg muscles, arthritis pain. (For information on two studies that document the improvement in local circulation brought about by contrast leg showers, see Chapter 12, partial-body tonic treatments.)

Contraindications

- For hot leg shower: acute joint sprain; acute bruise; lymphedema in leg; inguinal lymph nodes removed; peripheral vascular disease, including diabetes, Buerger's disease, and arteriosclerosis of the lower extremities; loss of sensation
- For short, cold leg shower: Raynaud's syndrome
- For long, cold leg shower: Raynaud's syndrome, chilled client
- For contrast leg shower: diabetes, lymphedema in leg, Raynaud's syndrome

Procedure

1. Check with client to make sure there are no contraindications to the leg shower.
2. Explain the use of the leg shower to the client and get his or her consent.
3. Place a bath mat in front of the bathtub or shower.
4. Have the client undress, or if preferred, put on a bathing suit or wrap a towel around the body.
5. Turn on the water in the shower, check the temperature with a thermometer, and adjust the flow as necessary to reach the desired temperature.
6. Spray the client's leg or legs for the desired amount of time. If the client prefers, demonstrate and then allow the client to do it. Include the feet in the shower.
7. Turn off water.
8. Have the client towel off and dress quickly to avoid chilling.

FOOT SHOWER

As Figure 9-6 shows, it is easy to spray the feet. Using a cold shower regularly can stimulate blood flow to the feet and diminish chronic coldness. The feet can also be sprayed with cold water at the end of any whole-body hot shower to prevent congestion of the head.

Temperature: 55° to 70°F

Time Needed: 30 seconds to 2 minutes

Equipment Needed: Water thermometer, handheld shower, towel, bath mat, bathtub or shower stall

Effect: Thermal and mechanical

Cleanup: Clean and sanitize tiled area or tub; launder used towel and bath mat.

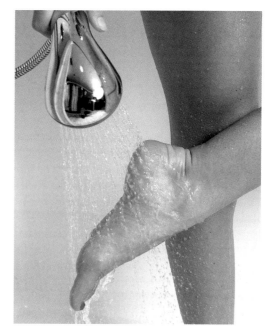

FIGURE 9-6 ■ Foot shower.

CASE HISTORY 9-1

Stimulating Local Circulation With a Contrast Leg and Foot Shower

Background

Katrina Johns is a 62-year-old retired bookkeeper who was diagnosed with multiple sclerosis (MS) 20 years ago. A determined and energetic person, Katrina continued to work and function fairly normally for many years after her diagnosis. As her MS progressed, however, Katrina's muscles became progressively weaker. While she still had full use of her upper extremities, she was not able to move her legs at all, and she used a scooter to get around. The circulation in her lower extremities was very poor for this reason. She frequently scraped her feet when transferring from scooter to bed, and because of the poor circulation in her lower extremities, the scrapes sometimes became infected and turned into large sores.

Treatment

Katrina received a massage twice a month because it helped her release muscle tension, maintain joint range of motion, and improve local circulation, particularly in her legs. However, because almost all of Katrina's waking hours were spent sitting upright in her scooter and her legs were not exercised at all, the improvement in the circulation to her legs lasted only a few hours. Her massage therapist suggested a daily contrast shower for her legs and feet to improve local circulation, and with the approval of her physical therapist, Katrina incorporated it into her daily bath routine. Normally, every morning her caregiver helped Katrina transfer from her scooter to a bath chair in her bathtub, and Katrina used a handheld sprayer to wash herself with warm water. Her massage therapist, who always treated her at home, taught Katrina how to perform the contrast shower at the end of her regular bath, using three rounds of hot followed by cold on her legs. After a few days of this routine, the color in Katrina's lower extremities began to improve. Her massage therapist and she discovered that when she performed the contrast treatment before her legs were massaged, her legs were warmer, pinker, and more relaxed for a full day rather than for just a few hours. As an added benefit, though she continued to get scrapes on her feet from transferring, they healed more quickly and no longer became infected.

Discussion Questions

1. How did the contrast leg shower improve the circulation in Katrina's legs?
2. What other hydrotherapy treatments could have been used to improve her circulation?

Indications: Chronically cold feet

Contraindications: Raynaud's syndrome, chilled client, menstruation

Procedure

1. Check with client to make sure there are no contraindications to the foot shower.
2. Explain the use of the foot shower to the client and get his or her consent.
3. Place a bath mat in front of the bathtub or shower.
4. Have the client remove shoes and socks, then sit on the edge of the bathtub or in the shower or other tiled area on a plastic stool or chair.
5. Turn on the water in the shower, check the temperature with a thermometer, and adjust the flow as necessary to reach the desired temperature.
6. Spray the tops and bottoms of both feet are with cold water for 30 seconds to 2 minutes. If the client prefers, demonstrate and then allow the client to do it.

7. Turn off the water; have the client dry the feet briskly, then don socks and shoes quickly to avoid chilling. The client should not step barefoot on the floor.

Variation

Cold foot spray to relieve congestion after whole-body hot shower. After a hot shower, quickly dry the rest of the body, then spray the feet for 30 seconds only.

WHOLE-BODY SHOWER

Whole-body showers (Fig. 9-7) are another useful water treatment for the massage therapist. Unlike the partial-body shower, which targets a specific area, a whole-body shower has a more general effect. Rather than delivering thermal or mechanical stimulation to just one area, the entire body is affected, but the effect is not as strong as

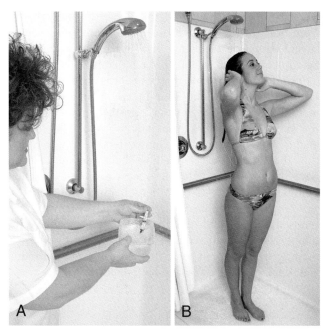

FIGURE 9-7 ■ Whole-body shower. **A.** Checking shower water temperature. **B.** Client in whole-body shower.

when the shower is applied to just one area. While showers can provide many of the same thermal effects as whole-body immersion baths, they are particularly suitable in certain situations. For example, people who are physically disabled, obese, or have difficulty moving generally find it easier to get in and out of a shower than a bathtub. In addition, showers take less time, since there is no waiting while a bathtub is filled, and at the end of a massage session, showering can quickly remove massage oil, creams, or other products which have been put on the skin.

Whole-body showers also provide the sensation of water striking the skin, which a great many people find relaxing and soothing. At Wildwood Hospital in Wildwood, Georgia, whole-body showers are given to a wide variety of patients, including patients who are hospitalized for serious illness. Under the direction of the hospital's physicians, patients are given contrast showers whenever possible to stimulate their bodies' vital functions. Water temperature and shower duration are carefully tailored to sick patients; someone who cannot tolerate cold water may receive a contrast shower using hot alternated with tepid water. Patients are given chairs to use in the shower stall if there is any chance they will be unsteady on their feet. Physicians prescribe these showers to make patients stronger and speed their recovery (E. Qualls, personal communication, December 1, 2006).

When deciding whether to employ showers with your clients, remember that they use a lot of water. A 10-minute shower will use 60 gallons of water or more, whereas a full hot bath uses only 30 gallons. Hot showers

also expose the client to more chlorine than does a hot bath, and you may wish to install a shower water filter to prevent this (see Appendix D for information).

HOT SHOWER

Many clients enjoy the sensation of a hot shower, either before or after a massage session. A hot whole-body shower can be used to raise the body's core temperature, depending upon how hot the water is and how long the shower lasts. This can be useful anytime a client is not warm enough, especially if the client enters your office chilled or will be receiving a cold treatment. One study comparing hot showers and baths found that both raised core temperature about equally when the shower water was 2°F higher than the bath water: in the tub, the subjects' bodies were completely surrounded by water and heat was transferred to the skin to a greater degree. (For this reason, the average person runs the shower hotter than the tub bath.) Since the skin was surrounded by water, skin temperature was slightly higher in the bath over the shower. The subjects' heart rates and blood pressures were slightly higher in the shower than in the bathtub, since they had to expend some energy just to stand up.(2) Blood flow to the skin is increased.(3) Muscle tension is reduced and connective tissue is made more elastic with a hot shower. (See Chapter 12 for a stretching routine for the upper body that is performed in a hot shower for these reasons.)

Water Temperature: Hot (102°–110°F)

Time Needed: 5 to 10 minutes

Equipment Needed: Shower stall with grab bar, water thermometer, bath towel, bath mat brush or loofah mitt for extra stimulation if desired

Effect: Thermal and mechanical

Cleanup: Clean, sanitize, and dry shower and bath chair if used. Launder used towel and bath mat.

Indications: When warming and softening of the connective tissue of the upper body is desired before massage; muscle tightness; nervous tension; musculoskeletal pain, including arthritis, gout, dysmenorrhea, back pain, arthritis, neuralgia, muscle spasm, muscle tension, sprains, strains, stiffness, bruises and contusions

Contraindications: Systemic or chronic conditions including cardiovascular problems, diabetes, hepatitis, lymphedema, multiple sclerosis, and seizure disorders; loss of sensation; great obesity; pregnancy; inability to tolerate heat; ingestion of alcohol or drugs; recent meal (wait at least an hour)

Cautions

1. Anyone who is at risk for lymphedema due to removal of lymph nodes should avoid prolonged hot showers (more than 15 minutes) or very hot showers.
2. Very frequent hot showers are not recommended for those with hypothyroid conditions.

Procedure

1. Check with client to make sure there are no contraindications to the whole-body shower.
2. Explain the use of the whole-body shower to the client and get consent.
3. Place a bath mat in front of the bathtub or shower.
4. Have the client undress or if preferred, put on a bathing suit.
5. Turn on the water in the shower, check the temperature with a thermometer (Fig. 9-7A), and adjust the flow as necessary to reach the desired temperature.
6. Have the client enter the hot shower (Fig. 9-7B).
7. Have the client remain in the water for at least 5 minutes, so that the body is thoroughly warm. If desired, begin with the water temperature at 102°F, then gradually increase the water temperature to 110°F.
8. Have the client towel off and dress quickly to avoid chilling.
9. The client may now lie down for a rest or a massage session if one is planned.

Variations

1. Hot shower to warm specific muscle areas (suitable for upper body only). Many stretching exercises for the upper body can be performed in a shower or bath after the application of hot water has relaxed chronically tight neck, back, or shoulder muscles. See Chapter 12 for instructions.
2. Warm shower. A warm shower may be used for relaxation, cleansing, and gentle warming, and it is suitable for many clients for whom hot showers are contraindicated, including clients with lymphedema and diabetes.(5) It will cause a mild vasodilation of the entire skin surface, and rubbing the skin with a brush or loofah can stimulate additional vasodilation without heat. Follow the procedure for the hot shower but use warm, not hot water (99° to 102°F). Warm showers are contraindicated for those with loss of sensation, great obesity, inability to tolerate heat, ingestion of alcohol or drugs, or having eaten a meal recently (wait at least an hour).

GRADUATED SHOWER

Graduated showers use water that gradually runs from hot to cold. They are excellent for clients who have just received a heat treatment, such as a hot bath or sauna, but who are not hardy enough to tolerate a quick change from hot to cold or for those who do not enjoy such a strong sensation. (A change in water temperature is felt far more acutely when the temperature is changed quickly from hot to cold than when it is changed slowly.) Rather than have clients step directly from a heat treatment into an 80° to 85°F shower, instead gradually lower the water temperature from hot to cool. The shower begins with the client standing under 102°F water, and then the temperature is raised (to client tolerance, but no hotter than 110°F), held there for 2 minutes, and then gradually lowered. If the client begins with a 102°F shower, after 2 minutes under the water, the temperature is raised to 106°F and kept there for 2 minutes. The water temperature is then reduced to 102°F, held there for 1 minute, then reduced to 98°F, held there for 1 minute, and so on, gradually working back to 80° to 85°F.

Temperature: Begins at 102°F and ends at 80° to 85°F

Time Needed: 10 minutes

Equipment Needed: Shower stall with grab bar, water thermometer, bath towel, bath mat, brush or loofah mitt if extra stimulation is desired

Effect: Thermal and mechanical

Cleanup: Clean, sanitize, and dry shower and bath chair if used. Launder used towel and bath mat.

Indications: Overheated client, gentle stimulation of the general circulation after a heat treatment, as part of a daily program to build tolerance to cold

Contraindications: Systemic or chronic conditions, including cardiovascular problems, diabetes, hepatitis, lymphedema, multiple sclerosis, seizure disorders; sedentary or frail person whose blood vessels may not react well to cold; advanced kidney disease; loss of sensation; great obesity; pregnancy; inability to tolerate heat; ingestion of alcohol or drugs; recent meal (wait at least an hour)

Procedure

1. Check with client to make sure there are no contraindications to the graduated shower.
2. Explain the use of the graduated shower to the client and get his or her consent.
3. Place a bath mat in front of the bathtub or shower.
4. Have the client undress or if preferred, put on a bathing suit.
5. Turn on the water in the shower, check the temperature with a thermometer, and adjust the flow as necessary to reach 102°F.
6. Have the client enter the hot shower.
7. Increase the temperature to maximum tolerance, but no hotter than 110°F.
8. After 2 minutes, decrease the temperature by 4°F.
9. After 1 minute, decrease the temperature by 4°F.

10. Continue decreasing the temperature in the same manner until the water is 80° to 85°F.
11. Have the client towel off and dress quickly to avoid chilling.
12. The client may now lie down for a rest or a massage session if planned.

NEUTRAL SHOWER

According to John Harvey Kellogg, a neutral shower for 3 to 5 minutes can produce the same calming effect as a 40- to 60-minute neutral bath and it may be preferred since it takes less time. One study explored the average person's sensitivities to water temperature and fluctuations of water temperature in the shower. Although a neutral shower temperature produced no discomfort, subjects preferred a warmer temperature, and when the shower was made hotter than neutral, it increased their own ratings of skin warmth and pleasantness of the shower.(5) The client must always be warm at the beginning of the neutral shower; if for some reason a client who is not completely warm is going to take a neutral shower, a hot footbath may be given first. If prolonged, a neutral shower may lower the systolic blood pressure 20 points in a person who is hypertensive. This shower is an effective way for a very tense client to relax before a massage, or you may suggest it to clients as part of home treatment in between massage sessions.

Temperature: Neutral (92° to 97°F)

Time Needed: 5 to 10 minutes

Equipment Needed: Shower stall with grab bar, water thermometer, bath towel, bath mat, brush or loofah mitt if extra stimulation is desired

Effect: Thermal and mechanical

Cleanup: Clean, sanitize and dry shower and bath chair if used. Launder used towel and bath mat.

Procedure
1. Check with client to make sure there are no contraindications to the neutral shower
2. Explain the use of the neutral shower to the client and get his or her consent.
3. Place a bath mat in front of the bathtub or shower.
4. Have the client undress or if preferred, put on a bathing suit.
5. Turn on the water in the shower, check the temperature with a thermometer, and adjust the flow as necessary to reach the desired temperature.
6. Have the client enter the neutral shower.
7. Have the client remain in the water for 5 to 10 minutes.
8. Have the client towel off and dress quickly to avoid chilling.
9. The client may now lie down for a rest or a massage session, if planned.

COLD SHOWER

The short, cold shower, along with the short, cold bath, is perhaps the most challenging as well as the most rewarding of all hydrotherapy treatments. Historically, it was one of the hydrotherapist's most important tools to build strength in a weak or ailing person. According to John Harvey Kellogg, the shock of a cold shower set up a "perfect cyclone of nerve impulses" and stimulated all general metabolic activity, especially the movement of lymphatic fluid. Today we know that the quick fall in skin temperature causes an initial gasp, and then, as the body tries to warm itself, a marked increase in blood pressure and breathing rate. Traditional hydrotherapists always gave the patient a heat treatment first, such as hot bath or a sweating body wrap, and patients were sometimes given their showers in a steam room to eliminate the chilling effects of evaporation and cold drafts.

Today we can use cold showers to cool overheated clients, to stimulate and tone their muscles and skin, and as a general tonic. On a hot day a client who is very warm may find a cold shower a welcome prelude to a massage. Another client with chronic cold feet may use a heat treatment followed by a cold shower and massage in order to address this problem. Unless a person is very hot, enduring a cold shower requires a certain amount of discipline. However, almost everyone agrees that the feelings of invigoration and warmth that follow a short, cold shower are worth the effort.

Never give a cold shower to someone with is chilled, or the person may have an entirely negative reaction: rather than being invigorated, the person will become more chilled. If there is any question about core temperature, give a short, hot footbath first. Cold showers longer than 1 minute should not be given without the advice of a physician. For more on the cold shower as a tonic treatment, see Chapter 12.

Temperature: About 55° to 65°F, ideally as cold as can be tolerated by the client, but no warmer than 65°F

Time Needed: 1 minute. A longer shower may cause the client's core temperature to fall too low.

Equipment Needed: Shower stall with grab bar, water thermometer, bath towel, bath mat, brush or loofah mitt if extra stimulation is desired

Effect: Thermal and mechanical

Cleanup: Clean, sanitize and dry shower and bath chair if used. Launder used towel and bath mat.

Indications: Body cooling (such as before a massage on a hot day or after a heating treatment); building resistance to cold; general tonic; stimulation of blood flow to the skin; general feelings of lethargy or fatigue for a client with no health problems, such as when a person has jet lag; to prevent muscle soreness after vigorous exercise

Contraindications: Chilled person; Raynaud's syndrome; sedentary or frail person whose blood vessels may not react well to cold; very fatigued person; cardiovascular disease, because a brief rise in systolic blood pressure (about 18 points) will occur when the person first goes into the shower; advanced kidney disease; great obesity

Caution: Very frequent cold showers are not recommended for those with hyperthyroid conditions.

Procedure
1. Check with client to make sure there are no contraindications to the cold shower.
2. Explain the use of the cold shower to the client and get his or her consent.
3. Place a bath mat in front of the bathtub or shower.
4. Have the client undress or if preferred, put on a bathing suit.
5. Turn on the water in the shower, check the temperature with a thermometer, and adjust the flow as necessary to reach the desired temperature.
6. Have the client enter the cold shower.
7. Have the client remain in the water for 1 minute.
8. Have the client towel off and dress quickly to avoid chilling.
9. The client may now lie down for a rest or a massage session if planned.

CONTRAST SHOWER

A contrast shower is a series of hot showers alternated with cold showers, with the hot phase always lasting longer than the cold phase. A person who is taking a contrast shower will experience great circulatory changes, because the body is stimulated to throw off heat during the hot phase and then stimulated to conserve heat during the cold phase. Typically, clients who take a contrast shower report that they are invigorated and alert and feel warm for a long time. Contrast showers are often used by athletes to prevent muscle soreness after exercise and to speed recovery after very vigorous exercise. They may also be successful at terminating a migraine headache if the shower is taken when very the first symptoms are noticed.

Although a contrast shower is not as extreme as a contrast bath, only the hardiest of clients can tolerate the temperature extremes of very hot alternated with very cold. Someone who would like to try a contrast shower but is unaccustomed to such a circulatory system challenge would do better to try a warm shower alternated with a cool shower at first. If a salt glow or dry brushing is performed first, the client will experience an even deeper sense of invigoration and well-being. This treatment is generally more suitable after a massage session than before one, because the client will feel wide awake and stimulated rather than in the mood to lie down and relax.

Temperature: Hot (102°–110°F) alternated with cold (65°F or less)

Time Needed: 10 minutes

Equipment Needed: Shower stall with grab bar, water thermometer, bath towel, bath mat, brush or loofah mitt if extra stimulation is desired

Effect: Thermal and mechanical

Cleanup: Clean, sanitize, and dry shower and bath chair if used. Launder used towel and bath mat.

Indications: Stimulation of blood flow to skin, general feelings of lethargy or fatigue when the client has no health problems, general tonic, prevention of soreness after vigorous exercise, to prevent development of a migraine headache, when training the circulatory system to react faster to heat and cold in order to stay warmer in the winter (see Chapter 12), as a finish for other hydrotherapy treatments

Contraindications: Systemic or chronic conditions, including cardiovascular problems, diabetes, hepatitis, lymphedema, advanced kidney disease, multiple sclerosis, seizure disorders; loss of sensation; great obesity; pregnancy; inability to tolerate heat; ingestion of alcohol or drugs; recent meal (wait at least an hour); chilled person; sedentary or frail person whose blood vessels may not react well to cold; very fatigued person

Cautions: Very frequent contrast showers are not recommended for those with hyperthyroid conditions.

Procedure
1. Check with client to make sure there are no contraindications to the contrast shower.
2. Explain the use of the contrast shower to the client and get his or her consent.
3. Place a bath mat in front of the bathtub or shower.
4. Have the client undress or if preferred, put on a bathing suit.
5. Turn on the water in the shower, check the temperature with a thermometer, and adjust the flow as necessary to reach the desired temperature.
6. Have the client enter the hot shower and remain for 2 to 5 minutes, until thoroughly warmed.
7. Change the water to cold for 30 seconds to 1 minute, checking temperature.
8. Change the water back to hot for 2 minutes, checking temperature.
9. Change the water to cold for 30 seconds to 1 minute, checking temperature.
10. Change the water back to hot for 2 minutes, checking temperature.
11. Change the water to cold for 30 seconds to 1 minute, checking temperature.
12. Have the client towel off and dress quickly to avoid chilling.

(continued on page 180)

BOX 9-1   *Point of Interest*

SPECIALTY SHOWERS

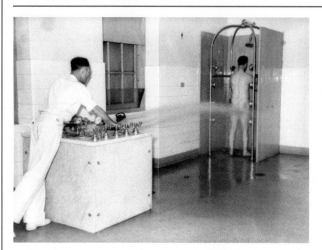

Percussion douche to the back. (Photo courtesy of the National Library of Medicine, Bethesda, Maryland.)

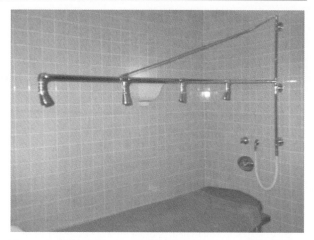

Vichy shower. (Photo courtesy of HEAT SpaKur Therapy Development Inc., Calistoga, California.)

Applying pressurized water to the body through showers, jets, sprays, and pours has long been a major part of European hydrotherapy, and this practice was introduced to the United States by the hydrotherapists of the nineteenth and twentieth centuries. Above, we see a **percussion douche**, a very strong spray of water, applied to the posterior aspect of a man's body. (Although there are many other specialized ways of applying water to the body, today's massage therapist is likely to use showers rather than jets, sprays, or pours.) Besides the standard full-body shower given with water coming out of one showerhead above the client's head, a number of specialty showers may be used to perform hydrotherapy treatments. Such specialty equipment is quite expensive and generally available only in spas. At the bottom left we see a tiled shower with extra showerheads on both the ceiling and the walls.

A **Vichy shower** (*top right*) is given with the client lying on a special waterproof table. Water showers down from a long pipe arm that has about seven jets in it, positioned about 4 feet above the table. Vichy showers can be given at hot, warm, cold, or contrast temperatures.

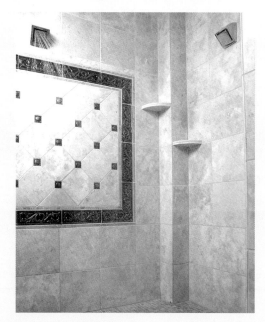

Spa shower with multiple heads.

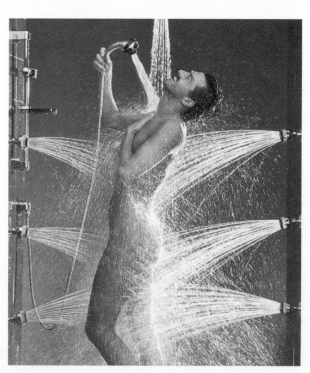

Swiss shower. (Photo courtesy of HEAT SpaKur Therapy Development Inc., Calistoga, California.)

A **Swiss shower** has multiple showerheads mounted in the shower wall at different levels and on all sides of the client. It sprays the entire body, from head to toe. Swiss showers may have pipes in all four corners of a shower stall, with 8 to 16 streams of water coming from each pipe.

13. The client may now lie down for a rest or a massage session if desired but often will feel too invigorated to by still.

Note: This contrast shower consists of three complete rounds, or cycles of hot and cold. The muscles of the blood vessels generally become fatigued after three or four rounds. To continue the treatment after that, it is necessary to increase the temperature of the hot water and decrease the temperature of the cold water so that the blood vessels continue to respond.

CHAPTER SUMMARY

This chapter discusses partial-body and whole-body showers, simple and popular hydrotherapy treatments. Showers are simple and practical ways to cleanse and stimulate the skin and tissues underneath. They can also be used to perform various hot, warm, cold, or contrast treatments, to target specific musculoskeletal problems, and as part of a general health program. For these reasons they may be appropriate for many of your massage clients. Now that you understand their benefits, you can use them before or after massage sessions and offer them to your clients as a home treatment for various musculoskeletal problems. You will also be able to use them with other hydrotherapy treatments. In the next chapter you will learn how to combine a whole-body salt glow with a whole-body shower.

REVIEW QUESTIONS

Short Answer

1. How can the mechanical effect of a shower be increased without altering the water temperature?

   _____

   _____

2. Explain how water pressure should be adjusted for an area that needs extra tactile stimulation.

   _____

   _____

3. Explain the effects of whole-body showers of different temperatures upon the client's circulation.

   _____

   _____

4. Describe and explain the effects of a hot chest shower on sore, tight, or aching chest muscles.

   _____

   _____

5. Explain why a contrast arm shower is contraindicated for a client with Raynaud's syndrome.

   _____

   _____

True/False

____ 6. Showers have the same effect whether they are targeted to a specific area or to the entire body.

____ 7. A hot leg and foot shower can be used to treat a migraine due to its derivative effects.

____ 8. A cold head shower can be used to treat a migraine headache due to its vasoconstricting effect.

____ 9. A neutral shower can have the same calming effect as a neutral bath.

____10. A graduated shower consists of hot water alternated with cold water.

REFERENCES

1. Keatinge W et al. Cardiovascular responses to ice cold showers. *J Appl Physiol* 1964;19:1145.
2. Ohnaka T, Tochihara Y, Kubo M, Yamaguchi C. Physiological responses to standing showers, sitting showers, and sink baths. *Appl Human Sci* 1995;14:235.
3. Charkoudian N. Skin blood flow in adult human thermoregulation: How it works, when it does not, and why. *Mayo Clin Proc* 2003;78:603.
4. Thrash A, Thrash C. *Home Remedies: Hydrotherapy, Charcoal, and Other Simple Treatments*, Seale, AL: Thrash, 1981, p 59.
5. Hermann C, Candas V, Hoeft A, Garreaurd I. Humans under showers: Thermal sensitivity, thermoneutral sensations, and comfort estimates. *Physiol Behav* 1994; 56:1003.

RECOMMENDED RESOURCES

1. Buchman D. *The Complete Book of Water Healing*. New York: Instant Improvement, 1994.
2. Kellogg JH. *Rational Hydrotherapy*. Battle Creek, MI: Modern Medicine, 1923.

10

BODY WRAPS

The wet sheet pack is one of the most useful of hydrotherapeutic procedures, as it combines at once very powerful effects, great convenience, universality of application, and remarkable flexibility to suit different pathological conditions.

—John Harvey Kellogg, Rational Hydrotherapy

Chapter Objectives

After completing this chapter, the student will be able to:

- Describe the effects of three full-body wraps.
- Explain the cautions and contraindications to full-body wraps.
- Name and describe different full-body wraps.
- Perform full-body wraps using the procedure included with each treatment.

Body wraps are hydrotherapy treatments in which the client is wrapped first in a sheet, then in layers of blankets. All body wraps use the client's own body heat to advantage, trapping the heat which would normally be lost through radiation. Although sometimes cumbersome to assemble, once wraps are in place, many clients enjoy the feeling of being warm and the sensation of being snugly enclosed reinforces their sense of body boundaries in a reassuring way.

Because body wraps can be performed without showers, baths, or elaborate hydrotherapy equipment, they may be easily incorporated into a massage therapy setting. Wraps can be used for a number of therapeutic purposes. For instance, a massage therapist might choose to use a moist or dry blanket wrap with a client who is hypersensitive to the touch, a client who would like to spend some quiet time absorbing the full effects of his or her massage session, or a chilled client who needs a heating treatment before a massage. The wet sheet wrap, on the other hand, because it uses an initial application of cold, is both more stimulating to the circulation and more difficult to tolerate than the moist and dry blanket wraps. Historically it was used for graver situations, such as influenza, pneumonia, drug and alcohol addiction, and mental illness

(see Chapter 1). It has continued to be widely used by naturopathic doctors as a way to encourage profuse sweating for detoxification.

Body wraps are often used at hot springs resorts, where therapists may simply wrap clients up in blankets after a warm soak for a period of relaxation before massage. Specialized body wraps are very popular in spas, and Anne Williams, author of *Spa Bodywork*, lists more than 40 ingredients (including herbs, food items such as oatmeal and coffee, salts, seaweeds, muds, and essential oils) that can be used to create wraps for specific conditions such as arthritis pain, muscle soreness, dry skin and body toxicity. Even melted paraffin can even be used to make a body wrap (Box 10-1).

Although body wraps have been seen as archaic by many health care professionals, they are being rediscovered for specific medical situations. For example, at the Center for Hyperthermia Cancer Treatment at the University of Texas Health Science Center in Houston, body wraps are being used to heat patients with cancer. Elevated body temperatures not only stimulate the immune system dramatically, they also weaken cancer cells, so it is believed that radiation or chemotherapy will be more effective when core temperature is high. In ongoing clinical trials at the center, one regimen includes

WHOLE-BODY PARAFFIN WRAP

Melted paraffin can deeply heat a painful or stiff body part to ease joint stiffness and pain. Paraffin can be used in dips, but it can also be painted directly onto the body. A whole-body application of paraffin and body wrap can be not only deeply warming and soothing but also an effective treatment for joint pain. However, full-body paraffin treatments can be messy and time consuming and can require a lot of equipment, some quite expensive.

To perform a paraffin wrap, the therapist brings a large-capacity paraffin tank to the massage table. The client wears little or no clothing. He or she lies upon the massage table while the skin is cleansed, and then at least three layers of paraffin are brushed onto the posterior surface of the body from the toes to the neck. The client is then covered with plastic wrap, wrapped in an electric blanket, and rests for 20 minutes. Massage may be performed on the head during this time. At this point, the client is unwrapped, all paraffin is removed from the skin, and the client turns over. Then paraffin is painted onto the anterior surface of the body in the same fashion, and the client is again covered and wrapped. After a 20-minute rest period, the paraffin is removed from the skin and massage can begin.

administration of chemotherapeutic medication along with body heating, or **pyrotherapy,** the treatment of disease by inducing an artificial fever in the patient. The core temperature of cancer patients is raised to 104°F using heat lamps, and then the patient is "wrapped like a mummy" in a cotton flannel blanket and an insulated space blanket to maintain the elevated temperature. Fluid is administered intravenously to avoid dehydration, and a sedative may be administered to help heat-sensitive or claustrophobic patients tolerate the prolonged wrap. At the end of 6 hours the patient is uncovered, given a complete washing with warm water, and left to cool until he or she is again at normal body temperature.(1–3) Other academic centers in Europe, Scandinavia, and Asia are researching similar thermal body wrap treatments for cancer.

Three body wraps are presented in this chapter: the moist blanket wrap, dry sheet wrap, and cold, wet sheet wrap.

MOIST BLANKET WRAP

As seen in Figure 10-1, the **moist blanket wrap**— essentially a hot compress for the entire body—consists of a cotton blanket wrung out in 110°F water and additional blankets to cover it plus external warming devices applied over the wrap. The client's body is thoroughly warmed before the wrap begins, using a hot footbath, hot shower, hot tub, aerobic exercise, heat lamp, or other form of body warming. Next the client is wrapped in a cotton blanket that is wrung out in 110°F water, then in one space blanket and two wool blankets, on top of which are laid external warming devices, such as fomentations, hot water bottles, or hydrocollator packs. This treatment is commonly used to stimulate circulation, detoxify, and help the client relax. Although it can be used as a general tonic, to be effective the wrap has to be performed on a regular basis. Since the treatment raises body temperature, it also increases the client's heart rate and blood pressure and so is not recommended for people with heart conditions or hypertension.

Temperature: Hot (110°F)

Time Needed: 20 to 30 minutes

Equipment Needed: Two wool blankets, one space blanket, and one cotton blanket; two sheets that will be used for massage after the body wrap is finished; warming device such as a hot water bottle, hydrocollator pack, or heating pad; small bath towel to wrap around the neck; large container of water at 110°F for wetting the blanket; bolster for client's knees; cup with drinking water and a straw

Effect: Thermal

Cleanup: Launder wet cotton blanket and small bath towel. Fold and put away the wool blankets. Spray the space blanket with alcohol, leave it to air dry, then fold it and put it away. Clean, disinfect, and dry the water container.

Indications: Detoxification; general tonic, often given to stimulate the immune system and increase energy; warming of a chilled client before massage; chronic muscle or joint pain, especially arthritis; sciatica; gout; emotionally upset client

Contraindications: Any condition that specifically contraindicates whole-body heating, such as cardiovascular problems, diabetes, hepatitis, lymphedema, multiple sclerosis, and seizure disorders unless treatments are specifically prescribed by a doctor; pregnancy; ingestion of alcohol and drugs; claustrophobic person

Cautions

1. Very frequent sweating body wraps are not recommended for persons with hypothyroid conditions.
2. Anyone who is at risk for lymphedema due to removal of lymph nodes should avoid prolonged sweating in wraps (longer than 15 minutes after the client begins sweating).

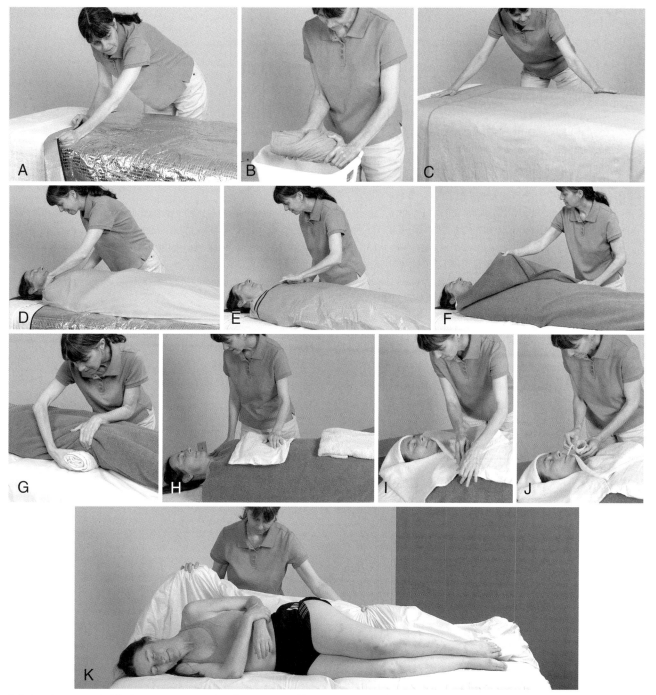

FIGURE 10-1 ■ Moist blanket wrap. **A.** Preparing the massage table. **B.** Wringing out hot, wet blanket. **C.** Laying out hot, wet blanket. **D.** Wrapping client in hot, wet blanket. **E.** Wrapping client in space blanket. **F.** Wrapping client in wool blanket. **G.** Placing a bolster under the client's knees. **H.** Applying external warming devices. **I.** Draping the head with a towel. **J.** Offering the client drinking water. **K.** Removing blankets with the client on the table.

Procedure
1. Check with client to make sure there are no contraindications to the use of the body wrap.
2. Explain the use of the body wrap to the client and get his or her consent.
3. Make sure that the client is warm, giving a hot footbath or other type of warming treatment if necessary.

4. Cover the massage table with one massage sheet, two wool blankets, and then a space blanket (Fig. 10-1A). Reserve the other massage sheet for covering the client at the conclusion of the body wrap.

(continued)

CASE HISTORY 10-1

Moist Blanket Wrap for a Client With Fibromyalgia

Background

Roberta was a healthy 62-year-old woman who had had **fibromyalgia** for many years. She was in a motor vehicle accident the day before her massage appointment and was bruised, sore over her entire body except her head, and upset. When she visited the emergency department at her hospital after the accident, Roberta was told she had no fractures or other major injuries. The next day she visited her daughter's massage therapist to receive the first massage she had ever had.

Treatment

As the massage therapist began to take Roberta's heath history, Roberta mentioned that she was cold. The therapist immediately gave her a footbath at 102°F; however, Roberta exclaimed that it was much too hot, so he added more cold water until it was at 99°F. As Roberta answered his questions, the therapist began to suspect that she was not only bruised from yesterday's accident but hypersensitive to touch as well. Roberta acknowledged that she could not tolerate wool on her skin, cut all the tags out of her clothing, felt any loose thread in her socks as a major annoyance, wore only very soft fabrics, could not tolerate very hot or very cold water, and disliked any touch on her abdomen and feet.

The therapist decided that massage, especially when she was bruised and sore, would likely be more stressful than relaxing to Roberta. He chose instead to administer a moist blanket wrap. He soaked a cotton blanket in warm water with a high concentration of Epsom salt, laid it on the massage table, and wrapped Roberta snugly in it. Then, while she was relaxing in the wrap, he performed very gentle massage of her head and neck along with energetic techniques. Roberta became not only comfortably warm but deeply relaxed. When she was dressed again at the end of the session, she told the therapist that she felt much better emotionally, and "it doesn't hurt so much when I move."

Discussion Questions

1. How did the moist blanket wrap relieve Rebecca's pain?
2. Why did the therapist use Epsom salt water for the wrap?
3. What other hydrotherapy treatments would have been appropriate for this client's needs?

5. Soak a cotton blanket in 110°F water and wring it out (Fig. 10-1B). Now lay it out upon the massage table, working quickly so it does not cool off (Fig. 10-1C). It should cover the space blanket completely, so that the space blanket never comes into contact with the client's skin.
6. Have the nude or partially dressed client lie on the sheet, and quickly wrap him or her in it. Tuck the sheet in snugly around the client's neck so that no air escapes (Fig. 10-1D). Next wrap the space blanket over the wet sheet (Fig. 10-1E), and over that wrap both wool blankets (Fig. 10-1F).
7. Place a bolster under the client's knees (Fig. 10-1 G).
8. Apply to the client's feet one external warming device, such as a hot water bottle, fomentation, or microwave hot pack. If the client is not warming up quickly, place one on the abdomen and/or chest as well (Fig. 10-1H).
9. Drape the head with a towel (Fig. 10-1I).
10. As the client begins to warm up, add a cold compress to the forehead (not shown).
11. Offer the client drinking water from a cup with a straw (Fig. 10-1J).
12. After 20 to 30 minutes, unwrap the client (remove all the blankets) and if desired, give a cold mitten friction.
13. Now the client may receive a massage. However, you want only one dry massage sheet remaining on the massage table. The wool blankets, space blanket, and wet blanket must all be removed. Have the client roll onto one side, bunch up the sheet and all the blankets up against the back, and then have the client roll to the other side. To do this, the client will have to roll over the bunched-up blankets, but then you may easily gather up all the linens and remove them (Fig. 10-1K). (Another option is to have the client get off the massage table momentarily while you remove all the blankets.) Now underneath the client is one clean massage sheet. Cover the client with the reserved massage sheet and the massage session may begin.

DRY SHEET WRAP

The **dry sheet wrap** consists of two blankets and a sheet, with external warming devices placed on top of the client's wrapped body. It is a simple treatment for body warming that provides a cocooned feeling loved by many. As seen in Figure 10-2, the client is simply wrapped snugly so that body heat is trapped, and then external warming devices are added. This wrap is excellent for warming a cold client before a massage or for providing a warm environment in which to relax after a massage. Although it is possible to overheat the client if this treatment is prolonged, this is unlikely; however, if the client begins to sweat, apply a cold compress to the forehead. Here we give directions for the dry blanket wrap to be used before a massage, but it may also be used afterward.

> **Temperature:** Warm. External heating devices provide heat through the blankets.
>
> **Time Needed:** 10 minutes or more, depending on the client's core temperature
>
> **Equipment Needed:** Two blankets; three sheets; warming device, such as a hot water bottle, hydrocollator pack, or heating pad; small bath towel to wrap around the neck; bolster for client's knees

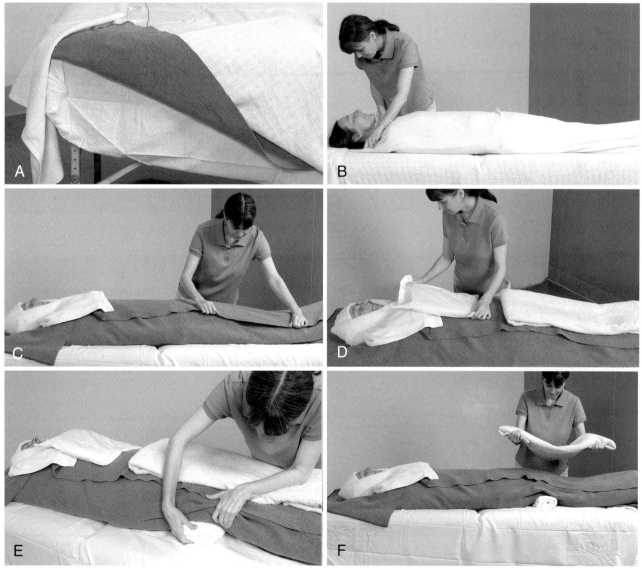

FIGURE 10-2 ■ Dry sheet wrap. **A.** Preparing the table. **B.** Wrapping the client in the dry sheet. **C.** Wrapping the client in the blankets. **D.** Placing warming devices. **E.** Placing a bolster under the knees. **F.** Removing warming devices.

Indications: Chilled or emotionally upset client

Contraindications: Because external warming devices will be applied to the legs and the skin cannot be directly monitored, compromised circulation to the lower extremities is a contraindication. This includes arteriosclerosis of the legs, Buerger's disease, or diabetes; lack of feeling in the legs; and claustrophobia.

Procedure

- Check with client to make sure there are no contraindications to the use of the body wrap.
- Explain the use of the body wrap to the client and get his or her consent.
- Cover the massage table with a massage sheet. Lay two wool blankets on top of that and finally another dry sheet. (Reserve the third sheet to cover the client at the conclusion of the body wrap.) Place the small bath towel at the head of the table (Fig. 10-2A).
- Have the client lie on the sheet, then wrap it around the client. Tuck the sheet in snugly around the client's neck so that no air escapes (Fig. 10-2B).
- Next wrap the blankets over the sheet-covered body (Fig. 10-2C).
- Place the small bath towel around the head and neck and lay warming devices, such as fomentations, hot water bottles, hydrocollator packs, and electric heating pads, on the client's legs. Add one over the chest if the client is very cold (Fig. 10-2D).
- Place a bolster under the knees (Fig. 10-2E).
- After 10 minutes or more, check to make sure the client is thoroughly warm. If so, remove warming devices, sheets, and blankets (Fig. 10-2F); then, if desired, perform a cold mitten friction.
- The client may now receive a massage. However, you want only one dry massage sheet remaining on the massage table. The wool blankets and the sheet that was covering the client must all be removed. Have the client roll onto one side, bunch up the sheet and both blankets against the back, and then have the client roll onto the other side. The client must roll over the bunched-up blankets, but then you may easily gather the bunched linens and remove them (Fig. 10-1K, page 184). Now underneath the client is one clean massage sheet. Cover the client with the reserved massage sheet, and the massage session may begin. Another option is to have the client get off the massage table momentarily while you remove all the blankets.

COLD WET SHEET WRAP

Observant people over the centuries have noticed that wrapping a person in cold linens and then covering him or her with blankets leads to profuse sweating. In 1697 English physician Sir John Floyer, author of *The History of Hot and Cold Bathing*, advised sportsmen who wanted their jockeys to lose weight to "Dip the rider's shirt in cold water; and after it is put on very wet, lay the person in warm blankets to sweat him violently, and he will after lose a considerable weight."(4) However, Vincent Priessnitz (1801–1851) invented the formal use of the cold, wet sheet wrap. In this wrap, the client is wrapped in one wet sheet and a few blankets and left for varying amounts of time to achieve a variety of therapeutic goals.

This treatment was a staple first of the water cure and then of classic naturopathic medicine. Different stages of the wet sheet pack were used for various conditions: stage 1 for fever, weakness, and as a tonic for convalescents; stage 2 for mental illness, anxiety, nervousness, and insomnia; stage 3 for pneumonia, certain digestive problems, and congestion of internal organs; and stage 4 for alcohol and drug addiction, general detoxification, or infectious illnesses such as bronchitis and influenza. Partial wraps were also popular; they included hip and leg packs for acute menstrual pain and arthritis, and heating trunk packs for digestive disturbances.

For today's massage therapist, the **cold, wet sheet wrap** (Fig. 10-3) can be an effective method of manipulating the client's core temperature without expensive or elaborate hydrotherapy equipment. It is also used to administer therapeutic substances, such as herbal preparations, salts, or essential oils, by adding them to the water in which the sheet is soaked.

The first stage of the wet sheet wrap has a cooling effect, since the client is surrounded by a sheet soaked in very cold water and then wrung out. (For this reason, it was once used as an antipyretic, or fever-reducing treatment.) The cold water strongly stimulates the cold receptors on the surface of the skin, causing blood vessels first to constrict strongly and then to dilate. As the body tries to defend against possible chilling, the flow of blood to the skin causes a burst of heat, much as do other short cold applications such as cold plunges or short cold showers. However, the extra blankets covering the client's sheet-wrapped body keep the burst of heat trapped, leading to a quick rise in core temperature.

In approximately 5 minutes, once the client's trapped body heat has warmed the wrap to a neutral temperature,

FIGURE 10-3 ■ Cold, wet sheet wrap. **A.** Preparing the table. **B.** Wringing out the cold sheet. **C.** Placing the cold sheet upon the blanket. **D.** Client laying supine upon sheet. **E.** Wrapping the client's body except the arms. **F.** Wrapping the entire body, including the arms. **G.** Tucking the bottom of the sheet snugly under the feet. **H.** Placing the small bath towel around the head and neck. **I.** Tucking blanket on the table around the client. **J.** Applying the second blanket to the client. **K.** Placing hot water bottle over the feet. **L.** Placing a bolster underneath the client's knees. **M.** Offering the client water. **N.** Removing the wet sheet. **O.** With the client rolled onto one side, bunching up the sheet and both blankets up against the back. **P.** Removing linens. **Q.** Covering client with reserved massage sheet.

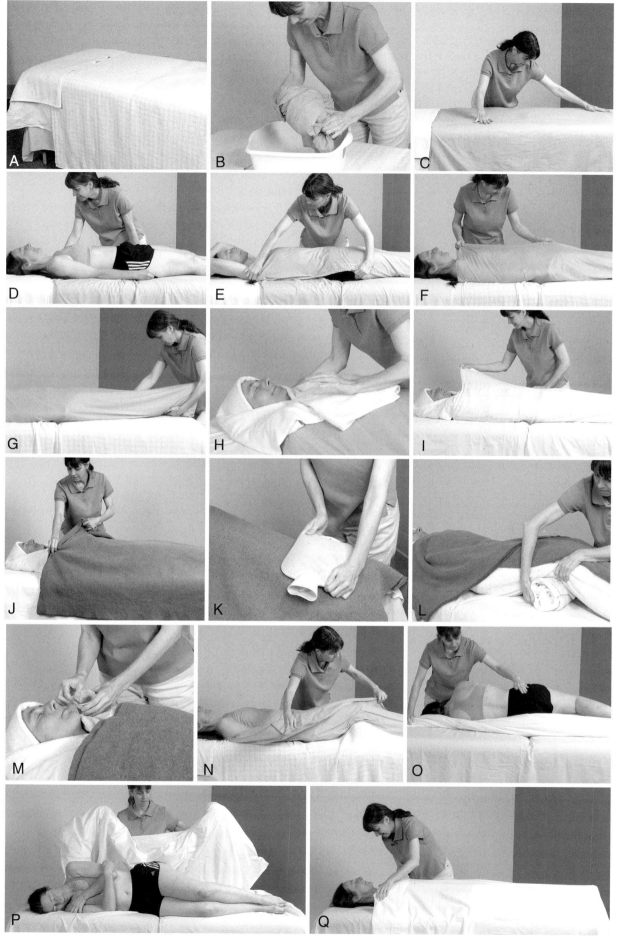

the second or neutral stage is reached. This neutral stage has a calming effect similar to that of the neutral bath.

After approximately another 15 minutes the third stage occurs when the client's trapped body heat has accumulated and raised the core temperature from neutral to hot. (A client can be warmed this way if he or she is chilled, or a client who cannot take a bath can still be warmed effectively.)

Finally, if the client continues in the wrap for 30 minutes or more, the fourth stage occurs: he or she becomes very hot and sweats profusely. This stage is better suited as a detoxification procedure under the supervision of a doctor than as a treatment performed in a massage session, since if detoxification is the goal, it may necessitate the client remaining in the wrap for another hour or more.

The wet sheet pack is soothing for most people, but for a claustrophobic person, it can be unpleasant instead. Be sure to ask clients if they are claustrophobic before giving any kind of body wrap. Polar fleece blankets may be substituted for wool blankets to make laundering easier.

Temperature: Cold (60–70°F)

Time Needed: Approximately 5 minutes or more for the first stage, 15 minutes or more for the second or neutral stage, 30 minutes for the heating phase, and 1 to 2 hours for the sweating stage. (Times are approximate because some clients generate body heat more easily than others.)

Equipment Needed: Water thermometer; plastic sheet to cover massage table; one cotton blanket and one wool blanket; a sheet to be wrung out in cold water; two sheets to be used for massage after the body wrap; small bath towel to wrap around the neck; large container of water at 60° to 70°F for wetting the sheet; warming device, such as a hot water bottle, hot footbath, or fomentation to the feet; bolster for client's knees; cup with drinking water and a straw

Effect: Thermal

Cleanup: Launder wet sheet, both blankets, and small bath towel. Clean, disinfect, and dry water container. Dispose of the plastic sheet or clean it as you would a space blanket.

Indications: Cooling (first stage only) and tonic; sedative for nervous or emotionally upset client (second and third stages); insomnia (second and third stages); warming (third and fourth stages); detoxification/sweating treatment if continued to fourth stage

Contraindications: Claustrophobic person; chilled client; ingestion of alcohol and drugs; any skin problem that is aggravated by excess moisture; when the wrap is taken to the third and fourth stages, any condition that specifically contraindicates whole-body heating, including pregnancy, cardiovascular problems, diabetes, hepatitis,

lymphedema, multiple sclerosis and seizure disorders, unless treatments are specifically prescribed by a doctor

Cautions
1. Very frequent sweating wraps are not recommended for persons with hypothyroid conditions.
2. Anyone who is at risk for lymphedema due to removal of lymph nodes should avoid prolonged sweating in wraps (for longer than 15 minutes once the sweating stage is reached).

Procedure
1. Check with client to make sure there are no contraindications to the use of the body wrap.
2. Explain the use of the body wrap to the client and get his or her consent.
3. Make sure that the client is quite warm, giving a hot footbath or other type of warming treatment if necessary.
4. Cover the massage table with one dry massage sheet, and cover that with a plastic sheet. On top of that place one blanket with its upper edge about 8 inches from the head of the table. The edge of the blanket should hang down farther on the far side of the table than on the side closest to you. Place the small bath towel at the head of the table (Fig. 10-3A). Reserve the second blanket for step 13 and the second massage sheet for step 19.
5. Soak one sheet in the cold water and wring it out (Fig. 10-3B).
6. Place the sheet upon the blanket with its upper end slightly below the upper edge of the blanket (Fig. 10-3C).
7. Have the client lie supine upon the sheet, with the shoulders about 3 inches below the top of the sheet (Fig. 10-3D).
8. Have the client hold the arms up while you wrap one side of the sheet around the body (away from yourself) and tuck it in under the opposite side (Fig. 10-3E).
9. Now have the client lower the arms, and wrap the opposite side of the sheet around the body (you will be bringing the sheet toward yourself) and tuck it in (Fig. 10-3F).
10. Tuck the bottom of the sheet snugly under the feet (Fig. 10-3G).
11. Place the small bath towel around the head and neck to protect the client's neck and keep out cold air (Fig. 10-3H).
12. Draw the shorter side of the blanket over the body and tuck it in, and then do the same with the wider side (Fig. 10-3I).
13. Lay the second blanket over the client and tuck it in (Fig. 10-3J).
14. Place a hot water bottle, hydrocollator pack, or other warming device on the feet to speed warming (Fig 10-3K).

15. Place a bolster underneath the client's knees (Fig. 10-3L).
16. Offer the client a sip of water from a cup with a straw as needed (Fig. 10-3M).
17. Remove the blankets and wet sheet when the client has reached the proper stage— neutral, hot, or sweating. (Fig. 10-3N).
18. When the pack is removed, give the client a cold mitten friction (see Fig. 11-1) if desired.
19. Now the client may receive a massage. However, you want only one dry massage sheet remaining on the massage table. The blankets and wet sheet must be removed. Have the client roll onto one side and bunch up the sheet and both blankets up against the back (Fig. 10-3O), and then have the client roll onto the other side over the bunched-up blankets. You may easily gather up the bunched linens and remove them (Fig. 10-3P). Now underneath the client is one clean massage sheet. Cover the client with the reserved massage sheet (Fig. 10-3Q). Now the massage session may begin. Another option is to have the client get off the massage table momentarily while you remove the blankets.

CHAPTER SUMMARY

In this chapter you have learned about another type of hydrotherapy treatment, the body wrap, which may be used to advantage by massage therapists. When the body wrap is properly done, clients will feel soothed, relaxed, and comfortably warm. You may perform these wraps without expensive equipment in your office and in other places, such as at your clients' home. Body wraps may also be combined with other treatments. For example, a client may receive a salt glow or take a full-body bath, sauna, hot shower, or steam bath before a wrap.

REVIEW QUESTIONS

Multiple Choice

1. The first stage of the wet sheet pack is
   a. Antipyretic
   b. Sedative
   c. Useful in detoxification

2. Blankets are used in body wraps for all but one reason:
   a. To keep the massage table dry
   b. To prevent claustrophobia
   c. To trap body heat
   d. To give clients an enclosed sensation

3. All but one makes a chemical application when added to the water used for a wrap:
   a. Oatmeal
   b. Sand
   c. Essential oil
   d. Seaweed

4. Body wraps may be combined with all but one:
   a. Steam bath
   b. Ice packs
   c. Sauna
   d. Full-body bath

5. A moist wrap is appropriate for all but one:
   a. Chilled client
   b. Hypersensitive client
   c. Overheated client
   d. Resting client

Fill in the Blank

6. Heating body wraps are being used for patients with cancer because they _____ the immune system and weaken _____.

7. The _____ wrap and the _____ wrap may be used for detoxification.

8. The moist blanket wrap is used for a general _____ and for chronic _____ or _____ pain.

9. The first stage of the cold wet sheet wrap has a _____ effect.

10. The second stage of the cold wet sheet wrap has a _____ effect.

REFERENCES

1. www.clinicaltrials.gov/ct/gvi/show/NCT00178802. Accessed December 1, 2006.
2. www.uth.tmc.edu/thermaltherapy. Accessed December 1, 2006.
3. Interview with Glenna Scott, RN, University of Texas Medical Center, December 1, 2006.
4. Floyer J. Quoted in Kellogg, JH. *Rational Hydrotherapy*. Battle Creek, MI: Modern Medicine,1923, p 28.

RECOMMENDED RESOURCES

1. Boyle W, Saine A. *Lectures in Naturopathic Hydrotherapy*, Sandy, OR: Eclectic Medical, 1988.
2. Peterson S. *Hydrotherapy in the Home*. Loveland, CO: Eden Valley Institute, 1973.
3. Shorter E. *From Paralysis to Fatigue: A History of Psychosomatic Illness in the Modern Era*. New York: Free Press, 1992.
4. Williams A. *Spa Bodywork*. Baltimore: Lippincott Williams & Wilkins, 2006.

FRICTION TREATMENTS

The cold-mitten friction is undoubtedly one of the finest hydrotherapy measures known for stimulating the circulation in the skin. . . For toning up the skin and as a general tonic this is better than any tonic one can take from a bottle.

—*Stella Peterson, RN, Hydrotherapy in the Home*

Chapter Objectives

After completing this chapter, the student will be able to:

- Describe the effects of friction treatments.
- Explain the indications, cautions, and contraindications for friction treatments.
- Name and describe different friction treatments, both partial body and whole body.
- Perform friction treatments using the procedure included with each treatment.

Friction treatments are a small but unique part of traditional hydrotherapy. When any area of the body is rubbed vigorously, blood vessels there open, so extra oxygen and nutrients are available in case of injury. Early hydrotherapists, who were deeply involved in manipulating blood flow to different parts of the body, discovered that chafing or rubbing parts of the body would stimulate local blood flow and make their treatments more effective. Friction was used to warm cold areas, bring water applications into closer contact with the skin, and stimulate the body's vital functions to heighten the patient's responses to other hydrotherapy treatments. Patients with very high fevers were doused with cold water while being vigorously rubbed: this caused the cold of the water to more thoroughly permeate the skin and encouraged dilation of skin blood vessels so more heat would be lost from the patient's skin. Cold mitten frictions were standard treatment for pneumonia, and in the days before antibiotics, when people might take many days or weeks to recuperate from an illness, convalescents received them daily to strengthen their constitutions. Salt glows were developed for patients who were too weak to tolerate a cold mitten friction, and

dry brushing became a method for patients to build up their immune system over time.

All friction treatments use a coarse-textured agent to vigorously stimulate the skin and its underlying blood vessels, which improves the circulation of blood and lymph, increases uptake of nutrients and excretion of wastes, and stimulates the nervous and immune systems. Frictions are relaxing as well, and salt glows in particular may leave the client feeling euphoric. Various friction treatments can be used to cool clients who are overheated, to stimulate function in a particular area, and to provide sensory stimulation to your clients.

Epsom salt, herbs, or essential oils may also be added to salt glows so their specific chemicals can be absorbed through the skin. In spas, some friction agents, such as salt and sugar, are also used for beauty effects because they exfoliate (remove the top layer of dead skin cells). This leaves the skin smoother, brighter, and better able to absorb creams and cosmetics.

Three friction treatments are presented in this chapter: cold mitten friction, salt glows, and dry brushing. Another treatment, the Swedish shampoo, is described briefly in Box 11-1. You will learn not only how to

BOX 11-1 *Point of Interest*

SWEDISH SHAMPOO

A Swedish shampoo is a stimulating and cleansing treatment that is more commonly found in a spa than in a massage therapist's office, since a sweat bath, a room with a tiled floor, and a shower are required. It is used for general cleansing after a massage and a sauna or steam bath and for pleasant stimulation of the skin. As a friction treatment, a Swedish shampoo is milder than either a cold mitten friction or a salt glow. Each part of the client's body is soaped and then rinsed in turn. The therapist scrubs with a circular motion, using a body brush dipped in soapy water to work up a lather, and then 105°F water is poured over the area to rinse off the soap. Each lower extremity is soaped and rinsed separately, followed by each upper extremity, the back, and finally the chest and abdomen. After the Swedish shampoo is concluded, the client takes a lukewarm shower and then lies down for a rest.

perform these treatments but how to use them appropriately in your massage practice.

COLD MITTEN FRICTION

The **cold mitten friction** is a whole-body friction performed with a terry cloth mitt or washcloth dipped in cold water. During the treatment, the entire body is draped, except for the area that is being frictioned. This simple but powerful treatment can be given to finish a whole-body heating treatment, when the client's blood vessels are widely dilated and massive heat loss from the skin could cause him or her to become chilled. It is also useful to stimulate blood flow to the skin, to train the skin to react to cold, and as a general tonic. The cold mitten friction is a good treatment for clients who are bedridden and not receiving any circulatory stimulation through exercise.

Your clients may also give themselves a cold mitten friction between office visits or daily as a long-term tonic. As you will learn in Chapter 12, regular applications of cold act as a form of exercise for the muscles that dilate and constrict the blood vessels of the skin. When the cold mitten friction is given over a long time, the temperature of the cold water can be gradually lowered as the blood vessels react more strongly. The cold mitten friction is the only friction treatment that is thermal as well as mechanical.

Never begin this treatment with a chilled client: if in doubt, give a hot footbath or another warming treatment first. To prevent chilling, the room in which the treatment is given should be at least 65°F. When the client is comfortably warm, the cold terry cloth will give a brief shock to the skin, but it should feel refreshing as well. Once the area is frictioned, dried, and draped, the client will have a comfortable feeling of warmth. As with other applications of cold given to a warm client, the cold receptors on the surface of the skin are stimulated, the blood vessels constrict strongly and then dilate, and the flow of blood to the skin causes a burst of heat there. The area is stimulated by the cold water, friction, and finally by brisk drying; quickly covering it retains the heat produced by the body.

For a client who is overheated after a heating treatment and needs to be cooled down, see the variation at the end of the instructions.

Temperature: 50° to 60°F. The colder the water, the greater the reaction. If repeated on a regular basis, colder water will gradually become more tolerable. If the water is too cold for the client, add hot water to raise the temperature to a tolerable level.

Time Needed: 15 to 20 minutes

Equipment Needed: Water thermometer, two sheets, washable blanket, container for water, 2 quarts of water, two or more towels, one or two friction mitts of coarse towel or loofah. A coarse terry cloth washcloth wrapped around the hand may also be used.

Effect: Thermal and mechanical

Cleanup: Clean, disinfect, and dry water container; launder mitts or washcloths.

Indications: Finish after a heating treatment; poor capacity of skin blood vessels of the skin to react to cold; skin stimulation, particularly for individuals who are sedentary, bedridden, wheelchair-bound or who have reduced sensation; general tonic; overheated client

Contraindications: Chilled person, because if the client is not warm before the treatment, the blood vessels will react weakly and the client will not enjoy the friction; open, infected, or damaged skin; advanced varicose veins; sunburned skin; skin rash; sensitive skin

Procedure
1. Check with client to make sure there are no contraindications to the use of the cold mitten friction.
2. Explain the use of the cold mitten friction to the client and get his or her consent.
3. Make sure that the client is warm, giving a hot footbath or other type of warming treatment if necessary.
4. Have the client, either nude or wearing only underwear, lie supine upon the table on top of one

sheet and covered by the other sheet and a blanket. For the treatment to be effective, only one part of the body should be exposed to cold at a time, and the rest of the body should be covered and warm. Each area must be treated, dried, and then covered without the bottom sheet becoming damp.

5. Expose one arm. Slide a towel underneath the arm all the way up to the shoulder. Dip the friction mitt in the cold water, wring it out, and begin on the arm (Fig. 11-1A). Start with the fingers. Use a brisk back-and-forth motion, and use light to moderate pressure. Move from the fingers to the top of the shoulder and back again. The skin

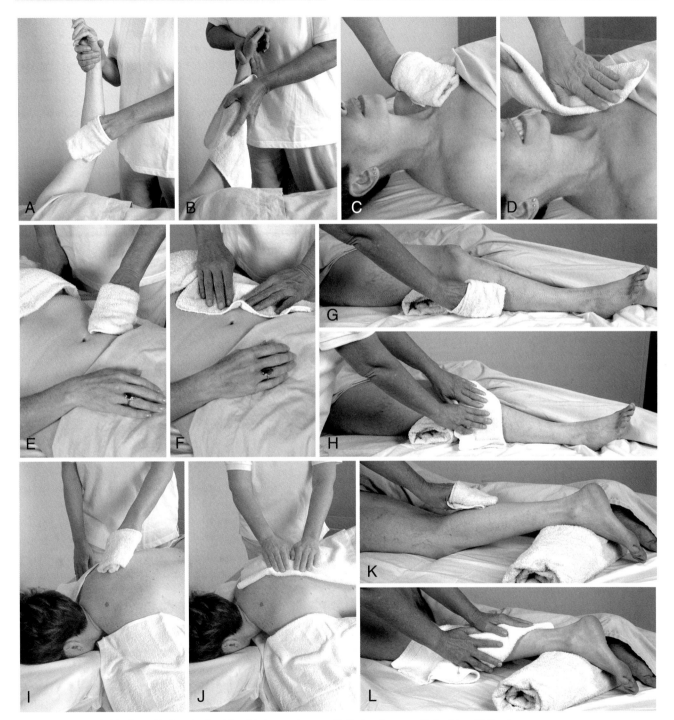

FIGURE 11-1 ■ Cold mitten friction. **A.** Applying friction to the arm. **B.** Drying the arm. **C.** Applying friction to the chest. **D.** Drying the chest. **E.** Applying friction to the abdomen. **F.** Drying the abdomen. **G.** Applying friction to the front of the leg. **H.** Drying the front of the leg. **I.** Applying friction to the back. **J.** Drying the back. **K.** Applying friction to the back of the leg. **L.** Drying the back of the leg.

should become pink. If not, repeat the friction. The more water that is left in the mitt, the greater the reaction will be; however, the client should not be extremely wet.

6. Remove the mitt from your hand and briskly dry the arm with a dry towel (Fig. 11-1B). Remove the first towel from under the client's arm, and put the arm back on the bottom sheet, which should be dry, and under the top sheet and blanket.

7. Repeat steps 5 and 6 with the client's other arm.

8. Uncover the chest.

9. Dip the mitts in cold water and wring them out. Do not have them dripping wet or water will run down the client's chest and wet the bottom sheet.

10. Ask the client to inhale deeply as you apply friction with the mitts. Move up the middle of the chest, across the shoulders, down the sides of the torso, and back to the midline (Fig. 11-1C). In a female client, do not apply friction over the breasts.

11. Remove the mitt from your hand and briskly dry the chest with a dry towel (Fig. 11-1D). Cover the chest with a towel so it will be warm as you treat the abdomen.

12. Dip the mitts in cold water and wring them out. Do not have them dripping wet or water will run down the client's abdomen and wet the bottom sheet.

13. Uncover and treat the client's abdomen (Fig. 11-1E).

14. Remove the mitt from your hand and briskly dry the client's abdomen with a dry towel (Fig. 11-1F). Now cover both chest and abdomen with the top sheet and blanket.

15. Repeat this procedure on the anterior surface of each leg, placing a towel under the leg before applying friction and removing it after drying the leg (Fig. 11-1, G and H).

16. Have the client roll over into the prone position, and treat the back in the same manner (Fig. 11-1I). Do not have the mitts dripping wet or water will run down the client's back and wet the bottom sheet.

17. Remove mitts from your hands, dry the back briskly, and then cover it with the top sheet and blanket (Fig. 11-1J).

18. Friction the posterior surface of each leg in the same manner, placing a towel under each leg before applying friction and removing it afterwards (Fig. 11-1, K and L).

19. The client will be warmed and relaxed, and a massage may now be performed if desired. If you have followed the directions correctly, both sheets will be dry.

Variation

Cooling friction suitable for an overheated client. Simply use plenty of very cold water (32°–50°F) and leave the client uncovered throughout the treatment.

SALT GLOWS

A **salt glow** is a friction treatment performed on the bare skin by rubbing it with moistened salt. During a salt glow, the skin turns pink, or glows, as blood vessels under the skin dilate. Traditionally, salt glows were used when patients were too weak to tolerate cold mitten frictions. However, so many people find them enjoyable that they are commonly used not only to increase blood flow to the skin but also as a pampering treatment. The skin feels softer after a salt glow, as the top layer of dead skin cells is removed by the friction of the salt crystals, and the skin absorbs substances such as herbal preparations, essential oils, and beauty products better. Of particular importance to the massage therapist, the salt glow prepares the client's tissues for massage. Local circulation will be much improved, the superficial muscles will be more relaxed, and the client will have a pleasant feeling of euphoria.

General tips on performing salt glows:

1. Salt is drying to the skin, so always apply some type of emollient lotion or oil to the client's skin afterward. If a massage is to be performed after the salt glow, the massage oil, cream, or lotion will serve this purpose.

2. Be careful not to use too much pressure, which can irritate the skin. Salt crystals have sharp edges and can feel unpleasant if too much pressure is used.

3. Do not use table salt. Coarser salts are better and give a greater reaction. Sea salt, kosher salt, pickling salt, Epsom salt, and Dead Sea salts are all good choices. When mixed with water, the chemicals in the salts will be absorbed to some extent through the skin.

4. Salt glows can be varied with additives. Whole and ground herbs, clays, creams, and essential oils can be added to salt glows for specific therapeutic purposes.

5. Salt glows can also be varied by changing the water temperature, In vigorous clients, very cold water will elicit a stronger reaction.

6. It is important to use good body mechanics. Follow directions carefully so you will not put yourself in awkward positions.

PARTIAL-BODY SALT GLOW

Partial-body salt glows increase local circulation, relax skeletal muscles, are very much enjoyed by some clients for the sensory stimulation they provide, and exfoliate the skin. Many clients also feel a pleasurable sense of being nurtured when salt is washed off of an area. Partial-body salt glows are performed in the much the same way as whole-body salt glows, and with care, they can be given on a massage table with little mess. Instead of the client sitting on a stool in a bathtub as for a whole-body salt glow, the client lies on a towel on the massage table. At the end of the salt glow, the towel, which will be coated with salt crystals, is removed so that the client is lying on a clean, dry sheet.

Temperature: Hot (110°F)

Time Needed: 5 minutes

Equipment Needed: Water thermometer, two containers of warm water, a few tablespoons of Epsom salt in a small container, two washcloths, one large towel. A plastic tub under the table may be used to dispose of linens during the massage.

Cleanup: Clean and sanitize containers; launder used linens

Effect: Primarily mechanical

Indications: Local muscle tension, poor local circulation, stress reduction, sensory stimulation

Contraindications: Open or damaged skin; eczema; fungal infection, such as ringworm, athlete's foot, or toenail fungus; advanced varicose veins; sunburned skin; skin rash; sensitive skin; skin that has just been shaved

Procedure
1. Check with client to make sure there are no contraindications for the salt glow.
2. Explain the use of the salt glow to the client and get his or her consent.
3. Place a towel under the part of the body that is to receive the salt glow.
4. Drip just enough water into the container of salt so that the granules clump together (Fig. 11-2A).
5. Inform the client that he or she will feel warm water on the area.
6. Gently wash the back, arm, or leg with warm water (Fig. 11-2B).
7. Take about 1 tbsp of the moistened salt in your hands and spread it on the back, arm, or leg. More salt may be needed, depending on the size of the area. Use a brisk upward movement with one hand while making a brisk downward movement with the other hand; as you alternate hands, you will be giving a friction type of massage. Move from one end of the area to the other and back again, using gentle pressure and always moving briskly (Fig. 11-2C).
8. Continue for 1 to 3 minutes, depending on the size of the area you are frictioning.
9. Ask the client to tell you when the salt starts to feel too scratchy; often the client will enjoy the abrasive and stimulating feel of the salt for a time and then will start to feel that it is too abrasive. Should the client complain that the salt glow is uncomfortable, stop immediately.
10. Gently wash the salt off with the wet washcloth, then dry the client with the dry one (Fig. 11-2D).
11. The towel underneath the body part will have salt crystals on it and should be removed before proceeding with the massage. Ask the client to roll first onto one side and then onto the other as you fold the towel in on itself and remove it.

WHOLE-BODY SALT GLOW

To perform the whole-body salt glow, apply friction to the entire body part by part and then rinse the client. Make sure that no salt remains on the client's skin at the end of the salt glow.

Indications: Poor circulation, stimulation of sweat glands before a whole-body heating treatment such as a sauna or steam bath, stimulation of the skin and muscles before massage, as a general tonic

Contraindications: Open, infected, or damaged skin; fungal infection such as ringworm, athlete's foot, or toenail fungus; skin rash; sensitive skin; skin that has just been shaved

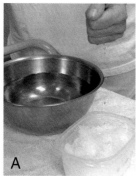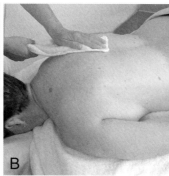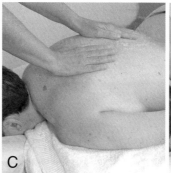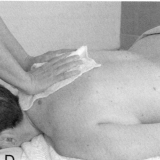

FIGURE 11-2 ■ Partial-body salt glow. **A.** Moistening the salt. **B.** Washing the back with a wet washcloth. **C.** Applying friction to the back with salt. **D.** Washing salt off the back.

Temperature: Pleasantly warm, about 95° to 100°F

Time Needed: 20 minutes

Equipment Needed: Bathtub; plastic stool, plastic bench, or bath chair; pitcher; two bath towels; water thermometer; 1 to 2 cups of salt moistened with just enough water so that the grains clump together. (Too much water will dissolve the salt.)

Effect: Primarily mechanical

Cleanup: Clean and sanitize tub, flushing the drain with extra water to make sure no salt water remains in the pipes. Launder used linens.

Procedure

1. Check with client to make sure there are no contraindications for the use of the salt glow.
2. Explain the use of the salt glow to the client and get consent.

3. Place a plastic stool, plastic bench, or bath chair in the bathtub or tiled area, and cover it with a towel. (Here we demonstrate the salt glow in a large shower stall, but if a bathtub is used, fill it with enough warm water to cover the client's ankles.)
4. Have the client undress and sit on the stool, bench, or bath chair. (The client may wear a bathing suit or disposable underwear, but this will reduce the amount of skin that can be treated.)
5. Add a little water to the container of salt, enough to make the grains clump together but not enough to dissolve the granules.
6. Pour warm water over the client's back. Now take a handful of the salt in your hands (Fig. 11-3A). Apply the handful of salt to the client's back, then, using a back-and-forth motion, rub briskly but gently. Cover the entire back from top to bottom (Fig. 11-3B). The trick is to use enough friction so that the

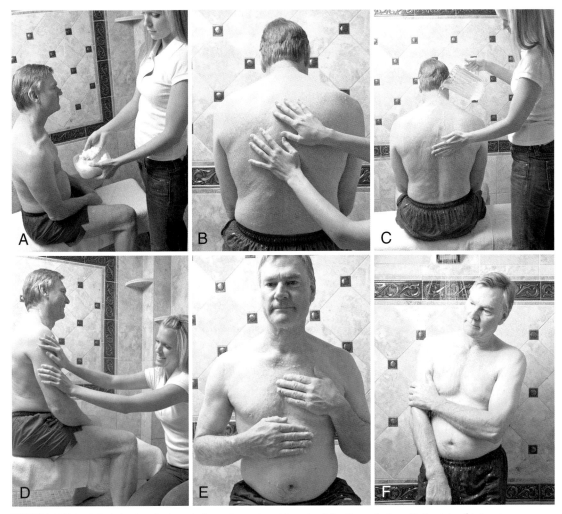

FIGURE 11-3 ■ Whole-body salt glow. **A.** Scooping out moistened salt for the salt glow. **B.** Applying friction to the back using the moistened salt. **C.** Washing salt off the back. **D.** Applying friction to the arm and leg on one side. **E.** Client applying friction to the chest and abdomen. **F.** Client rinsing salt off the chest and abdomen.

Whole-Body Salt Glow for Stimulation

Background

Alfredo was a 62-year-old schoolteacher who was generally in excellent health. He exercised regularly, was careful about his diet, and received massage therapy once a month to relieve muscle tightness and postexercise soreness. One day, however, he scheduled a massage for an entirely different reason. Ten days previously, he had surgery on his mid face area to remove a benign tumor behind his right eye and had been recuperating at home ever since. The surgery was successful and his recuperation was uneventful, but Alfredo was still not feeling well. The entire experience had been emotionally stressful, so he still felt very tense and, since he had not been able to exercise since the surgery, he also felt lethargic. Alfredo hoped that massage could address both of these problems.

Treatment

The massage therapist visited Alfredo at his home. Although there was considerable bruising on the right side of his face, Alfredo looked well otherwise. After discussion, the therapist considered what hydrotherapy treatments might be beneficial to him along with his massage. Something relaxing and gently stimulating seemed be ideal. Treatments on the head would have a tendency to affect blood flow there and were clearly contraindicated. Alfredo's doctor did not want him to exercise for at least 4 more days. Therefore, very hot or cold treatments that could move blood around the body as exercise would were contraindicated without his doctor's permission, which the therapist could not obtain at that time. While a neutral bath would have been a mild treatment, it is specifically designed to decrease stimulation, and so it was not suitable either. The therapist finally decided to perform a whole-body salt glow with warm (102°F) water.

   During the salt glow, Alfredo sat in his bathtub on a plastic stool covered with towels, with warm water up to his ankles. His body was treated using Epsom salt as described in the preceding section. The friction of the salt upon the skin felt pleasantly stimulating to him, and shortly after the salt glow began, he told the therapist, "My skin needed this!" After the salt glow was over, Alfredo showered briefly to remove all traces of salt, then moved to the massage table. As he lay down and the therapist prepared to begin the massage session, Alfredo told him that he felt more alive and more relaxed already.

Discussion Questions

1. Why would treatments on the head that would affect blood flow have been contraindicated?
2. What other hydrotherapy treatments might have been suitable in this situation?

skin glows pink and the client enjoys the sensation without having an overly abrasive effect. Use more salt if needed. When the client's back is thoroughly pink, use the pitcher to pour warm water over the back and rinse off the salt completely (Fig. 11-3C). Any time the friction begins to feel irritating to the client, stop and wash the salt off immediately.

7. After the back has been frictioned and rinsed, you are ready to continue with the legs and the arms. Apply salt to the arm and leg that are facing you (Fig. 11-3D), rub them with salt, and rinse the salt off. Now have the client stand up, turn 180° and sit down again. Help stabilize the client if needed to prevent slipping. The other arm and leg are now facing you. Apply salt to them and rub just as you did with the first arm and leg.

8. Now friction the torso and abdomen, or because the skin of the abdomen and chest is usually more sensitive, let the client do this (Fig. 11-3E).

9. Either pour water over the torso and abdomen to rinse the salt off, or if a shower is available, the client can rinse off (Fig. 11-3F).

10. Have the client dry briskly with a towel, and then lie down on the massage table for a session. If the client is not going to receive a massage, the skin should be moisturized with a cream or lotion.

DRY BRUSHING

Dry brushing, as the name implies, is a friction technique using a dry brush applied to the skin surface. The entire body is brushed, beginning with the feet and finishing with the back. Brushing stimulates the skin and its blood vessels, lymphatic vessels, and nerves, and consequently it is appropriate as a health-promoting technique for the skin and the immune system. Dry brushing can be performed during a massage session just before

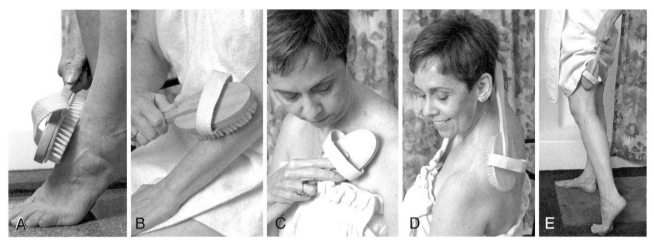

FIGURE 11-4 ■ Dry brushing. **A.** Dry brushing the foot and leg. **B.** Dry brushing the forearm. **C.** Dry brushing the chest. **D.** Dry brushing the back. **E.** Dry brushing the back of the leg.

each area of the body is massaged, adding to the sensory stimulation of the massage treatment. Dry brushing is also a treatment that a client can do to himself or herself between office visits, following the brushing with a shower to wash off dead skin cells and impurities that may have been scraped up. A contrast shower complements the toning action of dry brushing. As a self-treatment, dry brushing is best performed every day.

Time Needed: 5 to 10 minutes

Equipment Needed: Soft natural-bristle brush, loofah sponge, or coarse bath glove. (A softer brush should be used with clients who are new to this treatment; then, when the skin has become less sensitive, a coarser brush may be used.)

Effect: Mechanical

Cleanup: When treatment is given by a massage therapist in the course of a session, wash the brush afterwards with soap and hot water, then spray it with alcohol and air-dry before storing it. When a client is self-treating daily, the brush should be washed every few weeks with soap and hot water and then thoroughly air-dried.

Indications: General conditioning; skin stimulation, particularly for individuals who are sedentary, bedridden, or wheelchair-bound or who have reduced sensation; stimulation of blood and lymphatic vessels underneath the skin

Contraindications: Open, infected, or damaged skin; advanced varicose veins; sunburned skin; skin rash; sensitive skin; skin that has just been shaved

Procedure

1. Begin by brushing one entire foot and leg, starting with the sole of the foot and working up the leg (Fig. 11-4A). Brush vigorously in circular motions, keeping the brush in contact with the skin. Use the maximum pressure that is comfortable; over time, the skin will tolerate more pressure. Go more slowly and lightly over sensitive areas.
2. Repeat on the other foot and leg.
3. Brush one arm, starting with the hand and working up to the shoulder (Fig. 11-4B).
4. Repeat on the other arm.
5. Brush the abdomen and chest (Fig. 11-4C) with strokes moving toward the heart.
6. Brush the entire back (Fig. 11-4D) and the posterior surface of the legs (Fig. 11-4E).
7. Brush the neck, using slower and lighter pressure. Do not brush the face.
8. Take a shower of any desired length. All that is necessary is a brief shower to cleanse the skin, but a contrast shower enhances the toning effect of the brushing.
9. Towel off vigorously.
10. Moisturize the skin with an appropriate oil or lotion.

CHAPTER SUMMARY

This chapter discusses three classic hydrotherapy treatments that may be used to advantage by massage therapists, namely applications of friction using rough washcloths, moistened salt, or brushes. Frictions are easy to perform and enjoyed by massage clients, and they complement hands-on massage techniques. They can be easily integrated into your massage sessions and/or combined with other hydrotherapy treatments. You can also offer them to your clients as a home treatment to help promote their general wellness.

REVIEW QUESTIONS

Short Answer

1. The salt glow was originally seen as an alternative to what other friction treatment?

   _____

   _____

2. Why was the salt glow substituted for this treatment?

   _____

   _____

3. Explain the stimulating effect of a cold mitten friction.

   _____

   _____

4. Name two ways to vary the effects of a salt glow.

   _____

   _____

5. Why would a contrast shower add to the toning effect of dry brushing?

   _____

   _____

Multiple Choice

6. When performing a salt glow, use
   a. Slightly moistened salt
   b. Dry salt
   c. A 20% salt solution
   d. Salt water

7. All but one is an effect of a friction treatment:
   a. Stimulation of nerves
   b. Vasodilation of surface blood vessels
   c. Skin exfoliation
   d. Removal of wrinkles

8. Salt glows can be varied by using all these additives but one:
   a. Whole and ground herbs
   b. Sand
   c. Creams
   d. Essential oils

9. A cold mitten friction uses
   a. Sea salt or Epsom salt
   b. Terry cloth mitts
   c. Natural-fiber brush
   d. Soapy water

10. Local salt glows are contraindicated for all but one:
    a. Eczema
    b. Fungal infections
    c. Poor local circulation
    d. Sunburned skin

HYDROTHERAPY SELF-TREATMENTS FOR HEALTH AND WELLNESS

12

Cold mountain spring water sends our blood surging and crams every capillary with a belt of adrenaline.

— R. Deakin, *Waterlog: A Swimmer's Journey Through Britain*

Chapter Objectives

After completing this chapter, the student will be able to:

- Describe two types of detoxification treatments and explain how they work.
- Define and explain body hardening.
- Give specific examples of body-hardening treatments.
- Describe and perform tonic hydrotherapy treatments that are given to the whole body.
- Describe and perform tonic hydrotherapy treatments that are given to one part of the body at a time.
- Describe self-care treatments for the professional massage therapist.

In earlier chapters, you have learned how hydrotherapy can be an excellent adjunct to massage. When used as self-care, many treatments can also be used effectively as a stand-alone treatment for general health and wellness. In many cases they can also help your clients get faster and better results from their massage sessions. Specific self-treatments can detoxify, stimulate the body's functions, increase local circulation, and even help prevent repetitive strain injury. They are simple and inexpensive, and can make effective self-care treatments for the massage therapist. Because they stimulate the circulation of blood and lymph and speed the removal of metabolic wastes, these treatments all complement the effects of massage.

To be effective, the treatments in this chapter must be performed several times a week or even daily. As such, they are suitable for your clients who are interested in using hydrotherapy on a regular basis to improve their health and wellness. Self-treatment instruction sheets are provided in Appendix A for you to copy and pass on to your clients along with special instructions and a chart for your clients to record home treatments.

DETOXIFICATION TREATMENTS

Detoxification treatments are designed to assist the body in excreting **toxins.** Toxins from the external environment may be swallowed, inhaled, or absorbed through the skin, while metabolic wastes such as urea and lactic acid are produced by normal body processes. Both must be excreted or they can contribute to illness or chronic poor health. Two hydrotherapy treatments that are used for detoxification are whole-body heating and bathing in water with chemical additives. Other treatments for detoxification that are traditional but not practical for the modern massage therapist's practice are internal flushing with water and O. G. Carroll's **constitutional hydrotherapy** treatment, both discussed in Chapter 1.

WHOLE-BODY HEATING

Evaporation of sweat from the body surface is a powerful coolant, and so any hydrotherapy treatment that raises core temperature, such as a prolonged hot foot bath, hot sitz bath, hot full-body bath, sauna, steam bath, heating body wrap, or even a prolonged hot shower will cause sweating. As discussed in Box 12-1, a wide variety of toxic chemicals a person might be exposed to can be excreted in sweat. More everyday chemicals—including prescription medications such as antibiotics and anti-anxiety drugs and recreational drugs such as nicotine, marijuana, cocaine, and amphetamines—are also excreted in sweat.(1–5) So are metabolic wastes such as urea and lactic acid.

One dramatic example of detoxification using whole-body heating is the use of saunas to treat the rescue workers who responded to the destruction of the World Trade Center in New York City on September 11, 2001.

The attack on and subsequent collapse of the World Trade Center caused an enormous release of toxic substances into the air. Construction materials such as concrete, asbestos, and steel as well as office furnishings and equipment were pulverized or incinerated. Diesel and jet fuel burned in clouds. Asbestos, benzene, dioxins, mercury, manganese, lead, polychlorinated biphenyls (PCBs), fiberglass, silicon, and sulfuric acid and other chemicals were released and ingested, inhaled, and/or absorbed through the skin by the rescue workers.

As much as 7 years later, many of them had persistent, often worsening health problems. These included respiratory ailments, such as asthma and sinus problems; digestive

---

BOX 12-1 | *Point of Interest*

DETOXIFICATION THROUGH WHOLE-BODY HEATING

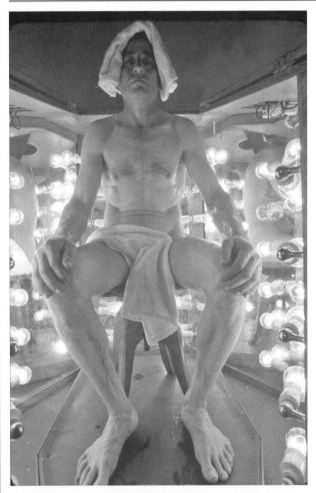

Mercury miner sweating out mercury in a hot box at the hospital at the world's oldest and largest mercury mine in Almadén, Spain, 1972. Miners who are sick from mercury vapors often exercise while in the sauna to raise their core temperatures even higher and encourage more sweating. (Reprinted with permission from Putman J. Quicksilver and slow death. *National Geographic,* October 1972, p 167.)

Many massage therapists are acquainted with the notion of sweating as a way to detoxify the body but have only a vague notion of what toxins are and how sweating might release them. A toxin is any substance that can cause illness or poor general health. Toxins from the external environment may be inhaled, swallowed, or absorbed through the skin. Many external substances are obviously toxic and can cause significant health issues. Arsenic, for example, can cause lowered immunity, some types of cancer, and poor respiratory or cardiovascular function. Lead can cause anemia, poor growth in children, encephalopathy, hyperactivity, learning problems, and infertility. In large enough amounts, both arsenic and lead can be fatal. Many chemicals that a woman accumulates in her body, such as dioxin and PCBs, can impair fetal brain development and harm the developing immune system, thyroid, and brain.

Exposure to toxins depends largely upon where a person lives. These toxins may be naturally occurring chemicals that end up in the water or food supply through erosion of local soils. For example, some parts of the world have bedrock that contains high levels of arsenic; their groundwater also has high levels of arsenic, which contributes to health problems peculiar to those areas. Toxic chemicals can also be introduced by human activities, such as farming, mining, and other industries. For example, living close to a copper smelter or mercury mine can expose one to high levels of copper or mercury in the soil, water, or air. A person who lives in a farming area is more likely to be exposed to pesticides, and a resident of an urban area could be exposed to heavy metals such as cadmium, chromium, or lead.(1,2)

Although the primary effect of sweating is to cool the body, it can also eliminate toxins. When core temperature rises and sweating begins, toxins are mobilized from fat tissues into the sweat. In a person with a high level of toxins whose other channels of excretion, such as the lungs or the kidneys, are not functioning properly, many other toxins can be excreted in his or her sweat. For example, if a person has longstanding kidney disease, the sweat glands will adapt by excreting more of the wastes the kidneys are unable to excrete. Because the detoxifying action of sweat can be so powerful, the skin is sometimes referred to as the third kidney and the sweat glands as miniature nephrons.

Environmental toxins which can be excreted through sweat include the following:

1. Pesticides
2. PCBs

3. Dioxin
4. DDE (a metabolite of DDT and a fat-soluble toxin)
5. Heavy metals such as cadmium, aluminum, lead, mercury, copper, and nickel.(3,4)

Mercury is a striking example of a dangerous toxin that can be excreted in sweat. Mercury poisoning generally has its most devastating effects on the central nervous system, but it is also toxic to other body systems. Women exposed to mercury during pregnancy are more likely than usual to have children with neurological and immune system problems. Excess mercury can be taken into the body by eating food with a high mercury content such as tuna fish, drinking water with a high mercury content, breathing mercury vapor, or absorbing it through the skin. At this stage, it is carried by the blood to cells in all organs of the body.

Normally, most of the mercury taken in by the body is excreted through the urine and the feces, but in cases of mercury toxicity, sweating treatments been used for hundreds of years to increase elimination of that mercury. In Almadén, Spain, site of the world's largest mercury mine, saunas have been used since 1752 to detoxify mine workers suffering from acute exposure, such as the miner shown here in a "hot box."(5) In 1979, daily saunas at 160° to 180°F were used by toxicologist W. Stopford, MD, to successfully treat a sick man who had been exposed to high levels of mercury.(6)

References

1. Alloway B. Bioavailability of Elements in Soil. In *Essentials of Medical Geology: Impacts of the Natural Environment on Public Health*. Burlington, MA: Elsevier, 2005, p 368.
2. Davies B. Medical geology: Perspectives and prospects. In *Essentials of Medical Geology: Impacts of the Natural Environment on Public Health*. Burlington, MA: Elsevier, 2005, p 2.
3. Sunderman FW. Excretion of copper in sweat of patients with Wilson's disease during sauna bathing. *Ann Clin Lab Sci* 1974;4:407.
4. Sunderman FW. Perils of mercury. *Ann Clin Lab Sci* 1988;18:89.
5. Putman J. Quicksilver and slow death. *National Geographic*, October 1972, p 167.
6. Stopford W. Industrial exposure to mercury. In *The Biogeochemistry of Mercury in the Environment*. New York: Elselvier/North Holland Biomedical, 1979, pp 375, 381.

tract problems, such as gastroesophageal reflux disease and severe stomach pain; and emotional issues such as depression, anger, and low motivation. Mainstream medical treatment has been unsuccessful in many cases. An alternative treatment, sauna detoxification, has been used by hundreds of the rescue workers. Sauna detoxification begins with aerobic exercise to warm the body, followed by a 2- to 5-hour sauna; this regimen is repeated daily for approximately 33 days (Fig. 12-1). Saunas are taken at temperatures between 140° and 180°F. Rescue workers go from sauna to shower and back again several times to prevent overheating and to wash off excreted substances. The effectiveness of this process as a way to excrete toxins is dramatically evident in the towels used to wipe off their sweat, which have been stained a variety of colors from brown to orange to blue to green to black. One such towel is shown in Figure 12-2, being held up by the firefighter who used it. A sample of the towel was cut off and sent for laboratory analysis. Tests revealed that his sweat was very high in metals, especially manganese. After the sauna treatment, most of the participants have had significant improvement in their vestibular and neurologic function, less need for medication, and fewer sick days. Blood samples taken before and after sauna treatment show greatly reduced levels of PCBs, more normal cholesterol levels, and improved thyroid function.(6–9)

In addition to detoxifying via the sweat glands, recently it has been realized that whole-body heating also detoxifies by moving toxic substances dissolved in fatty tissues back

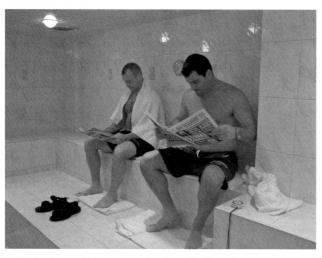

FIGURE 12-1 ■ Using saunas for detoxification. Sauna treatment of two New York City firefighters exposed to toxins at the World Trade Center, 2001. (Photograph courtesy of New York City Rescue Workers Detoxification Project.)

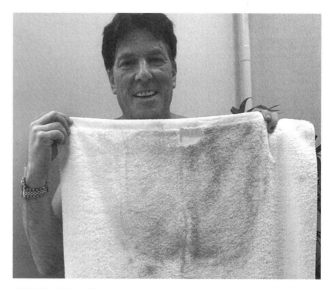

FIGURE 12-2 ■ Sweat excreted by one firefighter. A small piece of this towel was removed so the sweat it contained could be analyzed; tests found that it contained high levels of manganese and other heavy metals. Manganese was one of the components of the steel girders of the World Trade Center. (Photograph courtesy of New York City Rescue Workers Detoxification Project.)

into the bloodstream. As core temperature rises, blood flow to the fatty tissue increases and chemicals stored there return to the bloodstream, where they can pass through the liver to be broken down and finally excreted in the person's urine, bile, and feces. For example, environmental physician Jozeph Krop treated a patient who had been exposed to a variety of toxic solvents at her job in an appliance factory. By the time she saw Krop, she was ill with asthma, chronic fatigue syndrome, fibromyalgia, irritable bowel syndrome, chronic bladder infections, frequent upper respiratory infections, and allergies. Before treatment began, three solvents were detected in her blood. She then began taking daily 150°F saunas. After a week of saunas, the blood levels of those three chemicals had decreased—as they had been excreted—but three additional solvents that had never been detected before showed up in her blood samples. These solvents had moved out of her fatty tissues when her whole body was heated in the sauna. After 6 weeks, those new chemicals had also been detoxified and were no longer detected in her blood. While the chemicals were passing out of her system, the patient felt sicker than usual, but by the end of the sauna treatment, her health had improved dramatically.(10) Other patients with toxic exposures have used saunas with similar results.(11–14) Although these examples are extreme in terms of exposure to toxins, they demonstrate the effectiveness of sweating as a treatment for detoxification. You and your clients may use regular saunas to eliminate toxins or simply to prevent a buildup of them in the future. Some toxicologists now advise women to undertake detoxification before pregnancy.

SAUNA

Cross-Reference
See Chapter 8.

Duration and Frequency
Take for 15 to 30 minutes two or three times a week.

Cautions
1. To avoid dehydration, be sure to drink a cup of water before entering the sauna and 1 to 2 cups more during and after the sauna.
2. Do not take more than 2 or 3 saunas a week; too many heat treatments can actually weaken the system with water and electrolyte losses.
3. Until accustomed to taking saunas, stay in only 10 to 15 minutes. Leave the sauna immediately if not tolerating the heat well, that is, feeling lightheaded or weak.

Special Instructions
Take a shower immediately after the sauna to cleanse the body of any toxins excreted in the sweat and to prevent them from being reabsorbed. If more than one cycle of heating and resting is done, take a shower each time you leave the sauna.

BATHS WITH DETOXIFYING ADDITIVES

Another traditional hydrotherapy treatment that may be used for detoxification is a chemical bath, using baking soda, sea salt, or Epsom salt. As discussed in Chapter 7, when dissolved in bath water, the chemicals they contain may neutralize toxins, withdraw toxins from the body, or in the case of Epsom salt, enhance the body's ability to detoxify.(15) Baths need only be warm, not hot: although this mild body heating will stimulate only moderate sweating, that effect is combined with the detoxifying effect of the bath additives.

TREATMENT

BATHS WITH DETOXIFYING ADDITIVES

Cross-Reference
See Chapter 7.

Duration and Frequency
Take for 20 to 30 minutes two or three times a week.

Cautions
1. To avoid dehydration, be sure to drink a cup of water before entering the bath and 1 or 2 cups more during and after the bath.
2. Leave the bath immediately if not tolerating the heat well, that is, feeling nauseated or tired. However, if feeling lightheaded or weak, before you get out, let the water out of the tub and let your body cool down until you feel normal again.

Special Instructions
1. Here are three recipes for a detoxifying bath:
   - 1 cup sea salt, 1 cup Epsom salt, and $1\frac{1}{2}$ cups baking soda
   - $1\frac{1}{2}$ cups baking soda and 2 cups of sea salt
   - 4 cups of Epsom salt
2. Take a shower immediately after the bath to cleanse the skin of any toxins that have been excreted and to prevent them from being reabsorbed.

TONIC HYDROTHERAPY TREATMENTS

A tonic hydrotherapy treatment stimulates one or more body functions and helps to invigorate the client, increase physical vigor, decrease fatigue, make oneself more robust, or give a sense of well-being. Regularly exposing oneself to extremes of hot and cold or exercise to strengthen the body—sometimes called body hardening—is an ancient tonic used in many cultures. To the Spartans, for example, cold baths were regarded as a method to make oneself hardier, whereas warm-water bathing was regarded as a sign of weakness. Many of the early hydrotherapists also relied heavily upon whole-body cold treatments such as cold baths, showers, and walking in cold water or snow as well as whole-body heat treatments such as wet sheet wraps to treat the chronically ill. Local treatments, such as contrast baths, were commonly used to stimulate circulation or other functions in many specific areas (see Chapter 1).

Today we know that as the body recognizes both extreme cold and extreme heat as potential threats to core temperature and reacts defensively, various bodily functions are stimulated. Being exposed to whole-body cold, for example, causes a strong reaction as the body attempts to keep core temperature at a normal 98.6°F. The sympathetic nervous system is activated, various hormones are released, blood vessels under the skin are constricted, shivering begins, and a host of other reactions work together to increase heat production. When the skin blood vessels normally react weakly, repeated whole-body cold can train them to respond more forcefully; while for someone whose thyroid is underactive, very frequent whole-body cold can increase its activity. Repeated exposure to whole-body heat treatments also causes a strong reaction. Over time the blood vessels will react more strongly and the person will sweat more. Tonic treatments for individual areas of the body can cause local blood vessels to contract more quickly and more forcefully, increasing local blood flow, which will supply bones, arteries, muscle, organs, or other cells with additional oxygen and nutrients.

In summary, this is a list of key points to remember about tonic hydrotherapy treatments so you can use them yourself or recommend them to your clients:

1. They challenge the body to adapt to differing temperatures and can have powerful short-term effects on the body, particularly upon the circulatory system. They complement the circulation-enhancing effects of massage.
2. Their effects are not permanent, so they must be done on a regular basis to be effective.
3. Although any healthy individual can benefit from these tonic treatments, those with a weak constitution, low energy and endurance, and poor resistance to infection can benefit the most.
4. Anyone not accustomed to extremes of heat or cold should begin with a mild treatment and gradually increase (or decrease) the water temperature. Stop any treatment immediately in the event of a bad reaction, such as feeling nauseated or lightheaded. The body will adapt to different temperatures over time.
5. It is important to observe the contraindications given with each treatment, as some of them can be a significant strain on the body's adaptive powers.
6. Tonic treatments provide various sensations. Some, such as saunas and warm baths, are soothing and relaxing, while others, such as contrast treatments and cold baths or showers, are invigorating. As such, they complement the relaxing and invigorating sensations that our clients receive from massage therapy.
7. Many different cultures, from Native America to Scandinavia to the Far East to the Mediterranean, have used these treatments to treat illness and keep the body strong and healthy. Many experienced hydrotherapists and wholistic practitioners believe these tonics can be a significant part of a health-promoting lifestyle. Try them, use them safely, and see for yourself what effect they have.

WHOLE-BODY TONIC TREATMENTS

Although little research has been conducted on the effectiveness of whole-body hydrotherapy tonic treatments, studies do support several benefits, including boosting immunity, affecting basal metabolic rate, increasing tolerance to both cold and heat, and stimulating healthy functioning of blood vessels. Examples of these benefits are discussed below:

■ Exposure to both extreme cold and extreme heat causes increased numbers of white blood cells to be pulled into the general circulation. Thus, taking contrast showers or saunas on a regular basis has been shown to decrease the incidence of the common cold, (16,17) and regular swimming in very cold water significantly increases concentrations of plasma interleukin, leukocytes, and monocytes in the blood.(18)

■ Short, intense exposures to whole-body cold such as bathing, showering, or swimming in cold water, or simply being outside in very cold air stimulates heat production and raises the basal metabolic rate. In one study, both men and women who were immersed in 75°F water up to their neck for 90 minutes had a metabolic rate (internal heat production) that was three times their resting rate before beginning the bath.(19) Many other studies, including some with experimental animals and people who work in cold temperatures, have found similar results.(20,21) In 1998, the Thrombosis Research Center in London carried out a study investigating the effect of cold baths on high levels of cholesterol. In that study, 68 patients with high cholesterol took regular cold baths over 3 months. Blood samples taken before the study began and then after 3 months of baths showed that subjects had an increased metabolic rate, double the amount of the hormone noradrenaline, increased levels of free thyroid hormone, and a significant drop in blood cholesterol. Low levels of free thyroid hormones are associated with chronic feelings of coldness.(22,23) Many people who take regular contrast showers, which feature short cold exposures, feel warmer in the winter than they would otherwise.

- Many studies have found that after repeated short exposures to intensely cold air or cold water, the individual's feelings of coldness decrease and he or she is more tolerant of cold.(24,25) One study looked at how well men who had been exposed to cold fared when they went to a cold climate. Before traveling, the men took very cold baths for 3 weeks. Tests showed increased activity of their sympathetic nervous system, higher basal metabolic rates, and higher body temperatures. The men then spent 16 days in the Arctic, along with another group of men who had not taken the cold baths. Those in the cold bath group were able to tolerate the extreme cold (−80°F) much better than the others.(26)
- Regular whole-body heat exposures can increase tolerance to heat. Every year, as winter ends and summer begins, the body, ever vigilant to the danger of a change in core temperature, quickly adjusts from the task of keeping warm to the task of keeping cool. Within 2 weeks of hotter weather, remarkable adaptations are made: metabolic rates drop, sweating begins sooner, people sweat more, and salt is reabsorbed from the sweat on the skin at a higher rate to conserve it. In a similar fashion, someone who is exposed to brief, intense heat by taking regular saunas begins sweating faster and also sweats more when exposed to heat.(27)
- After a series of regular saunas, the blood vessels and heart become better at adapting to intense heat. In the sauna, the person's heart rate does not increase as much, blood vessels actually dilate and constrict better, and over time there can be a significant decrease in his or her systolic blood pressure. Some researchers now advocate using saunas to treat conditions involving poorly functioning blood vessels.(28–31) However, more research is needed before this can be safely recommended.

The following are a number of tonic whole-body treatments that you can recommend to your clients. Each of these treatments is also used as a specific tonic for the immune system.

TREATMENT
CONTRAST SHOWER

Cross-Reference
See Chapter 9.

Duration and Frequency
Three rounds of 2 minutes in a hot shower followed by 1 minute in a cold shower, for a total time of 9 minutes. Perform once a day.

CONTRAST COLD WATER TREADING

Cross-Reference
See Chapter 7.

Duration and Frequency
Do 10 rounds of a hot footbath for 30 seconds followed by cold water marching for 10 seconds. Perform once a day.

Special Instructions
The client will need a hot footbath and a bathtub partly filled with cold water. He or she then performs 10 rounds of immersing the feet in the hot footbath for 30 seconds while moving the feet and wiggling the toes, then carefully transferring to the cold bathtub to march in place for 10 seconds.

Cautions
The client must be very careful not to slip while transferring from the hot water to the cold and back again. A nonskid mat or a towel should be placed under the hot footbath.

COLD SHOWER

Cross-Reference
See Chapter 9.

Duration and Frequency
Total time in the shower is 1 minute. Perform once a day.

WHOLE-BODY SALT GLOW

Cross-Reference
See Chapter 11.

Duration and Frequency
Total time for the salt glow is 10 to 15 minutes. Perform one to three times per week.

Special Instructions
Moisturize the skin well after the salt glow.

COLD MITTEN FRICTION

Cross-Reference
See Chapter 11.

Duration and Frequency
Total time for the cold mitten friction is 5 to 10 minutes. Perform once a day.

BATH WITH VASODILATING ADDITIVES

Cross-Reference
See Chapter 7.

Duration and Frequency
Total time for the bath is 20 minutes. Take the bath two or three times a week.

CASE HISTORY 12-1

Contrast Showers Increase Resistance to the Common Cold

Background

In 1987, Edzard Ernst, a professor of medicine at the Hanover Medical School in Munich, Germany, investigated the effect of contrast showers on the incidence of the common cold. Ernst selected contrast showers because he wanted to find a simple, practical, and inexpensive therapy that could be performed in anyone's home. In the study, 25 people participated by taking regular contrast showers, and a similar group of 25 people acted as controls and took no contrast showers. The average age of both the shower and control group was 28 years, and no one with circulatory or respiratory disease was allowed to partici-pate. Whenever any of the 50 participants had a cold, blood samples were taken to confirm the diagnosis, and everyone kept a diary of any cold symptoms during the 6 months of the study.

Treatment

The 25 members of the test group performed contrast showers five times a week for 6 months, for a total of 137 showers. Subjects were introduced gradually to the complete hot and cold procedure. For the first week, they took a whole-body warm shower (96°–104°F) for 5 minutes, followed by a 30-second cold shower (65°–75°F) to the arms and legs only. The second week, subjects took a whole-body warm shower for 5 minutes followed by a whole-body shower cold shower for 30 seconds. The third week, and for the final 25 weeks of the study, the subjects took a whole-body warm shower for 5 minutes followed by a whole-body cold shower, then repeated the sequence another time for a total of two rounds. After the first 3 weeks, the time in the cold shower was gradually increased to 2 minutes, and the water temperature gradually became colder (52°–65°F).

At the end of the experiment (6 months of showers), Ernst examined blood samples and cold diaries from both groups. He found that the shower group's colds were significantly fewer, significantly milder, and slightly shorter. This effect took 3 months to become apparent, which suggests that the showers induced a slow adaptive process of strengthening the immune system, and it is possible that the improvement might have been even greater if the entire experiment had lasted longer than 6 months.(16)

Special Instructions

1. Add 5 tablespoons of powdered ginger, 5 tablespoons of ground mustard seed, or 2 teaspoons of cayenne pepper to the warm bath water. Begin with slightly less than these amounts, since some people's skin may be particularly sensitive, then increase if there is no stinging sensation.
2. Finish the bath with a 1-minute shower as cold as can be tolerated.
3. Drink water before, during, and after the bath.

DRY BRUSHING

Cross-Reference
See Chapter 11.

Duration and Frequency
Total time for dry brushing is 5 to 10 minutes. Perform once a day.

SAUNA

Cross-Reference
See Chapter 8.

Duration and Frequency
Take 15- to 30-minute saunas two or three times per week.

Cautions

1. To avoid dehydration, be sure to drink a cup of water before entering the sauna and 1 to 2 cups more during and after the sauna.
2. Do not take more than two or three saunas a week; too many heat treatments can actually be weakening to the system due to water and electrolyte losses.
3. Until accustomed to taking saunas, stay in only 10 to 15 minutes. Leave the sauna immediately if not tolerating the heat well, that is, feeling lightheaded or weak.

Take a shower at the end of the sauna for 1 minute, as cold as can be tolerated.

PARTIAL-BODY TONIC TREATMENTS

Tonic treatments for individual areas of the body actually exercise local blood vessels, conditioning them to contract more quickly and more forcefully, thereby improving local circulation. Gradually increasing responses to hot and cold temperatures have been demonstrated by many researchers. For example, when local cold treatments are given on a regular basis, such as a hand being regularly immersed in cold water, local arterioles begin to contract sooner and with greater force.(27) Regular exposure to hot water can even train the arterioles in the fingers of patients with Raynaud's syndrome to dilate when they would normally constrict. Usually, when those with Raynaud's are exposed to cold temperatures, the arterioles in their hands spasm, and this can lead to abnormally low blood flow to the hands. Because of the reduced blood flow, they have pale skin, uncomfortably cold hands, and in extreme cases, tissue damage. However, three separate studies have found that patients who regularly immerse their hands in hot hand baths while they sit in a very cold room have a more normal response to cold. Stimulating the arterioles of the hands to dilate while the person was exposed to cold induced a normal response and by the end of the studies, blood flow to the patients' fingers had greatly improved. Researchers were able to measure a 3° to 6°F increase in the temperature of the patients' fingers, even when they were in cold air.(33–35)

By alternating maximum vasodilation with maximum vasoconstriction, local contrast treatments cause significant fluctuations in local blood flow that can be not only measured (36,37) but also seen with the naked eye (the skin turns bright red). The muscles in the person's arterial walls may function better for some time after a series of contrast treatments is over. Both improved local blood flow and increased muscle performance can be significant for someone with a circulatory problem.

For example, patients with varicose veins who received alternating hot and cold showers to the legs for 25 days experienced significant improvement in the circulation to their legs. In people with advanced varicose veins, blood tends to pool in the lower legs, causing an increase in leg and ankle circumference. However, the volume of blood and circumference in the lower legs and ankles was significantly reduced in patients who received alternating hot and cold applications to the legs, compared to a group that received no hydrotherapy. More important to the patients, their leg pain discomfort and pain were also significantly decreased.(38)

At modern Seventh-Day Adventist hospitals, doctors commonly prescribe hot and cold whirlpools to the lower legs and feet for poorly healing wounds such as varicose and diabetic ulcers: they believe the increase in local blood flow speeds healing. A group of elderly patients with **intermittent claudication** received great benefit from contrast treatments to the legs. In this condition, blood pressure in the legs is low because the arteries to the legs are partially blocked. When walking, patients have extreme pain because local blood flow is not sufficient to meet the leg muscles' demands. As part of a research study, the elderly patients were given a 25-minute contrast treatment every other day for 3 weeks, for a total of 10 treatments. Each contrast treatment consisted of alternating streams of hot

and cold water directed over the legs and feet. All patients had a significant increase in the systolic blood pressure in their legs and toes immediately after the study and a month later as well. Seventy percent of the patients also reported less pain when walking and they could walk for a longer period of time before they felt pain. A year after the study, some of them still had higher blood pressure and less pain when walking, indicating that their blood vessels were still functioning better than before.(39)

Below are a number of partial-body tonic treatments that you can use with your clients.

Tonic Treatments for Poor Local Circulation

Common symptoms of poor local circulation include cold hands and feet and poorly healing scrapes, cuts, or other wounds. The following tonic treatments will help increase blood flow in these area, and you and your clients are likely to find that their hands or feet feel warmer in the wintertime.

TREATMENT

LOCAL CONTRAST BATH FOR THE HAND, ARM, FOOT, OR LEG

Cross-Reference
See Chapter 7.

Duration and Frequency
Begin by immersing the part in hot water (104°–110°F) for 3 minutes and cold water (55°F) for 1 minute. Perform three to six rounds, ending with cold. Perform the contrast bath once a day.

Special Instructions
If desired, add vasodilating herbs to the hot water: use 1 teaspoon of ginger, mustard powder, or cayenne, or mix 1/3 teaspoon of each, and add to 1 gallon of the hot water.

LOCAL CONTRAST SHOWERS FOR THE HAND, ARM, FOOT, KNEE, OR LEG

Cross-Reference
See Chapter 9.

Duration and Frequency
Use 3 minutes of hot water on small areas, such as the feet, but up to 5 minutes of heat for larger and denser areas, such as the arms. Alternate the hot shower with a 1-minute cold shower, and perform a total of three to six rounds. Use the contrast shower once a day.

Special Instructions
Use water from the showerhead as hot and as cold as can be tolerated.

LOCAL COLD FOOT SHOWER

Cross-Reference
See Chapter 9.

Duration and Frequency

Spray the tops and bottoms of both feet are with cold water for 30 seconds to 2 minutes and use this shower once or twice a day.

Special Instructions

1. Make sure you are warm before performing this shower.
2. At the end of the shower, do not step barefoot on the bathroom floor. Dry the feet briskly, then quickly put on socks to avoid chilling.

Tonic Treatments for the Digestive System

Local treatments improve blood flow to the digestive organs and can stimulate tone in sluggish conditions such as atonic constipation.

TREATMENT
LOCAL CONTRAST APPLICATION OVER THE ABDOMEN

Cross-Reference

See Chapters 5 and 6.

Duration and Frequency

Place large hot compresses, hot fomentations, or hydrocollator packs over the entire abdomen for 3 to 5 minutes. Follow that with an ice water rub over the abdominal area for 30 seconds. Perform a total of three or more rounds. Use at least once a day.

Special Instructions

1. This treatment is contraindicated during pregnancy.
2. This treatment is sometimes given as a liver tonic. In this case the heat application and ice rub are performed over the upper abdomen only. Then, if possible, a whole-body contrast shower is taken afterward.

Tonic Treatments for the Eyes

Improving the circulation over the eyes can relieve eyestrain and give the client a very refreshing sensation.

CONTRAST APPLICATIONS OVER THE EYES USING HOT AND COLD COMPRESSES OR HOT AND COLD GEL PACKS

Cross-Reference

See Chapters 5 and 6.

Duration and Frequency

Use 2 minutes of hot compresses followed by 30 seconds of cold compresses. Repeat three times. Perform once a day.

Tonic Treatments for Skeletal Muscles

Because the strength of muscles is temporarily increased by cold applications, cold water baths may be used as a muscle tonic before exercising. For example, a 30-minute leg bath at 54°F increases the maximum lifting strength of the legs and delays the onset of fatigue; vasodilation and increased blood flow last up to 6 hours. This effect is due to increased blood flow to deeper muscles, as peripheral blood flow is restricted by vasoconstriction during the cold immersion.(40) Interestingly, acute heat exposure has the opposite effect on skeletal muscles. One study found that muscular endurance in both the leg press and the bench press was significantly decreased after 30 minutes in a 160° to 175°F sauna.(41) To take advantage of this stimulating effect of cold baths, use water as cold as can be tolerated and submerge the part in the water for at least 5 minutes.

TREATMENT
PARTIAL-BODY COLD BATH

Cross-Reference

See Chapter 7.

Duration and Frequency

Take the cold bath for 5 minutes before vigorous exercise.

Special Instructions

1. Make sure you are warm before taking the cold bath.
2. At the end of the partial-body bath, dry the part briskly, cover with clothing, and begin exercising immediately.

PARTIAL-BODY COLD BATH FOR WEAK OR SPASTIC MUSCLES

Cross-Reference

See Chapter 7.

Duration and Frequency

The hand, arm, foot, or leg is immersed in 35°F water for 3 seconds, then removed for 30 seconds, for six rounds. Use once daily as a tonic, or use whenever the weak or spastic muscles or groups of muscles are to be given exercises.

Special Instructions

1. Make the client is warm before using the cold bath.
2. Alternatively, an entire extremity can be immersed in 50°F water for 10 minutes or a body part can be wrapped in an ice pack made with crushed ice for 10 minutes.

Tonic Treatments for the Respiratory System

Local treatments improve blood flow to the chest muscles and lungs and make breathing easier.

LOCAL CONTRAST APPLICATION OVER THE CHEST

Cross-Reference

See Chapters 5 and 6.

Duration and Frequency

Place large hot compresses, hot fomentations, or hydrocollator packs to cover the entire chest for 3 to 5 minutes. (Be sure to place the heat so it covers the sides of the chest as well as the front.) Next give an ice water rub over the entire chest for 30 seconds, and perform a total of three or more rounds. Perform once a day.

HEAT-TRAPPING COMPRESS TO THE CHEST

Cross-Reference

See Box 6-2.

Duration and Frequency

The compress is to be left on all night while the person sleeps. Perform three to five times a week.

Procedure

1. Make sure you are warm before applying the compress.
2. Dip a cotton T-shirt in water as cold as can be tolerated, adding ice to the water if tolerable.
3. Put the T-shirt on.
4. Take a large plastic trash bag and cut holes for your arms and head.
5. Put the plastic bag on over the T-shirt.
6. Put a dry shirt or sweater on over the plastic bag.
7. Leave on all night, or if it is uncomfortably warm, take off after no less than 1 hour.
8. Give a cold mitten friction to your chest and as far around the back as you can reach.
9. Dry yourself well and dress immediately.

Tonic Treatments for the Anterior Cervical Muscles and Throat

A contrast treatment to the throat will improve blood flow to the anterior neck muscles and the throat, which is especially helpful if the muscles are extremely tight and circulation is poor (Fig. 12-3).

LOCAL CONTRAST APPLICATION OVER THE THROAT

Cross-Reference

See Chapters 5 and 6.

Duration and Frequency

Place a hot compress, moist heating pad, or small hot water bottle over the throat for 3 to 5 minutes. Next place an iced compress or very cold compress over the throat for 1 minute (Fig. 12-3) or do an ice water rub over the throat for 30 seconds. Give a total of three or more rounds. Perform once a day.

Tonic Treatments for the Skin

Tonic treatments for the skin increase circulation and nutrition to the skin and stimulate its nerve endings.

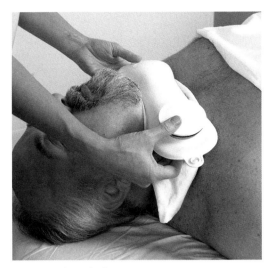

FIGURE 12-3 ■ Throat ice bag.

TREATMENT
CONTRAST SHOWER

Cross-Reference

See Chapter 9.

Duration and Frequency

Three rounds of 2-minute hot shower followed by 1 minute cold shower, for a total time of 9 minutes. Perform once a day.

WHOLE-BODY SALT GLOW

Cross-Reference

See Chapter 11.

Duration and Frequency

Total time for the salt glow is 10 to 15 minutes. Perform one to three times per week.

Special Instructions

Moisturize the skin well after the salt glow.

DRY BRUSHING

Cross-Reference

See Chapter 11.

Duration and Frequency

Total time for dry brushing is 5 to 10 minutes. Perform once a day.

SELF-CARE TREATMENTS FOR THE MASSAGE THERAPIST

In addition to enhancing clients' health and wellness through massage and hydrotherapy, massage therapists can take care of their bodies as well. One way to do this is to take measures to prevent **repetitive strain injury (RSI)**, a general term that denotes damage to muscles, tendons, ligaments, nerves, bursae, and/or joints. RSI is initiated when one or more parts of the body are used intensively without sufficient recovery time, such as performing the same massage techniques for many hours without enough rest between sessions. There is a significant correlation between RSI and jobs that require the hands to use a lot of force and to repeat the same movements many times. This is true regardless of the person's age and sex.(42) RSIs can affect any of the structures that are involved in movement. Types of RSI include myofascial pain and tendonitis; carpal tunnel syndrome or thoracic outlet syndrome; arthritis of the shoulder, elbow, hand, or wrist; and bursitis of the shoulder. Work that requires repetitive bending and twisting of the hand is especially correlated with hand and wrist arthritis.(43)

Because massage therapists work their hands and arms intensively—not only for prolonged periods but often while using great pressure—they are particularly at risk for some type of RSI. Many massage therapists work in pain because of RSIs, and some have even had their career ended by them. Even the most conscientious massage therapist, mindful of proper posture and use of the body and careful to take breaks or rest between massage sessions, must be constantly vigilant to avoid this occupational hazard.

Below are several local hydrotherapy treatments that can help prevent RSIs by stimulating local circulation. They can be used to relieve muscle fatigue by increasing local blood flow, help minor injuries heal before they become major ones, and facilitate stretching of chronically tight tissues, which in turn helps maintain normal flexibility and range of motion.

LOCAL TREATMENTS FOR THE HANDS, FOREARMS, AND UPPER BODY

Use these when your hands, arms, or other parts of your upper body feel tired or achy, or to stimulate local circulation before or after giving a massage.

CONTRAST HAND BATHS OR FOREARM BATHS

Cross-Reference
See Chapter 7.
These treatments can be used to increase local circulation and to relieve fatigue, pain, and swelling.

Duration and Frequency
Three rounds of immersing the hands in hot water for 2 minutes, then immersing the hands in cold water for 1 minute, for a total of 9 minutes. This treatment can be performed as many times as needed during the day, especially before or after massage.

Special Instructions
Contrast baths are an excellent preparation for stretching of the hand and wrist muscles.

EPSOM SALT HAND BATH

Cross-Reference
See Chapter 7.

Duration and Frequency
Take for 20 minutes. Use anytime the hands are inflamed or cold or you wish to warm the muscles before stretching them.

Special Instructions
1. Finish with a brief splash of cold water.
2. As shown in Figure 12-4, the hand muscles may be stretched while your hands are in the bath water.

ICED COMPRESS USING GLOVES FOR TIRED, ACHING, OR INFLAMED HANDS

Cross-Reference
See Chapter 6.

Duration and Frequency
Take for 10 to 15 minutes. This treatment can be performed as many times as needed during the day, especially before or after performing massage.

Special Instructions
Soak a pair of thin cotton or wool gloves in water, wring them out, and place in a zipper bag in the freezer. They will be very cold and stiff when taken out of the freezer, so run a little cold water over them and wring them gently so they are flexible enough to slip on your hands.

ICE PACKS AND ICE WATER BATHS FOR INFLAMED MUSCLES IN THE HANDS OR ARMS

Cross-Reference
See Chapter 7.

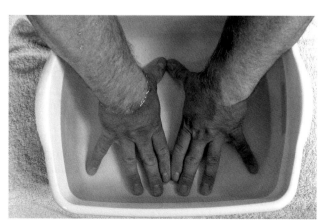

FIGURE 12-4 ■ Epsom salt hand bath with stretching of hand muscles.

Duration and Frequency

Take for 20 minutes. This treatment can be performed as many as three times during a day, especially before or after performing massage.

PARAFFIN HAND BATH FOLLOWED BY A COLD DIP OF 30 SECONDS OR LESS

Cross-Reference

See Chapter 7.

Duration and Frequency

Take for 15 minutes. May be repeated as often as three times daily.

Special Instructions

1. After the hands have been dipped and covered, wait 10–15 minutes. Remove the paraffin and perform stretching exercises if desired.
2. Paraffin hand baths can be part of a contrast treatment: dip the hands in cold water for 30 seconds after removing the paraffin. Do three rounds of hot paraffin followed by cold water.

HEAT-TRAPPING COMPRESS FOR THE HANDS OR ARMS

Cross-Reference

See Box 6-2.

Duration and Frequency

The compress should be left on 1 to 8 hours, ideally all night. This compress can be used every night or as desired.

STRETCHING AND RANGE-OF-MOTION EXERCISES IN A HOT SHOWER

When you are in a hot shower, the heat will penetrate and warm your muscles, making stretching easier. A hot shower is an excellent place to stretch the muscles of the upper body, not only because stretching is easier when muscles and fascia are warm, but because it is a convenient way to add stretching to your daily routine. Be especially careful not to slip. You may wish to install a grab bar and some nonslip tape on the shower floor to prevent falls. Also take care that any area with a condition contraindicating local heat is kept out of the shower. For example, an acute shoulder sprain or an acute whiplash injury should not be under the hot water for long periods.

The following sequence takes about 10 minutes. When you first get in the shower, you can perform gentle range-of-motion exercises while the hot water warms your tissues. To learn more about stretching in hot water, whether in a shower, hot bath, or bath tub, see *Hot Water Therapy* by Patrick Horay, DC.

RANGE-OF-MOTION EXERCISES

Procedure

1. Slowly trace the letters of the alphabet with your nose. As you form each letter, you will be making many subtle movements that help free the joints of the cervical spine. Trace all 26 letters.
2. Roll the shoulders up, back, down, and forward to make a circular movement 10 times. Now roll the shoulders in the opposite direction: up, forward, down, and then back to form a circle in the opposite direction, 10 times.
3. Straighten the arm, then alternate fully pronating and fully supinating the palm, 10 times.
4. Make circles with the wrists in a clockwise direction 10 times, then in a counterclockwise direction 10 times.

UPPER BODY STRETCHES

Hold each area directly under the hot spray, then perform each stretch gently until you feel a mild tension. As you hold the stretch, that mild tension will subside. Never stretch to the point of pain.

Procedure

1. Lift your chin toward the ceiling, then turn your head to one side to stretch the front of the neck. Hold for 15 seconds (Fig. 12-5A). Repeat on the opposite side.
2. Tucking your chin to your chest, stretch the back of the neck. Hold for 30 seconds (Fig. 12-5B).
3. Placing one hand over your head and on the opposite ear, gently stretch the upper trapezius and hold for 15 seconds (Fig.12-5C). Repeat on the opposite side.
4. Extend your upper arm to stretch the biceps and hold for 15 seconds (Fig. 12-5D). Repeat on the opposite side.
5. Bend your arm. With your elbow pointed toward the ceiling, touch your scapula. This stretches the triceps. At the same time, with your other arm, bring your hand back behind you and try to touch that same scapula. This stretches the anterior shoulder muscles of the other arm (Fig. 12-5E). Hold for 15 seconds. Repeat on the opposite side.
6. Cross your arms behind your back, then bring your shoulders back until you feel a mild tension in the pectoral muscles, then hold that stretch for 15 seconds (Fig. 12-5, F and G). Repeat on the opposite side.
7. Lean to the side until you feel a stretch along the side of the torso but not down into the side of the leg. Hold for 15 seconds (Fig. 12-5H). Repeat on the opposite side.
8. Twist the spine and hold for 15 seconds (Fig. 12-5I). Repeat on the opposite side.

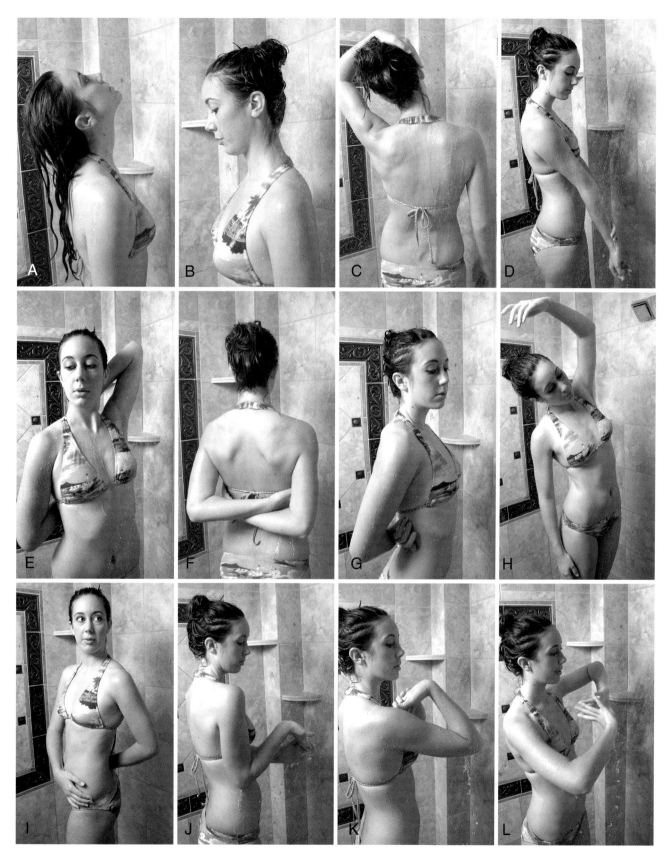

FIGURE 12-5 ■ Stretches in a hot shower. **A.** Front of neck. **B.** Back of neck (tuck chin). **C.** Trapezius. **D.** Biceps.
E. One hand up, one hand down (stretches triceps and front of shoulder at the same time). **F** and **G.** Pectoral muscle.
H. Side of torso. **I.** Spinal twisting. **J.** Wrist flexors. **K.** Wrist extensors. **L.** Fingers.

9. Bring the wrist back, and holding it with your other hand, gently stretch the wrist flexor muscles. Hold for 15 seconds (Fig. 12-5J). Repeat on the opposite side.

10. Bring the wrist down, and holding it with your other hand, gently stretch the wrist extensor muscles. Hold for 15 seconds (Fig. 12-5K). Repeat on the opposite side.

11. Place the tips of your fingers together, bring the palms towards each other, and gently stretch the fingers. Hold for 30 seconds (Fig. 12-5L).

INCREASING JOINT RANGE OF MOTION THROUGH SWIMMING

Using the body in repetitive and effortful ways tends to decrease joint range of motion, but swimming in warm water is an excellent way to retain and increase range of motion. Participating in water fitness classes, swimming laps, or simply moving for pure enjoyment in the water can be a fun way to keep your body healthier and your joints freer.

CHAPTER SUMMARY

This chapter explains how many hydrotherapy treatments can be used to promote health and wellness. Classic detoxification treatments, tonic treatments which stimulate the body's functions, and treatments to help you keep your upper extremities healthy all encourage good health. Using the hydrotherapy treatments for self-care can help your clients get faster and better results with their massage treatment. And now our final two chapters explain how you can use hydrotherapy in conjunction with massage to help treat injuries and a wide variety of chronic diseases and disorders.

REVIEW QUESTIONS

Multiple Choice

1. A short exposure to whole-body cold does all but one:
   a. Heightens the body's activities
   b. Stimulates the body to try to keep warm
   c. Is relaxing
   d. Increases the body's basal metabolic rate

2. A person who takes regular saunas experiences
   a. Regular feelings of warmth and relaxation
   b. Decrease in systolic blood pressure
   c. Loss of fluid and electrolytes
   d. All of the above

3. Massage therapists are prone to repetitive strain injury if they do which of the following?
   a. Take regular breaks between massages
   b. Have good posture
   c. Use their hands improperly
   d. Have a table at the proper height

4. Detoxifying bath additives work by doing all but one of the following:
   a. Neutralizing toxins
   b. Withdrawing toxins from the body
   c. Enhancing the body's ability to detoxify
   d. Warming the body from within

5. All but one statement about tonic treatments is correct:
   a. Stimulate local function
   b. Must be done regularly
   c. Can be used by weak persons without modifying them
   d. Provide different sensations

Fill in the Blanks

6. Stretching should be performed _____ and never to the point of _____.

7. When a local area is exposed to cold over time, the blood vessels are able to contract _____ and _____.

8. This occurs because the _____ of the vessels are _____ to increase their contractions.

9. When toxins are _____ in the body, they can contribute to _____ or chronic _____ health.

10. Symptoms of poor local circulation include _____ hands and feet and poorly healing _____ and _____.

REFERENCES

1. Hoigy N et al. Excretion of β-lactam antibiotics in sweat: A neglected mechanism of antibiotic resistance? *Antimicrob Agents Chemother* 2000;44:2855.
2. James R, Cohn MS, Emmett E. The excretion of trace metals in human sweat. *Ann Clin Lab Sci* 1978:270.
3. Liberty HJ, Johnson BD, Fortner N. Detecting cocaine use through sweat testing: Multilevel modelling of sweat patch length of wear data. *J Anal Toxicol* 2004;28:667.
4. Saito T et al. Validated gas chromatographic-negative ion chemical ionization mass spectrometric method for delta (9)-tetrahydrocannabinol in sweat patches. *Clin Chem* 2004;50:2083.
5. Vree TB. Excretion of amphetamines in Human Sweat. *Arch Clin Pharmodyn Ther* 1972;199:311.
6. Cecchini M, Root D, Rachunow J, Gelb P. Chemical exposures at the World Trade Center: Use of the Hubbard sauna

detoxification regimen to improve the health status of New York City rescue workers exposed to toxicants. *Townsend Lett Doctors Patients*, April 2006, p 58.

7. Root D. Downtown Medical: A detox program for World Trade Center responders. *Fire Engineering*, June 2003, p 12.

8. www.nydetox.org. Accessed November 2006.

9. Dahlgren J, Schecter A, Cecchinin M, et al. Persistent organic pollutants in 9/11 rescue workers: Reduction following detoxification. *Chemosphere* 2007, Jan 16.

10. Krop J. Chemical sensitivity after intoxication at work with solvents: response to sauna therapy. *J Altern Complement Med* 1998;4:77.

11. Tretjak Z, Shields M, Beckmann S. PCB reduction and clinical improvement by detoxification: An unexploited approach. *Hum Exper Toxicol* 1990;9:235.

12. Schnare D, Ben M, Shields M. Body burden reductions of PCB's, PBB's and chlorinated pesticides in human subjects. *Ambio* 1984;13:378.

13. Kilburn KH et al. Neurobehavioral dysfunction in firemen exposed to polychlorinated biphenyls (PCB's): Possible improvement after detoxification. *Arch Environ Health* 1989;44:345.

14. Rhea W. *Chemical Sensitivity: Tools of Diagnosis and Methods of Treatment*, vol 4. Boca Raton, FL: Lewis, 1997.

15. Schecter S. *Fighting Radiation and Chemical Pollutants with Food, Herbs and Vitamins*. Escondido, CA: Vitality, 1990.

16. Ernst E. Prevention of common colds by hydrotherapy. *Physiotherapy* 1990;76:207.

17. Ernst E. Regular sauna bathing and the incidence of common colds. *Ann. Med*

18. Adaptation related to cytokines in man: Effects of regular swimming in cold water. *Clin Physiol* 2000;20:114.

19. LeBlanc J et al. Autonomic nervous system and adaptation to cold in man. *J Appl Physiol* 1975;39:181.

20. Tikusis P et al. Comparison of thermoregulatory responses between men and women immersed in cold water. *J Appl Physiol* 2000;89:1403.

21. Radomski MW. Hormone response of normal and intermittent cold-preadapted humans to continuous cold. *J Appl Physiol* 1982;53:610.

22. DeLorenzo F, Sharma V, Scully M, Kakkar VV. Central cooling effects in patients with hypercholesterolemia. *Clin Sci* 1998;95:213.

23. DeLorenzo F et al. Haeomodynamic responses and changes of haemostatic risk factors in cold-adapted humans. *Q J Med* 1999;92:509.

24. Leppaluoto J, Korhonen I, Hassi J. Habituation of thermal sensations, skin temperatures and norepinephrine in men exposed to cold air. *J Appl Physiol* 2001;90:1121.

25. Smith E et al. Thermal sensation and comfort in women exposed repeatedly to whole-body cryotherapy and winter swimming in ice cold water. *Physiol Behav* 2004;82:691.

26. Hannuksela M, Ellahham S. Benefits and risks of sauna bathing. *Am J Med* 2001;110:118.

27. Ogilvie R. Benefits and Risks of Sauna Bathing. *Hypertens Can* Bull 74, March 2003, p 7.

28. Masuda A et al. Regular sauna use reduces oxidative stress. *Jpn Heart J* 2004;45:297.

29. Biro S, Masuda A, Kihara T, Tei C. Clinical implications of thermal therapy in lifestyle-related diseases. *Exper Biol Med* 2003;228;1245.

30. Hooper P. Hot tub for diabetes. *N Eng J Med*

31. Kihara T et al. Effects of repeated sauna treatment on ventricular arrhythmias in patients with chronic heart failure. *Circ J* 2004;69:1146.

32. Geurts C. Local cold acclimation of the hand impairs thermal responses of the fingers without improving hand neuromuscular function. *Acta Physiol Scand* 2005;183:117.

33. Jobe JB, Sampson JB, Roberts DE, Beetham WP Jr. Induced vasodilation as treatment for Raynaud's disease. *Ann Intern Med.* 1982;97:706.

34. Jobe JB et al. Induced vasodilation as a home treatment for Raynaud's disease. *J Rheumatol* 1985;12:953.

35. Jobe JB, Sampson JB, Roberts DE, Kelly JA. Comparison of behavioral treatments for Raynaud's disease. *J Behav Med* 1986;9:89.

36. Fiscus KA. Changes in lower-leg blood flow during warm-, cold-, and contrast-water therapy, *Arch Phys Med Rehabil* 2005;86:1404.

37. Rudofsky G et al. Changes of venous hemodynamics by thermic stimuli. *Med Klin* 1977;72:1639.

38. Saradeth B et al. A single blind, randomized, controlled trial of hydrotherapy for varicose veins. *Vasa* 1991;20:147.

39. Elmstadhl B. Hydrotherapy of patients with intermittent claudication: A novel approach to improve systolic blood pressure and reduce symptoms. *Angiol* 1995;14:3899.

40. *Physical Therapy Review* 1959;39:598.

41. Hedly AM et al. The effects of acute heat exposure on muscular strength, muscular endurance, and muscular power in the euhydrated athlete. *J Strength Cond Res* 2002;16:353.

42. Silverstein BA, Fine LJ, Armstrong TJ. Hand wrist cumulative trauma disorders in industry. *Br J Indust Med* 1986;43:799.

43. Dillon C, Petersen M, Tanaka S. Self-reported hand and wrist arthritis and occupation: Data from the U.S. National Health Interview Survey—Occupational Health Supplement. *Am J Indust Med* 2002;42:318.

RECOMMENDED RESOURCES

1. Horay P. *Hot Water Therapy*. Oakland, CA: New Harbinger, 1991.

2. Merendez N. The history of the Almadén mine hospital. *Quad Int Stor Med Sanita*. 3:51.

3. Mochizuki S. *Hand Maintenance Guide for Massage Therapists*. Boulder, CO: Kotobuki, 1999.

4. Prevention and treatment of cold-weather injuries. *TB Med Bulletin 500*. www.usareim.army.mil. Web site of the U.S. army's research in environmental medicine. Accessed September 2005.

5. Root-Bernstein R, Root-Bernstein M. *Honey, Mud, Maggots and Other Medical Marvels: The Science Behind Folk Remedies and Old Wives' Tales*. Boston: Houghton Mifflin, 1997.

6. Simon R, Aleskovsky R. *Repetitive Strain Injury Handbook*. New York: Henry Holt, 2000.

13

HYDROTHERAPY AND MASSAGE FOR MUSCULOSKELETAL INJURIES

Injuries are an inevitable part of any athletic program if an athlete remains in the sport for any length of time . . . a moist heat pack or heat rub can soothe aching muscles and help to loosen them prior to working out, and ice following the workout [can be used] if you are still sore or aching or have any pain.

—Trish Bare Grounds, Bare Essentials Guide for Martial Arts Injury Care and Prevention

Chapter Objectives

After completing this chapter, the student will be able to:

- Explain the most common types of musculoskeletal injuries and their causes.
- Describe the inflammatory process.
- Explain the rationale for using hydrotherapy to treat each injury in this chapter.
- Explain the difference between hydrotherapy for acute injuries and hydrotherapy for long-term effects of injuries.
- List five common injuries and the appropriate hydrotherapy treatments for each.

Perhaps the single most common reason for clients to seek out massage therapy, other than for relaxation, is for help with the aftermath of a musculoskeletal injury. Problems from poorly healed old injuries or new ones are common in people of all ages, and so it is vitally important that massage therapists have many tools at their disposal to help injured clients. This chapter explains how hydrotherapy can be one of the best tools for treating them.

Musculoskeletal injuries are common in everyday life. In the United States alone, traumatic injuries result in 26 million visits to hospital emergency departments and 55 million visits to doctors' offices each year.(1) Repetitive strain injuries, although not as sudden or dramatic, are responsible for about 60% of all workers compensation claims. They are so common that 1 in 10 people will develop a repetitive stress injury in his or her lifetime.(2) Sports injuries are also common, especially in competitive sports and among long-time athletes.

Recent injuries can cause acute pain, reduced range of motion, stiffness, edema, and muscle guarding. Massage therapy can relieve symptoms and promote complete healing by increasing local circulation, reducing muscle tension, and relieving muscle spasm and pain. Old, improperly healed injuries may feature excess scar tissue, latent or active trigger points, restricted movement, and musculoskeletal pain. Dysfunctional patterns of compensation, such as favoring an injured area when walking, make it more likely that a person will injure the area again or develop other problems due to poor body mechanics. (Box 13-1 has specific examples of the long-term effects of poorly healed injuries.) Massage therapy can address all of these issues by reducing muscle tension and pain, releasing fascial restrictions and excess scar tissue, and helping clients avoid dysfunctional patterns of compensation. Hydrotherapy treatments can add to the effects of massage by improving circulation and reducing pain, inflammation, and muscle tension. It can even be used when the injured area cannot be touched, such as in acute bursitis or joint dislocation. This chapter offers numerous specific examples of how hydrotherapy treatments can work together with massage to make treatments more effective and enjoyable for injured clients.

As you read this chapter, you will notice times when different massage modalities are mentioned to demonstrate

BOX 13-1 | *Point of Interest*

POORLY HEALED INJURIES CAN HAVE LONG-TERM EFFECTS ON THE BODY

Traumatic injuries that are not properly healed can cause long-term effects on the body. Below are some examples, each of which highlights the importance of proper healing to prevent future problems.

- Leg length inequality—the condition in which one leg is shorter than the other—can cause an uneven gait, a limp, hip and knee pain, and chronic low back problems. It can also lead to osteoarthritis both in the spine and in the hip of the longer leg. Poorly healed injuries can cause this condition in more than one way. For example, a femur fracture that heals poorly can cause one leg to be structurally shorter than the other one. However, leg length inequality can also be functional, that is, not caused by a structural problem. Instead, injuries can lead to soft tissue tightness that causes one leg to be held in such a way that is functionally shorter. For example, trigger points in the quadratus lumborum are often activated by trauma from motor vehicle accidents. When there are active, untreated trigger points in one quadratus lumborum muscle, that hip can be pulled up, secondary trigger points can occur in nearby muscles, lumbar scoliosis ensues, and the normal lumbar curve is flattened. Over time, the changes which begin in the injured muscle cause long-term problems in alignment, accompanied by uneven wear and tear on joints and musculoskeletal pain.

- At 8 years of age, massage therapist Genie Martin fell 20 feet out of a tree, striking branches on the way down and hitting her head hard enough to be knocked unconscious. Although Martin suffered only soft-tissue damage, she stopped breathing and lost consciousness, and she had to be given artificial respiration. Once she was breathing again, she was taken home. As she tells it, "My life was given back to me, though I was not aware of it for many hours. And when I did become aware of it, I no longer wanted it. Pain, heretofore unknown to me except for little hurts, was now my constant companion. A more nagging, convulsive, ruthless and demanding companion I had never known about in all my small life. Pain kept me awake at night—made my head ache with every move—burned my chest with fire, so

much that I squeezed my arms tightly around to smother the flames." From that time on, Martin carried a great deal of tension in her chest and experienced chest pain when she was anxious. Many negative emotions were carried in her chest, including a fear of falling, a fear of trying new things, and a fear of recurring pain. As an adult, Martin slept with her arms so tightly gripped over her chest that sometimes when she awoke they were numb. While receiving massages, she had to make a tremendous effort to stop her arms from springing over her chest to protect it. It was not until she was attending massage school as a middle-aged woman and receiving massage therapy that she began to heal from the emotional and physical effects of the injury.

- Football great Joe Namath was injured numerous times in his career—bruises, torn muscles, dislocations, sprains, torn cartilage and ligaments, fractures, and concussions. Namath frequently played even when he had new, unhealed injuries. This not only increased the chances of making the original injuries worse but also made it more likely that another area close by would be injured as well, because favoring an injured area causes other anatomical structures around it to be under increased stress. Namath began to have severe, ongoing knee pain as early as age 20, developed bursitis and severe swelling in both knees by age 24, and underwent many surgeries on his knees in an attempt to repair damage to tendons, cartilage, ligaments, and bursae. Although his physical problems forced him to retire at age 34, he continued to pay the price for playing with poorly healed injuries. At age 37 he had severe osteoarthritis in his fingers and spine, and at age 47 had joint replacement surgery on both knees. Unfortunately, knee replacement surgery was not able to eliminate his pain and even standing is painful for him now.

References:
1. Krieger M. *Namath: A Biography.* New York: Viking, 2004.
2. Martin G. Trauma and recall in massage: A personal experience. *Massage Therap J* Winter 1985, p 35.
3. Travell J, Simons D. *Myofascial Pain and Dysfunction: The Triggerpoint Manual,* vol 2, 2nd ed. Baltimore: Williams & Wilkins, 1999, p 49.

the pairing of hydrotherapy and massage, but these are not guidelines for what type of massage techniques to use. Specific massage techniques, including stretching and range-of-motion exercises used for injuries, are outside the scope of this book.

TYPES OF INJURIES

Before we turn to actual hydrotherapy treatments, first we discuss the three types of musculoskeletal injuries.

TRAUMATIC INJURY

Physical trauma to the body can cause a variety of injuries, including skin wounds, muscle strains, fractures, sprains, dislocations, tears in cartilage or ligaments, contusions,

back injuries, and even amputations. These injuries cause 27% of all visits to hospital emergency departments. Motor vehicle accidents and falls are the two most common traumatic injuries. Bicycle accidents, assaults, fires, recreational accidents, domestic violence, child abuse, suicides, homicides, and accidents while operating machinery are other significant causes of injury. On the job, traumatic injuries can include sprains, strains, muscle tears, fractures, and back injuries.

SPORTS INJURY

Sports injuries may be acute, such as a muscle strain, fracture, or dislocation which occurs while playing a sport. However, they can also be chronic, such as inflammatory conditions from overuse. Muscle injuries can result from poor conditioning, muscular imbalance, excessive muscle

HYDROTHERAPY AND MASSAGE USED IN INTENSIVE TREATMENT OF AN ATHLETIC INJURY

The following excerpt from the *Columbia* [Missouri] *Daily Tribune,* while it does not involve a massage therapist, illustrates the effectiveness of hydrotherapy for treating sports injuries.

When Corby Jones suffered a significant toe sprain in University of Missouri's football game against Northwestern on October 3, 1998, the clock began ticking for the Missouri sports medicine staff. The staff had seven days to improve Jones's condition and keep him in football-playing shape so that he could take the field next Saturday at Iowa State. As Jones' toe became the favorite topic of sports pages around the state, Rex Sharp, MU's head athletic trainer, knew the pressure was on his staff to heal the ailing digit. "It was probably the most well-publicized toe injury I'd ever seen," Sharp says. Monday, Tuesday and Wednesday, Jones spent the majority of his time in the Dr. Glenn L. McElroy Medicine and Rehabilitation Center, the new MU sports medicine facility that had opened late in the summer. Sharp treated Jones for

10 hours a day—heating the injury in the whirlpool, running him in the Swim Ex pool [rehabilitation pool with a current that the athlete can swim against], having him ride the stationary bikes and exercise on the stair stepper. Sharp coated Jones' toe in a paraffin bath and treated the toe with ultrasound and massages. However, when Friday came, and the team made the trip to Iowa State, Sharp was still unsure of success. "We did everything we could, but on Friday I still did not know whether he'd be able to play," Sharp said. The line for Jones on Saturday in an MU win—9 for 15 passing for 176 yards and two touchdowns, along with one rushing touchdown."When people come to a football game, all they see are the players running out on the field," Sharp said. "Then they go home. They have no idea of what goes on all week long."

—*Luke Vilelle, Heal Thyself With Help.* Columbia Daily Tribune, *June 16, 1999*

tension, or inadequate healing of a previous injury. The most common sports injuries are muscle strains, tendonitis, and joint sprains. (As shown in Box 13-2, hydrotherapy techniques can accelerate healing of injuries.)

REPETITIVE STRESS INJURY

Repetitive stress injuries are caused by the physical strain of performing the same movements for many hours, particularly if the person is in an awkward position or having to use great force to perform the task. Any repetitive activity—from typing to heavy lifting—can initiate an injury in a particular part of the body. Common injuries include tendonitis, bursitis, carpal tunnel syndrome, and disc herniation.

HYDROTHERAPY AND INJURIES

Massage therapists do not treat or evaluate injuries when they occur. When clients are injured, it is important that they consult with their doctor, go to the hospital, or even call 911 to ensure that their injuries are properly diagnosed and treated. Then, as long as the doctor has approved massage, clients may be treated whether their injury is **acute** (sudden onset and not prolonged), subacute (less than completely acute, between acute and chronic), or **chronic** (lasting 3 months or more and showing virtually no change).

HYDROTHERAPY AND PAIN FROM INJURIES

When a musculoskeletal structure is injured, **nociceptors,** receptors on the skin or in deeper structures that carry pain signals to the brain, are stimulated. This pain helps alert us

to threats against our body and also promotes healing by forcing us to rest. Pain gets our attention! When it is properly used, hydrotherapy can promote healing and alleviate much of the short-term discomfort and pain of recent musculoskeletal injuries. According to Agatha Thrash, MD, who has 40 years of experience in this area, "The application of heat or cold to relieve the pain of acute or chronic inflammatory disorders has been used for centuries, and is still a method without peer in the area of pain control. No other method is so effective, so safe and easy, and so free from side effects and expense."(3) Muscle spasm and pain are common after both acute and subacute injuries, and for those who cannot take medications such as pain relievers or antispasmodics, hot and cold treatments can offer great relief. Heat relaxes muscles and slows conduction of pain messages to the brain. In one study, researchers found that local heat applied over the palm could even relieve the pain of a mild electric shock.(4) Recent research with heat wraps worn continuously for hours has found that they can relieve both neck and low back pain better than ibuprofen or acetaminophen.(5) Cold applications, on the other hand, numb muscles and also relieve pain by overriding or bypassing pain messages to the brain. Contrast treatments, however, appear to relieve pain by greatly increasing local circulation.

Hydrotherapy can also help prevent long-term tissue dysfunction by promoting proper healing. Treating the long-term consequences of various musculoskeletal traumas often requires myofascial work or breaking up of old adhesions, and heat can relax and warm soft tissues, making deep work much easier. Heating treatments such as paraffin or moist hot packs can help soften old scar tissue so that massage techniques are less painful and more effective.

HYDROTHERAPY AND INFLAMMATION

As shown in Figure 13-1, injuries are almost always accompanied by inflammation. Because massage therapists perform massage with many clients with both recent and old injuries, it is important for them to understand this process. (Box 13-3 has more about the stages of inflammation.) To reduce inflammation, musculoskeletal trauma is generally treated with cold applications for the first 48 hours after an injury. Cold causes local blood vessels to constrict, which reduces bleeding from any blood vessels that are still not sealed off. It also reduces inflammation. However, after 48 hours, the application of cold packs and ice packs will continue to inhibit the circulation, thereby decreasing arterial blood flow, soft tissue blood flow, and local metabolism. After that point, contrast, not cold, applications are recommended, because they not only increase circulation to specific areas and ease pain, they also keep edema at bay. Various anti-inflammatory medications may be used at this stage of an injury, but because much research indicates that they can actually delay or inhibit healing, contrast treatments that stimulate blood flow and bring extra oxygen and other nutrients to the injured tissues are generally preferred.(6) After the first 48 hours, a contrast treatment followed by lymphatic drainage techniques can be used in the earlier stages of an injury, while contrast treatments may be combined with circulatory massage and other techniques in the later stages of an injury.

A very important benefit of early treatment with hydrotherapy and massage is the healing of an injury with appropriate scar tissue. In the subacute phase of an injury, cells which produce collagen fibers form scar tissue around the injury to knit the damaged area back together. Initially,

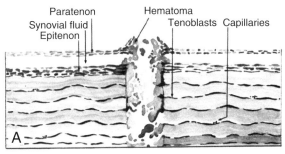

SEVERED TENDON

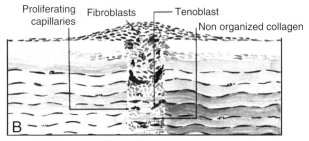

REPAIRING TENDON

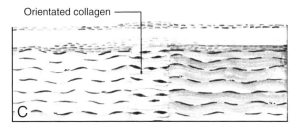

HEALED TENDON

FIGURE 13-1 ■ Tendon healing. **A.** Acute phase of repair of a torn tendon. **B.** Subacute phase of repair of a torn tendon. **C.** Healed tendon. (Reprinted with permission from Bucholz RW, Heckman JD. *Rockwood and Greens Fractures in Adults.* 5th ed. Baltimore: Lippincott Williams & Wilkins, 2001.)

BOX 13-3 | *Point of Interest*

THE BODY HEALS THROUGH INFLAMMATION

Inflammation is the body's defensive response to injury. The four main signs are redness, swelling, heat, and pain. Let's consider what happens when the body sustains an injury in which a lot of force is applied to an area, such as a shoulder dislocation. At the moment of injury, not only are blood vessels and nerves torn, but muscle and connective tissue cells may be ripped open. As seen in Figure 13-1A, the body responds to the injury with many protective responses, including the following:

Initially, local blood vessels constrict to prevent blood loss. Soon afterward, many more local capillaries than usual dilate, and as they open wide the area is flooded with fresh blood. Fibrin and blood platelets collect in the blood vessels at the site of the injury and gradually close off the damaged vessels. (Heat applied to the area in the very early stages after an injury, before the small capillaries are closed off, increases the chance that they will leak blood and plasma into the soft tissues around the injury. Heat should not be applied until the capillaries have been sealed and have stopped leaking, which usually requires a maximum of 24 hours except in the case of very severe injuries.)

Because there is a sharp increase in the number of active capillaries, a significant increase in their diameter, and blood leaking

out of broken vessels and pooling, blood flow to the area increases. However, with many vessels wide open, the blood actually flows more slowly, and this allows more **macrophages** to get into the area. Their job is to remove damaged tissue. More heat-carrying blood that is flowing more slowly creates some of the cardinal signs of inflammation—redness and heat, swelling because there is more fluid in the area, and pain because extra fluid puts pressure on nerve endings. If there is enough inflammation to limit movement, loss of function, the fifth sign of inflammation, can result.

Leukocytes concentrate where the tissue damage is the greatest, engulfing and destroying the tissue debris that was created by the rupture of individual cells, along with any pathogens that are present. At the same time, if there is any bleeding, this debris and a mass of red blood cells form a **hematoma,** a local mass of blood. Pressure on pain nerves causes additional pain.

In the subacute phase, as seen in Figure 13-1B, tissues are beginning to heal; ruptured small blood vessels have closed, white blood cells are cleaning up debris, blood flow has returned to its normal state, and cells which produce collagen fibers are forming scar tissue around the injury to knit the damaged area back together.

new collagen fibers form without having any direction or grain (Fig. 13-2A), and without proper treatment, they may either form in the wrong direction or attach to the structures that they should be gliding over. If not aligned with the other tissues, they can adhere to structures such as fascia or muscle, and then they have a restricting, not reinforcing, effect. These scar tissue fibers are not as elastic as muscle fibers, and they have a tendency to restrict free movement and to tear when they are exposed to stress. Many chronic musculoskeletal problems can result from excessive or poorly aligned scar tissue. Massage treatment of many subacute injuries focuses on helping the area heal without this type of scar tissue. Exercise is important at this stage, for the injured part will heal best when the person moves it actively but gently, allowing it to remain pliable and healthy, and ensuring that scar tissue fibers are properly aligned (Fig. 13-2B). Once pain relief is achieved with contrast treatments and massage, gentle exercise promotes this optimum healing. Exercising while the part is in a contrast bath increases local circulation even more.

A traditional adjunct to hydrotherapy for injuries is the use of herbal preparations: as explained in Box 13-4, herbs have been used for centuries to treat muscle soreness and

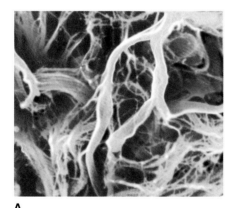

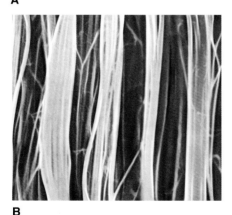

FIGURE 13-2 ■ Ligament fiber organization. **A.** Incompletely healed ligament with disorganized fibers. **B.** Fully healed ligament with well organized fibers. (Reprinted with permission from Archer M. *Therapeutic Massage in Athletics*. Baltimore: Lippincott Williams & Wilkins, 2004: 104, Fig. 6-4.)

aching, inflammation, muscle spasm, poor local circulation, and poorly healing wounds.

AMPUTATION

An amputation is the cutting off of a limb or a part of a limb. It is performed when it would be dangerous to leave that part of the body because of life-threatening infection, irreversible damage to local blood vessels, tissue damage beyond the hope of repair, or advanced loss of function. As a result of increasing rates of diabetes in the United States, amputations are an injury you are likely to encounter among your clients. As of 2007, 20 million Americans had diabetes, and of the 82,000 amputations performed in the United States each year, 70% are due to diabetes. Most of the rest are the result of musculoskeletal trauma or cancer.(7,8) Accidents such as injuries from lawnmowers or gunshot wounds cause most amputations in children, whereas diseases cause most of them in adults. Individuals with advanced diabetes have to have amputations when sores on their feet will not heal. Gangrene in the foot that spreads to the rest of the person's body can be fatal, so instead the foot is sacrificed.

Hydrotherapy can be a helpful treatment for clients with amputated limbs, in particular when the amputation stump is sensitive to touch or local circulation is poor. Hydrotherapy is an excellent way to improve the client's tolerance for tactile stimulation, improve circulation to the stump, soften adhesions, and begin the massage experience in a soothing fashion. Warm-water whirlpools, for example, are sometimes used by physical therapists to desensitize amputation stumps, increase local circulation, and possibly relieve phantom pain. Besides helping the amputation stump itself, using hydrotherapy treatments such as moist hot pack applications can help relieve discomfort and tension in muscles in other parts of the body, such as the back or extremity, which are compensating for the missing part. For example, with one leg amputated above the knee, compensations may cause muscle tightening and discomfort at the hip directly above the stump, in the entire other leg, and/or in the back.

TREATMENT

Below are two hydrotherapy treatments that are useful for treating clients with amputations.

CONTRAST TREATMENT OF THE STUMP

The contrast treatment may be extended to the entire extremity by using more than one hot pack or heating pad. A moist hot pack can be applied by itself but will not stimulate the circulation as much as a contrast treatment.

(continued)

BOX 13-4 *Point of Interest*

HERBS TRADITIONALLY USED WITH HYDROTHERAPY TO TREAT INJURIES

Herbal preparations have been used for centuries along with hydrotherapy treatments for many injury-related problems. These include soreness, aching and inflammation, muscle spasms, poor local circulation, and wounds caused by physical trauma. Massage therapists who use herbal preparations in their clients' hot and cold compresses, local baths, fomentations, ice massage plasters, and other water treatments feel that it deepens the effectiveness of hands-on techniques.

HERBS FOR MUSCLE SORENESS, ACHING, AND INFLAMMATION

Herb	Bruise	Edema	Eye Inflammation	Ligament Tear	Muscle Aching	Muscle Soreness	Plantar Fasciitis	Sinus Inflammation	Sprain	Strain
Arnica	X	X		X					X	
Calendula	X									X
Chamomile			X					X		
Comfrey							X			
St. John's wort	X				X	X				
Witch hazel	X				X	X				

HERBS FOR MUSCLE SPASMS AND MUSCLE TIGHTNESS

Herb	Muscle Cramps	Flu Aches and Pains	Rheumatic Pain	Sleep Aid and Relaxant	Spasmodic Asthma
Blackhaw	X				
Chamomile	X	X		X	
Cramp bark	X				
Ginger	X	X			
Lavender			X	X	
Lobelia					X
Mullein					X

HERBS WHICH TREAT INJURIES BY IMPROVING LOCAL CIRCULATION

Herb	Fibrositis	Fracture (delayed union)	Frozen Shoulder	Low Back Pain	Migraine	Muscle Strain	Poor Circulation	Rotator Cuff Tear
Cayenne					X		X	
Ginger	X	X	X	X	X	X	X	X
Mustard			X	X	X			X

HERBS FOR WOUNDS

Herb	Delayed Union of Fractures	Damaged Joints and Muscles	Pulled Tendons
Arnica		X	
Comfrey	X	X	X
St. John's wort		X	

References
1. Treasure J. MNIMH, AHG, Course notes from class "Herbs and Massage," Eugene, Oregon, Feb 28, 2004.
2. Ody P. *The Complete Medicinal Herbal.* London: Dorling Kindersley, 1993.

Duration and Frequency

10 to 12 minutes. This may be performed as many as three times a day.

Cautions

If the stump is sensitive, hot applications may have to be relatively cool and cold applications relatively warm. Ask the client to tell you what feels right. Clients with diabetes should have the heating pad set on medium, not high, or hydrocollator packs covered with extra towels so they are warm, not hot, on the skin.

Procedure

1. Apply a moist heating pad, fomentation, or hydrocollator pack to the amputation stump for 3 minutes.
2. Wring out a washcloth in ice water and rub the stump for 30 seconds, or perform ice massage for 1 minute. Brisk rubbing will help desensitize sensitive tissues.
3. Repeat steps 1 and 2 two more times, for a total of three rounds.

CONTRAST PARTIAL SHOWER

Cross-Reference
See Chapter 9.

Duration and Frequency
10 to 12 minutes. May be performed as many as three times a day.

Cautions
Diabetics should have water no hotter than 102°F.

Procedure
1. Spray the amputation stump with hot water for 2 minutes.
2. Spray the stump with cold water for 30 seconds.
3. Repeat steps 1 and 2 two more times for a total of three rounds.

WHIRLPOOL BATH FOR AN AMPUTATION STUMP

Cross-Reference
See Chapter 7.

Duration and Frequency
15 to 20 minutes. This may be performed before a massage session.

Special Instructions
Water can be warm to hot (98°–105°F), whatever is comfortable. Diabetics should receive whirlpool baths no hotter than 102°F.

BURSITIS

Another common injury you are likely to see in your practice is **bursitis,** the inflammation of a **bursa.** This can occur after repetitive stress or trauma, because of inflammation in a specific area or due to rheumatoid arthritis. The subacromial bursa of the shoulder is the most common bursa to become painfully inflamed in this fashion. Sedentary workers and workers at jobs requiring heavy lifting are prone to bursitis of the shoulder, and women are more prone to it than men. However, bursitis can occur at many other joints, including the elbow, hip, knee, and ankle. Bursitis is extremely painful, and that pain is aggravated by almost any movement of the joint. However, should someone stop using the affected joint because it hurts, **adhesive capsulitis** (extreme stiffness caused by adhesions between the joint capsule and the bone) can develop. Below we discuss the hydrotherapy treatment of both acute and subacute bursitis.

Acute Bursitis

In recently developed or acute bursitis, hydrotherapy and massage can be used to reduce the client's pain and to prevent the joint stiffness that can occur when pain causes a person to stop moving. Hydrotherapy applications can relieve pain, enabling clients to perform their regular activities and even gentle range-of-motion exercises that cause very limited discomfort, so that they do not lose range of motion and flexibility in the muscles around the painful joint. In some cases, contrast treatments can also relieve inflammation. Massage is contraindicated on or near the inflamed bursa in the acute stage, but it can be helpful in other parts of the body during that time.

A good way to combine treatments is to apply a hydrotherapy treatment on the area with the bursitis, while performing actual massage techniques on other parts of the body. Cold applications may relieve pain for some clients better than heat, but for some people, cold may cause the muscles to seize up. Clients may need to experiment at home to find out whether hot or cold relieves their symptoms better. Since it is the joint most commonly affected with bursitis, the shoulder is used here for an example, but the following treatment can be performed over any joint with inflamed bursa.

TREATMENT
UPPER HALF-BODY PACK

Cross-Reference
See Chapter 5.

Duration and Frequency
30 to 45 minutes, depending upon how many fomentations are used over the shoulder.

Caution
All fomentations should be well covered with towels so there is no risk of burning the client.

Special Instructions
This treatment can fit into a massage session if you perform massage on the other parts of the body while the client is in the half-body pack, and then remove the

pack and perform massage on or around the painful area at the end of the session.

Procedure

1. Place two fomentations on the massage table so that they will cover the area from neck to waistline. Have the client lie on them, and then place one more hot fomentation over the front of the shoulder. Proceed with massage of other areas of the body.
2. Replace the fomentation of the front of the shoulder with a fresh one every 15 minutes. At the end of the treatment, remove all fomentations, then briefly rub the shoulder and the back with a washcloth dipped in cold water. Cover the shoulder. The client may perform gentle range-of-motion exercises at this time.

LOCAL SALT GLOW FOLLOWED BY APPLICATION OF CASTOR OIL AND HEAT-TRAPPING COMPRESS

Cross-Reference
See Chapters 5 and 11.

Duration and Frequency
20 minutes, ending with wrapping the joint after heat application and salt glow have been performed. Then the compress may be left on 1 to 8 hours. May be performed daily.

Caution
Remember that massage is contraindicated in acute bursitis, so do not perform massage techniques. Wrap the compress snugly but not tightly enough to cut off the local circulation.

Special Instructions
This treatment may be performed at the very beginning of a massage session but will be more effective if the heat-trapping compress is left on overnight. After you have demonstrated it to a client during a session, it can be performed at home.

Procedure

1. Apply moist heat over the joint for 10 minutes.
2. Perform a salt glow with Epsom salt over the joint.
3. Gently rub a generous amount of castor oil into the skin over the joint.
4. Apply a heat-trapping compress over the joint and leave it in place for 1 to 8 hours.
5. Gentle range-of-motion exercises may be safely performed after the compress is removed.

APPLICATIONS OF COLD

Cross-Reference
See Chapter 6.

Duration and Frequency
15 minutes. Can be performed every 1 to 3 hours.

Special Instructions
Instead of ice massage, apply an ice-water compress or ice pack over the shoulder joint for 20 minutes.

Procedure

1. Perform ice massage over the shoulder joint for about 5 minutes, then take the ice off for 1 minute. Massage around the painful area during the rest period.
2. Repeat step 1 twice more.
3. Have the client perform gentle range-of-motion exercises at this time.

CONTRAST TREATMENT FOR THE SHOULDER JOINT

Cross-Reference
See Chapters 5 and 7.

Duration and Frequency
10 minutes. This contrast treatment can be performed as many as three times a day.

Procedure

1. Place moist heat over the joint, as hot as can be tolerated. Leave it on for 3 minutes.
2. Place an ice pack, ice cold compress, or cold gel pack over the joint for 30 seconds.
3. Repeat steps 1 and 2 twice for a total of three rounds of hot followed by cold. The client may perform gentle range-of-motion exercises at this time.

Subacute Bursitis

For subacute bursitis, which normally occurs after a few days or weeks of acute bursitis, heating treatments such as mustard plasters, hydrocollator packs, or paraffin baths may be used prior to massage. Then circulatory, myofascial, and deep friction massage can be used to release chronic tension and possible muscle compensation patterns.

TREATMENT
PARAFFIN BATH

Cross-Reference
See Chapter 7.

Duration and Frequency
15 minutes. Use before or during a massage session.

Special Instructions
Joints that cannot be immersed in paraffin may be treated with a hot moist application for at least 1 minute and then painted with paraffin. Cover the joint well and leave the paraffin on for at least 10 minutes before massage and exercise.

Procedure

1. Dip the joint in warm water for at least 1 minute.
2. Dry briskly.

3. Dip at least six times in hot paraffin.
4. Wrap the area well to keep it warm, and leave the paraffin on for at least 10 minutes before massage and exercise.

HOT, MOIST APPLICATIONS

Cross-Reference
See Chapter 5.

Duration and Frequency
30 minutes. Use before or during a massage session.

Special Instructions
Vasodilating herbs such as mustard, ginger, or cayenne may be added to the compress water.

Procedure
1. Apply a hot fomentation, moist heating pad, or hot compresses over the joint for 30 minutes.
2. Replace with another one after 15 minutes if it cools off.
3. Finish with a 1-minute ice application (ice pack or ice massage) over the joint.

CARPAL TUNNEL SYNDROME

Carpal tunnel syndrome is a common and painful condition caused by the entrapment of the median nerve as it passes through the carpal tunnel. It causes wrist pain and symptoms of nerve compression such as tingling, pain, or numbness in the forearms, wrists, or hands. Like so many repetitive stress injuries, this overuse syndrome can be caused by a poor work environment (the user's computer or chair not ergonomically correct) and too many hours of doing the same activity, such as typing, massaging, or playing a musical instrument. The first reported cases of carpal tunnel syndrome were in workers who rolled cigars by hand all day.

Treatment for carpal tunnel syndrome most often involves physical therapy, a change in work environment, and decreasing or stopping the activity that caused the injury.

As part of the client's health care team—including the client's doctor and physical therapist—the massage therapist can use hydrotherapy techniques to ease pain and facilitate exercise. Robert Simon, MD, a specialist in repetitive strain injuries, believes that local contrast baths are the most effective home treatment for reducing pain.(9) Massage may or may not be indicated, depending on the individual and the type of carpal tunnel syndrome, and the therapist should consult with the client's doctor or physical therapist to find out whether it is indicated. Massage in related muscle groups may be indicated, and massage in other parts of the body can be helpful with stress. Below are several hydrotherapy treatments you can use with clients who have carpal tunnel syndrome.

TREATMENT
HOT HAND AND FOREARM SOAK

Cross-Reference
See Chapter 7.

Duration and Frequency
12 to 15 minutes before a massage session, and as many as three or four times daily in between sessions

Procedure
1. This hot soak can be performed three to four times a day.
2. Soak the hands and forearms in water as hot as can be tolerated (approximately 110°F) for 12 to 15 minutes.
3. Have the client exercise the hand or stretch the hand and forearm muscles during this time.
4. Immerse the hands and forearms in water as cold as can be tolerated (approximately 55°F) for 5 seconds.
5. Dry the hands well so they do not become chilled.

TREATMENT
CONTRAST HAND AND FOREARM BATH

Cross-Reference
See Chapter 7.

Duration and Frequency
10 minutes

Special Instructions
Gentle, painless movements performed while the hands are in the water will further increase local circulation.

Clients may also use a handheld shower attachment and spray hot water followed by cold water to perform a contrast treatment. The spray should cover the entire arm and hand, and the client should do one side at a time.

Procedure
1. Immerse the hands and forearms in hot water (approximately 110°F) for 2 minutes.
2. Immerse the hands and forearms in cold water (approximately 55°F) for 1 minute.
3. Repeat steps 1 and 2 twice for a total of three rounds.

ICE MASSAGE FOLLOWED BY EXERCISE

Cross-Reference
See Chapter 6.

Duration and Frequency
3 to 8 minutes before exercise and massage

Procedure
1. Gently massage over the painful area and above and below the wrist with an ice cup or ice cube.

2. Stop as soon as the area is numb.
3. Allow time for the client's hands and wrists to warm.
4. Have the client perform gentle exercises as prescribed by the doctor or physical therapist.
5. Begin hands-on massage.

DISLOCATIONS

When force applied to a joint wrenches the bones out of their normal relation to each other, it is said to be dislocated. For example, in an anterior dislocation of the shoulder (the most common dislocation in adults), the head of the humerus is forced completely out of the glenoid fossa and lies anterior to it. Figure 13-3 shows this type of dislocation and how the humerus and scapula have been wrenched apart. This occurs when the shoulder is in an abducted, externally rotated position and a blow is received somewhere along the arm. The next most common adult dislocation is at the elbow, which is most often dislocated from a fall onto an outstretched hand.

When an area has been struck with enough force to dislocate a bone, other soft tissues around the joints can also be injured. Tearing or bruising can occur in the joint capsule, ligaments, periosteum, muscles, tendons, blood vessels, nerves, and nearby bursae. Some of this damage may not be apparent until years later. (For example, large rotator cuff tears can begin as small tears that occur along with a shoulder joint dislocation, and they may not progress to a full-thickness tear until later.) Treatment by the client's health care team includes manipulating the bone back into position as quickly as possible, followed by a period of immobilization and then by rehabilitation that includes range-of-motion and muscle-strengthening exercises. Immobilization of the injured joint, while necessary, carries its own hazards—activation of trigger points, joint contracture, and/or frozen shoulder.

NOTE: Massage therapists should never work with clients with dislocated joints until the client has been treated by a doctor who has approved massage.

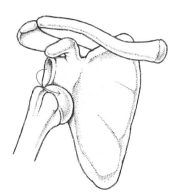

FIGURE 13-3 ■ Subglenoid shoulder dislocation. (Reprinted with permission from *Stedman's Medical Dictionary*. 27th ed. Baltimore: Lippincott Williams & Wilkins, 1999: 525.)

Ice is generally applied to dislocations as a first-aid measure for a few hours, since swelling can interfere with reducing the dislocation. While massage is contraindicated until the dislocation has been reduced and massage has been approved by a doctor, contrast treatments well above (proximal) to the injury can be used anytime to improve local circulation, decrease swelling and muscle spasm, and ease discomfort. Hydrotherapy treatments to the corresponding joint on the uninjured side can be used to improve circulation in the injured joint, by causing a reflex vasodilation (known as the contralateral reflex effect). At the same time, gentle circulatory massage in the surrounding areas can be done to enhance the circulation, ease muscle spasm, and promote general relaxation, as long as the dislocated joint is not massaged or moved in any way. Once the sling or other immobilization is removed and the client's physician has been consulted, massage therapists can use contrast treatments directly over the dislocated joint to improve local circulation and relieve pain. Hot applications relieve discomfort or pain and improve circulation, and gentle exercise of the extremity in a whirlpool will improve range of motion and muscle strength around the joint. Circulatory, myofascial, or trigger point massage can be used to prevent muscle guarding in the area, treat trigger points, release any fascial restriction or contractures caused by immobilization, prevent scar tissue buildup in the soft tissues around the joint, and improve the circulation of blood and lymph. Here we use the knee to demonstrate hydrotherapy treatments, but these treatments are effective with any dislocated joint.

TREATMENT
CONTRAST TREATMENT OVER A PREVIOUSLY DISLOCATED KNEE

Cross-Reference
See Chapters 5 and 6.

Duration and Frequency
15 minutes, to be performed before or during a massage session, and up to two or three times daily as a home treatment

Cautions
Do not put pressure on the joint when performing this treatment.

Special Instructions
- A handheld shower sprayer may also be used for this treatment, alternating between very hot and very cold water.
- Another way to perform this treatment is to use hot and cold applications at the same time for the same intervals. Heat and cold are applied both over and under the knee at the same time for 3 minutes and then switched so the heat is where the cold was and the cold is where the heat was. After 3 minutes, switch them again, and leave on for 3 more minutes.

Procedure

1. Have the client lie supine on the table. Extra pillows may be needed to support painful areas and make the client position comfortable.
2. Apply a hot fomentation or other moist heat around the joint for 3 minutes.
3. Apply an ice pack or cold gel pack over the knee (Fig. 13-4) or perform ice massage over the joint for 1 minute.
4. Repeat steps 1 and 2 twice, for a total of three rounds of hot followed by cold.

CONTRAST TREATMENT OVER THE CORRESPONDING JOINT ON THE UNINJURED SIDE OF THE BODY

Alternating heat and ice is used to induce reflex vasodilation (the contralateral reflex effect) on the injured side.

Cross-Reference
See Chapters 5 and 6.

Duration and Frequency
12 minutes. Perform before or during a massage session. As a home treatment, it may be performed two or three times daily.

Special Instructions
A handheld shower sprayer may also be used for this treatment, alternating between very hot and very cold water. Joints that can be immersed in water, such as the wrist or ankle, can also be treated with contrast baths to produce this effect.

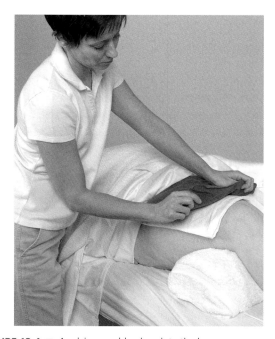

FIGURE 13-4 ■ Applying a cold gel pack to the knee.

Procedure

1. The client may lie supine, prone, or in side lying position, as long as the knee is completely supported.
2. Apply moist heat to the uninjured knee for 3 minutes.
3. Apply an ice water compress or perform ice massage on the uninjured knee for 1 minute.
4. Repeat steps 2 and 3 twice more for a total of three changes.

EXHAUSTION FROM OVEREXERTION

Exercising too hard with too little rest may cause extreme fatigue. Assuming the client's doctor has ruled out any other problems that could cause fatigue, hydrotherapy techniques can be used to help rejuvenate and invigorate the client.

Two hydrotherapy treatments are especially effective in reviving an exhausted person. The cold mitten friction is a classic treatment for fatigue, especially if followed by massage. The contrast shower is also effective because a short hot shower stimulates the circulation and the metabolism, as does a short cold shower. By alternating the two showers, the person who is exhausted can be reinvigorated, then circulatory massage can help stimulate the flow of blood and lymph and ease any musculoskeletal discomfort. Even a short massage, using tapotement and other stimulating techniques, can help stimulate the exhausted person.

TREATMENT
COLD MITTEN FRICTION

Cross-Reference
See Chapter 11.

Duration and Frequency
15 to 20 minutes before or during a massage session

Caution
Do not perform this treatment with a client who is chilled. Warm the client first with a hot footbath; an application of moist heat, such as multiple fomentations or hydrocollator packs; or other heating treatments. Make sure the room is warm.

CONTRAST SHOWER

Cross-Reference
See Chapter 9.

Duration and Frequency
10 to 15 minutes. Perform before a massage session.

Procedure

1. Have the client take a short (2 minutes) hot shower followed by a short (1 minute) cold shower. The hot shower should be as hot as the client can tolerate, short of burning, and the cold one as cold as the client can tolerate.

Repeat the hot and cold shower two to five times.

FRACTURE

A bone break, or **fracture,** can range from a small crack in the bone to a breaking of the bone into two parts to a complete shattering of the bone. Treatment varies according to how severely the bone is broken and what part of it is broken. Sometimes a standard cast is sufficient to repair a fracture, but in other cases, pins or plates may be required to stabilize the bone. Some types of fractures, such as a tibial fracture, can be treated by casting them, whereas others, such as a rib fracture, cannot be put in a cast at all. After a broken bone has healed and its cast (if any) has been removed, the muscles around the break are usually quite stiff and weak. There may be soreness and edema in the tissues around the fracture site and general stasis. At this time, hydrotherapy may be combined with massage to improve circulation of blood and lymph, ease soreness and pain, and reinvigorate an area that has deteriorated from a general lack of use during bone healing time.

A contrast treatment can be used to improve the circulation in an area that has been put in a cast and is not directly accessible, or blood flow to a casted left foot can be stimulated by a contrast treatment to the uninjured right foot through the *contralateral reflex effect.* Using this approach, blood flow in the right foot can be doubled, while that of the left foot can be increased by about 25%.

Warm whirlpools and pool therapy are also effective after a fracture has healed and the client's cast has been removed. Whirlpools are used to soften dead skin, reduce stiffness and edema, and improve local circulation. Pool therapy can be used to decrease muscle weakness (due to atrophy) and joint stiffness (due to immobilization or to damage at the time of the fracture) after the cast is removed. Fibrous adhesions in joint capsules can be stretched, range of motion increased, and apprehension about moving a limb reduced.

A massage therapist should delay treatment related to a fracture until after the client's cast is removed, unless massage is approved by the client's doctor. One of the most important benefits of massage is to reduce muscle tightness which began at the time of the injury or during the healing process. For example, a rib fracture can be very painful, as respiratory motions cause a constant grating of bone ends, which are very sensitive. Trigger points can be activated when the client tries to breathe shallowly.(10)

CONTRAST TREATMENT OF A FRACTURE IN A WATERPROOF CAST OR KEPT COMPLETELY DRY USING PLASTIC BAGS

This treatment should be performed only with the physician's approval.

Use a standard contrast bath as described in Chapter 7 and do three or more rounds of hot followed by cold. A waterproof cast or one that can be kept completely dry may be immersed in contrast water baths.

Cross-Reference

See Chapter 7.

Duration and Frequency

10 to 15 minutes. Perform before or during a massage session.

Caution

The cast must be kept entirely dry. It is possible to perform this treatment by putting the entire extremity into a large plastic bag and covering that with another plastic bag so that the cast stays perfectly dry when it is immersed.

Procedure

1. Immerse the casted area in hot water (approximately 110°F) for 3 minutes.
2. Immerse the casted area in cold water (approximately 55°F) for 1 minute.
3. Repeat steps 1 and 2 twice for a total of three rounds.

CONTRAST TREATMENT OVER THE SAME BONE AS THE FRACTURED BONE ON THE UNINJURED SIDE OF THE BODY

Alternating heat and cold, using baths, local showers, or compresses, can be used to produce reflex vasodilation (the contralateral reflex effect) on the injured side. For example, if the left ankle is in a cast, perform a contrast treatment on the right ankle.

Cross-Reference

See sections on contrast local baths, contrast local showers or contrast compresses in Chapters 5 to 7 and 9.

Duration and Frequency

10 to 15 minutes. Perform before or during a massage session. As a home treatment, it may be performed two or three times daily.

Special Instructions

A handheld shower sprayer may also be used for this treatment, alternating between very hot and very cold water. Contrasting hot and cold compresses may also be used.

Procedure

1. Immerse the area on the opposite side in hot water (approximately 110°F) for 3 minutes.
2. Immerse the area on the opposite side in cold water (approximately 55°F) for 1 minute.
3. Repeat steps 1 and 2 twice for a total of three rounds.

CONTRAST SHOWER TREATMENT OVER HEALED FRACTURE SITE

After the cast is removed, contrast treatments using baths, showers, or compresses are all effective, but a handheld shower attachment, which is described here, is ideal because it gives mechanical stimulation to the skin and superficial nerves as well as improving blood flow.

Cross-Reference

See sections on contrast local showers in Chapter 9.

Duration and Frequency

10 to 15 minutes. Perform before a massage session. As a home treatment, it may be performed two or three times daily.

Procedure

1. Spray the area with water as hot as tolerated for 2 minutes.
2. Spray the area with water as cold as tolerated for 30 seconds.
3. Repeat steps 1 and 2 twice for a total of three rounds of hot followed by cold.

PARAFFIN BATH FOR JOINT STIFFNESS AFTER CAST IS REMOVED

Cross-Reference

For full instructions and contraindications, see the section on paraffin baths, Chapter 7.

Duration and Frequency

10 to 15 minutes. Perform before a massage session.

Special Instructions

Therapeutic exercises and stretching may be performed after the paraffin is removed and before massage is performed, while the joint is still very warm.

KNEE INJURIES IN THE SUBACUTE STAGE

Knee injuries such as muscle strains, torn cartilages, and sprains of the knee ligaments are common in many sports. Once the injury is no longer acute and the danger of bleeding is past, using deep heat in combination with massage will encourage healing by promoting blood flow to the knee and surrounding tissues, as well as easing discomfort. NOTE: Massage therapists should not work with clients with knee injuries until their injury has been diagnosed and treated by a doctor.

TREATMENT

WHOLE-BODY HEATING FOLLOWED BY MOIST HEAT TO THE KNEE

Cross-Reference

See the sections on fomentations in Chapter 5 and the sections on full-body baths, steam baths, and saunas in Chapters 7 and 8.

Duration and Frequency

45 minutes. The client may take the bath, steam bath or sauna just before a massage session, then go directly to the massage table for the application of local heat to the knee.

Procedure

1. Have the client take a whole-body steam bath, sauna, or full hot bath for 15 minutes.
2. Have the client dry off quickly and dress warmly to avoid chilling.
3. Apply a hot fomentation to the knee, wrap it snugly around the entire knee, and leave it on for 30 minutes. Monitor carefully for burning. A moist heating pad set on low or medium may also be used.
4. Remove the fomentation or heating pad and quickly give an ice rub or cold mitten friction to the heated area.
5. Begin massage of the knee itself.

MUSCLE STRAINS

Muscle strains are tears in muscle fibers caused when they are not properly conditioned for a particular activity. Muscle strains in the lower extremities include groin pulls and torn hamstrings, while in the upper extremities, the deltoid and biceps muscles are some of the most frequently strained. The muscles of the chest and back can be strained by heavy lifting and in sports. Even a one-time illness can initiate a muscle strain, such as repeated vomiting from a digestive problem or violent coughing with a cold. Among athletes, common causes of muscle strains include failure to warm up adequately before exercise, overly intensive workouts with lack of rest for fatigued muscles, and continued use of an injured muscle. Another frequent cause of muscle strain is the stretching of a muscle or tendon beyond its normal length. Shortened, tight muscles cannot absorb normal amounts of stress and will strain and tear more readily than usual.

Strains are classified as mild, moderate, or severe by the amount of damage to the muscle fibers. Mild strains involve a minimal amount of torn fibers, minor discomfort, no loss in strength, and normal range of motion. In moderate strains, a significant amount of muscle fibers are torn and there is pain, swelling, and loss of strength and flexibility. Severe muscle strains, which are much rarer, are actually ruptures of the muscle–tendon unit, accompanied by significant weakness and pain.

Furthermore, although muscle strains that occur as a one-time event—such as a strain of the back muscles from lifting a single heavy object—are usually obvious, a greater number appear from repeated overuse of muscles, and they often have no specific onset. Such a strain can result from habitual overuse such as operating a cash register or computer, giving massages, or walking with very poor alignment for many hours every day.

A person with an acute muscle strain will experience stiffness and mild to severe pain in the strained muscle. In the long term, scar tissue fibers that form within and around the injured muscle as a result of the healing process can lead to increased likelihood of future tears and can limit the mobility and flexibility of the muscle in the future. (Repeated muscle strains can affect more of the body than the individual muscles themselves: prior injury may cause muscles not normally used for routine activities to be substituted.)

Rehabilitation for muscle strains focuses on helping restore the muscle to its normal flexibility, endurance, and strength. This is done through treating inflammation, stopping the activity that strained the muscle originally, and performing cautiously applied therapeutic exercises. When pain begins to go away, exercise may be cautiously resumed. Lymphatic massage in the early stages of rehabilitation of an injury, followed by circulatory, cross-fiber, and deep friction techniques in the later stages, can help the muscle heal without adhesions and with full mobility.

As a massage therapist, you can use a variety of hydrotherapy treatments along with massage to increase circulation to the injured area.

TREATMENT

ICE MASSAGE OF A STRAINED MUSCLE

Ice massage may be performed in the first 24 hours after a muscle strain.

Cross-Reference
See Chapter 6.

Duration and Frequency
5 to 10 minutes. Perform during a massage session, or as a home treatment, two or three times daily.

Special Instructions
Using the ice, massage gently on the entire length of the muscle and for a few inches all around it.

CASTOR OIL PACK APPLICATION

Cross-Reference
See Chapter 5.

Duration and Frequency
30 minutes or longer before or during a massage session. The client may use castor oil packs as a home treatment at least twice a day.

Special Instructions
Apply castor oil pack directly over the strained muscle for at least 30 minutes.

HOT MOIST APPLICATION

Apply moist heat in the form of hot local baths or showers, hot moist compresses or hot fomentations. Paraffin baths may be used for the muscles of the hands, forearms, lower legs or feet. Follow the hot application with a short (1 minute) cold pour, ice water bath, or ice massage over the muscle.

Historically, vasodilating and anti-inflammatory herbs and anti-inflammatory essential oils have been used in the water used in baths, compresses, and fomentations.

Cross-Reference
See Chapter 5.

Duration and Frequency
20 minutes before or during a massage session

Special Instructions
If the strained muscle is in a hot bath, you may perform ischemic compression or gentle stretching in the water.

CONTRAST TREATMENT USING ALTERNATE HOT AND COLD

Besides the specific hot and cold methods used in the following procedure, additional modes of hot and cold may also be used: alternating hot and cold compresses, hot and cold partial baths, hot fomentations alternated with ice massage, or a handheld shower attachment for alternating hot and cold sprays.

Cross-Reference
See Chapters 5 to 7 and 9.

Duration and Frequency
15 minutes. Perform during a massage session or as a home treatment three times daily.

Special Instructions
If the strained muscle is in a hot bath, you may perform ischemic compression or gentle stretching in the water.

Procedure
1. Apply a moist heating pad or hydrocollator pack to the strained muscle for 3 minutes.
2. Wring out a washcloth in ice water and briskly rub the area that was covered by the moist heat for 1 minute or perform ice massage over it for 1 minute.
3. Repeat hot and cold twice more for a total of three rounds.

MUSTARD PLASTER

Cross-Reference
See Chapter 5.

Duration and Frequency
20 minutes. Perform during a massage session.

Procedure
1. Prepare the mustard plaster and place it over the strained muscle.
2. Cover the plaster with the plastic, small towel, and heat source.

3. Leave the plaster on for 20 minutes, monitoring the client's skin for burning, then remove it.
4. Wipe off the client's skin to remove all traces of mustard.
5. Begin massage.

TREATMENT
STEAM BATH FOLLOWED BY BRIEF COLD

The steam bath may be given in a steam room or individual steam cabinet. At the end of the steam bath, perform ice massage on the strained muscle and a few inches all around it for 1 minute.

Cross-Reference
See Chapter 6 for ice massage and Chapter 8 for steam baths.

Duration and Frequency
20 to 25 minutes. Perform before a massage session.

PLANTAR FASCIITIS

Plantar fasciitis, or inflammation of the plantar fascia, can cause significant pain on the underside of the foot, most often in the heel or arch areas. The immediate cause of plantar fasciitis is extreme fatigue in the muscles of the feet. When these muscles can no longer perform their job of supporting the arch of the foot due to fatigue, the plantar fascia has to support more weight, but it is not really a weight-supporting structure and so it tears and becomes painful and inflamed. Risk factors for plantar fasciitis include flat feet, high arches, inflexible feet, weak calf muscles, and for runners, increasing the distance or intensity of their workout too fast. Being overweight or having deep tension in the calf muscles also puts more strain on the plantar fascia. Treatment for plantar fasciitis can include a consultation with a podiatrist, stretching and strengthening exercises, wearing proper shoes, receiving **prolotherapy,** and possibly wearing arch supports or orthotics (custom-made foot supports). The most radical medical treatments, should these conservative measures prove unsuccessful, are injections of cortisone into the fascia or surgical release of the fascia.

As a massage therapist, you can help relieve discomfort and promote healing with massage techniques, and you can add hydrotherapy treatments that decrease inflammation and relieve pain. Self-massage using a soda bottle filled with ice can relieve inflammation and stretch tight tissues, and contrast treatments can relieve inflammation and promote healing. Massage performed after ice massage or contrast treatments will increase circulation and release deep tension in the calf muscles. However, even if hydrotherapy and massage are helpful at reducing

pain and muscle tension, the real cause of this injury must be addressed by the client and his or her doctor for permanent healing to occur.

TREATMENT
SELF-MASSAGE USING AN ICE-FILLED SODA BOTTLE

Cross-Reference
See Chapter 6.

Duration and Frequency
10 minutes. Perform before a massage session. As a home treatment, it can be performed two or three times daily.

Procedure
1. Fill a 20-oz plastic soft drink bottle with water and freeze it.
2. Have the client roll his or her foot back and forth over the bottle for 10 minutes. Rather than leaning the entire body weight onto the bottle, the pressure should be no more than will gently stretch the muscles, tendons, and fascia.
3. Begin massage.

CONTRAST FOOTBATH

Cross-Reference
See Chapter 7.

Special Instructions
Gentle, painless movements performed while the feet and ankles are in the water will further increase local circulation.

Duration and Frequency
10 minutes. Perform before or during a massage session. As a home treatment, it can be performed two or three times daily.

Procedure
1. Fill two deep buckets or washtubs with water, one at 110°F and the other at 50°F.
2. Put both feet in the hot water for 3 minutes.
3. Put both feet in the cold water for 30 seconds.
4. Repeat steps 2 and 3 twice more, for a total of three rounds of hot followed by cold.

ROTATOR CUFF TEAR

The rotator cuff muscles consist of the supraspinatus, infraspinatus, teres minor, and subscapularis muscles. Together, these four short muscles that originate on the scapula pass around the shoulder, and their tendons come together to form the rotator cuff. They work together as a single unit, helping to stabilize the humeral head in the glenoid fossa by controlling its internal and external rotation. The supraspinatus is the most commonly torn of the rotator cuff muscles, most often due to repetitive strain, followed by the infraspinatus and then the teres minor. The subscapularis is rarely torn, usually only when excessive force is used to reduce anterior shoulder dislocations. Most rotator cuff tears occur in people over 40 years of age, when direct trauma or mechanical stress on an aging or degenerated tendon leads to a tear. However, direct trauma, such as an anterior shoulder dislocation, a fall onto an outstretched hand, or a humeral fracture, can cause them even in younger people. Throwing too hard whole playing baseball or serving too hard while playing tennis or volleyball can also cause rotator cuff tears. Dizzy Dean, the famous Hall of Fame baseball pitcher, even tore his rotator cuff muscles by pitching with a broken toe. He could not push off on his injured foot as he would normally, which increased the load on his shoulder and led to a career-ending injury.

In roughly half of cases, surgery is not necessary because more conservative treatment can heal the tear. Small rotator cuff tears are treated by immobilization in a sling for a few days or weeks, applications of cold or heat, massage, acupuncture, and gentle exercises to maintain and even increase the range of motion. Secondary changes that can take place if the tear does not heal properly include scarring, thickening of the involved tendon, chronic inflammation, and irritation of the overlying bursae. Large rotator cuff tears often require surgery.

Hydrotherapy treatments can help address the inflammation that so often accompanies rotator cuff tears and relax the muscles around the shoulder. Ice massage can numb the shoulder temporarily so that gentle range-of-motion exercises can be performed. It is particularly important that the client regain full range of motion as soon as possible, so that a frozen shoulder (adhesive capsulitis) does not develop. NOTE: Rotator cuff injuries should be treated only after the client has been evaluated by a physician and massage has been approved.

TREATMENT
ICE MASSAGE

Cross-Reference
See Chapter 6.

Duration and Frequency
8 to 10 minutes. Perform during a massage session, or the client may perform this as a home treatment two or three times daily.

Procedure
1. Massage with the ice over the length of the torn muscle and a few inches all around it.
2. Continue for 8 to 10 minutes.
3. Let the area warm up briefly, then perform very gentle shoulder range-of-motion exercises followed by massage.

CONTRAST TREATMENT

Cross-Reference
See Chapters 5 to 7 and 9.

Duration and Frequency
15 minutes. Perform during a massage session.

Special Instructions
Besides the specific hot and cold methods used in the following procedure, additional modes of hot and cold may also be used: alternating hot and cold compresses, hot and cold partial baths, hot fomentations alternated with ice massage, or a handheld shower attachment for alternating hot and cold sprays.

Procedure
1. Apply a moist heating pad or hydrocollator pack to the entire shoulder joint, front and back, for 3 minutes. Use two moist heat sources, one on top and one underneath, if needed to cover the entire joint.
2. Wring out a washcloth in ice water and briskly rub the area that was covered by the moist heat for 30 seconds or do ice massage for 1 minute.
3. Repeat steps 1 and 2 twice more for a total of 3 rounds.

MUSTARD PLASTER

Cross-Reference
See Chapter 5.

Duration and Frequency
20 minutes. Perform during a massage session.

Procedure
1. Prepare the mustard plaster and place it on the client's shoulder over the strained muscle.
2. Cover the plaster with plastic, small towel, and heat source.
3. Leave the plaster on for 20 minutes, monitoring the client's skin for burning, then remove.
4. Wipe the client's skin off to remove all traces of mustard.
5. Begin massage.

STEAM BATH FOLLOWED BY BRIEF COLD TO THE TORN MUSCLE

The steam bath may be given in a steam room or individual steam cabinet. At the end of the steam bath, perform ice massage on the strained muscle and a few inches all around it for 1 minute.

Cross-Reference
See Chapter 6 for ice massage and Chapter 8 for steam baths.

Duration and Frequency
20 to 25 minutes. Perform before a massage session.

SCAR TISSUE

Scar tissue is made up of collagen fibers that the body makes to replace damaged or destroyed tissue. The body makes scar tissue after injuries such as cuts, burns, or trauma to muscles, ligaments, and fascia. Within 1 to 6 weeks after injury, there are higher levels of certain enzymes and an increased number of collagen-forming cells already in place. Collagen fibers, which are denser than normal skin and muscle tissue, orient themselves around the injury and grow together, forming a thick, firm scar. Unfortunately, collagen is also laid down randomly without a definite orientation or grain (Fig. 13-2A). Over about a year, scars begin to soften and fade somewhat as the enzyme collagenase digests extra collagen in the area of the scar. The old wound is now as flexible as it will ever be without outside intervention. However, scar tissue is not the same as the tissue it replaces. Compared with normal skin cells, scar tissue cells are denser, have fewer blood vessels supplying them, are less sensitive, do not contain sweat glands or hair follicles, and are less resistant to ultraviolet radiation. Scar tissue can create problems when collagen fibers from the injury site adhere to many layers of tissue below or trigger points in the scar refer burning, prickling, or lightning-like jabs of pain to adjacent tissues. Scar tissue in deeper tissues, such as muscles, can also cause problems, because it is less elastic than muscle and tears more easily when stretched. If scar tissue is deep enough or large enough, it can cause decreased muscle strength and prevents optimum contraction of muscle fibers.

Concentrated moist heat can relax the soft tissues around the scar and make scar tissue softer and more elastic. As mentioned in Chapter 7, using a paraffin bath before stretching scar tissue from a burn can yield significant, measurable increases in local freedom of movement. Beginning a session with the client's scar tissue warmer and more elastic means that many types of massage, especially cross-fiber friction, can be performed more effectively and with less discomfort. (Massage techniques aim to soften scar tissue by loosening restricting fibers and adhesions between fibers by forcibly broadening the tissues, which can produce a more parallel fiber arrangement.)

TREATMENT

MOIST HEAT APPLICATION

Apply a hot water bottle with a wet cloth underneath, moist heating pad, hot compress, or hydrocollator pack to the area for 10 to 15 minutes before massage, until the tissue is thoroughly warm.

Cross-Reference
See Chapter 5.

Duration and Frequency
10 to 15 minutes. Use before or during a massage session.

PARAFFIN BATH FOR SCARS ON THE WRISTS, HANDS, ANKLES, OR FEET

Perform a standard paraffin bath treatment of the area containing the scar before massage.

Cross-Reference
See Chapter 7.

Duration and Frequency
20 minutes. Use during a massage session. Perform a standard paraffin bath treatment of the area with the scar before hands-on massage.

LOCAL WHIRLPOOL

Have the client immerse the body part in warm water (98°–105°F) for 15 to 20 minutes before massage. Gentle exercises may be performed in the water if desired.

Cross-Reference
See Chapter 7.

Duration and Frequency
15 to 20 minutes. Use before a massage session.

SHIN SPLINTS

Shin splints is a catchall term for a variety of lower leg problems that are characterized by aching pain along the medial or lateral border of the tibia. The basic cause of this injury is strenuous use of the legs combined with poor foot alignment. Running and dancing on a hard surface are the most common activities that lead to shin splints, but a client of the author's developed shin splints from walking on a treadmill after being completely inactive for a long time. Muscle fibers, particularly those of the tibialis anterior and posterior, may tear and become inflamed, and the periosteum may become inflamed as well. A person with shin splints has tender, painful, and swollen pretibial muscles and discomfort while performing the aggravating activity. If the person continues the activity, shin splints may progress to **stress fractures** or **lower leg compartment syndrome.**

The treatment for mild shin splints includes rest from the aggravating activity, light stretching, contrast treatments followed by simple exercises, and possibly orthotics to correct the alignment of the foot. More extreme cases, such as those that have progressed to compartment syndrome, may require more medical intervention including surgery.

Hydrotherapy, particularly contrast treatments, can help increase circulation to injured muscles and relieve pain. Deep friction and massage can follow hydrotherapy treatment for mild shin splints, but massage is not suitable for advanced cases, which may actually be compartment syndrome. The client should consult a physician before receiving massage for shin splints.

TREATMENT

CONTRAST BATH TREATMENT OF THE LOWER LEG

Cross-Reference
See Chapter 7.

Special Instructions
Gentle, painless movements that are performed while the ankles and feet are in the water will further increase local circulation.

Duration and Frequency
15 minutes. Perform during a massage session, or the client may perform this as a home treatment two or three times daily.

Procedure
1. Fill two buckets or washtubs with enough water to immerse the lower legs, one at 110°F and the other at 50°F.
2. Have the client put both lower legs and feet in the hot water for 3 minutes.
3. Have the client put both lower legs and feet in the cold water for 30 seconds.
4. Repeat steps 2 and 3 three times, for a total of four rounds of hot followed by cold.
5. Remove the feet from the water and dry them thoroughly.

ICE MASSAGE OF THE LOWER LEG

Perform a standard ice massage treatment, moving over the entire length of both pretibial muscles for 8 to 10 minutes before beginning local hands-on massage.

Cross-Reference
See Chapter 6.

Duration and Frequency
8 to 10 minutes. Perform during a massage session, or the client may perform this as a home treatment two or three times daily.

SORENESS AFTER EXERCISE

Muscle soreness caused by strenuous exercise is generally felt for about 24 to 36 hours afterwards. Working muscles very vigorously causes microscopic tears to muscle fibers, along with local swelling, and then pain messages are sent from the nerves in the muscles to the brain. Soreness after exercise can be prevented by warming up the muscles that are to be used and then stretching them, gradually increasing the frequency and intensity of workouts, stretching again after exercising, and then cooling down completely. Sometimes, however, it is not possible to avoid muscle soreness when exercise comes in unexpected ways. For example, the intercostals, pectorals, and even the diaphragm itself can become sore

after violent coughing. When muscle soreness is felt after strenuous exercise, partial-body showers, Epsom salt baths and gentle circulatory massage will increase the circulation to sore muscles, help relieve swelling and pain, and help the muscles repair themselves.(11)

Hot whirlpools and ice massage are not effective for muscle soreness(12), but contrast treatments and cold whirlpools have been found effective. Many collegiate and professional long-distance runners take a cold lower-leg whirlpool bath after long runs; because peripheral blood vessels are constricted and blood flows to deeper vessels, the cold water helps prevent fatigue and soreness to deeper leg muscles. Heat-trapping compresses can also soothe muscle aches and pains.

TREATMENT

HOT PARTIAL-BODY SHOWER

Cross-Reference
See Chapter 9.

Duration and Frequency
5 minutes. Perform before a massage session, or the client may perform this as a home treatment three or four times daily.

Procedure
1. Using a handheld shower massager, spray the sore area with water that is as hot as the client can tolerate for about 5 minutes.
2. Have the client dry off and proceed with massage.

TREATMENT

EPSOM SALT BATH

Cross-Reference
See Chapter 7.

Duration and Frequency
20 minutes. Perform before a massage session, or the client may perform this as a home treatment three or four times daily.

Procedure
1. Add 2 pounds Epsom salt to a full tub of water at 98° to 104°F.
2. Have the client soak in the tub for 20 minutes.

SPINAL CORD INJURIES

Spinal cord injuries occur when strong forces applied to the spinal cord damage some or all of its fibers. Figure 13-5 shows a 12th thoracic level spinal cord injury caused by a crushing blow. Almost all of these injuries happen during motor vehicle accidents, falls, or some type of violence, and they happen almost exclusively to single males aged 16 to 30. The force that tears, bruises,

CASE HISTORY 13-1

Muscle Soreness and Bruises After a Fall out of a Tree

Background

David was a healthy and active 11-year-old boy who was climbing a fir tree one day and fell 15 feet. He landed on a few large branches on the way down, then hit the ground, and his entire back was severely bruised. David was examined by his physician and told that he had no fractures or other serious musculoskeletal injuries. Although this was welcome news, David was in a lot of pain, and he felt stiff and sore whenever he tried to move around. On his doctor's advice, he rested quietly, and his mother began applying ice packs over his bruises at intervals of 20 minutes on and 20 minutes off. However, 3 days later, David's mother called and scheduled a massage for him because, despite using ice and resting, his body still felt stiff and sore, and the bruise itself was still painful.

Treatment

Although the therapist felt that massage was likely to relieve much of David's discomfort, she was not sure he could tolerate being touched, and therefore, she suggested he try several 20-minute warm Epsom salt baths, using 2 pounds of salt in the tub each time. The next day, David's mother called to say that the Epsom salt baths had relieved much of his pain and he could still come in after school for a massage. During the session, the therapist planned to use alternating compresses in remaining areas of muscle soreness and even over David's bruise, to make massage more tolerable for him.

Discussion Questions

1. What made the Epsom salt baths effective?
2. Why would alternating compresses be appropriate during the massage session?

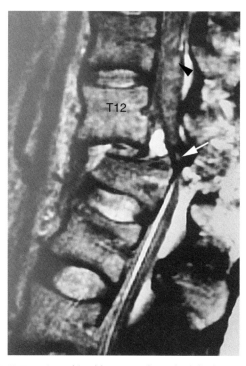

FIGURE 13-5 ■ A crushing blow caused vertebral displacement and compression of the spinal cord at the T12 level (*white arrow*). (Reprinted with permission from Yochum TR, Rowe LJ. *Essentials of Skeletal Radiology*. 2nd ed. Baltimore: Lippincott Williams & Wilkins, 1996: 398, Fig. 6-38.)

or severs the spinal cord is generally powerful enough to cause many musculoskeletal injuries at the same time. When the cord is damaged, sensation as well as controlled movement may be partially or completely lost below the level of the injury. Common problems associated with spinal cord injuries include pain so severe that it interferes with daily life; development of contractures and scoliosis from spasticity or from continual sitting in a wheelchair; pressure sores in body areas where feeling has been lost; urinary infections; decalcification of the leg bones from lack of exercise; and lack of stimulation to the circulation that exercise provides. Persons with spinal cord injuries also have difficulty controlling their body temperature in hot weather.

Massage therapists should work with patients who have acute or subacute spinal cord injuries only after they have been treated by a physician and massage has been approved. Hydrotherapy can help persons with spinal cord injuries get the most out of their massage therapy in a variety of ways. Applications of moist heat can prepare the person's tissues for massage by increasing local circulation and relaxing muscles. Contrast applications will also stimulate local circulation. Cold footbaths can reduce the body temperature up to 4°F when a client is in danger of becoming overheated on a hot day. (See the section on cold footbaths, Chapter 7.) Muscle strength may be temporarily stimulated (for about 20 minutes) with the immersion of different parts of the body in cold water. This helps the client with an incomplete lesion, which leaves some function and sensation intact below the level of the injury, to perform exercises to build muscle strength. And finally, hydrotherapy can be an important source of sensory stimulation for the skin and for the entire body. Pool therapy is a wonderful way for a person with a spinal cord injury to exercise without fighting gravity, improve the circulation as a whole, decrease muscle spasms, and receive sensory stimulation.(14) (See Appendix A for more information.) Besides promoting general relaxation, massage is helpful in addressing a range of problems associated with spinal cord injuries, including chronic pain, constipation, lack of sensory stimulation, and overuse of some parts of the body coupled with underuse of other parts.

Because paralyzed areas may be numb, all hydrotherapy applications must be very carefully monitored. Observe and feel the client's skin more often than usual to prevent burns from hot applications and frostbite from cold applications. Begin by making hot applications cooler and cold applications warmer than usual until you can see how the client responds.

TREATMENT

MOIST HEAT APPLICATION

Cross-Reference
See Chapter 5.

Duration and Frequency
10 minutes over each body area that will be massaged. Perform during a massage session.

Caution
Do not let the client become overheated. If this should occur, either discontinue heat applications, or add a cold application on another part of the body.

Special Instructions
Apply a moist hot pack, a compress (washcloth wrung out in very hot water), or a hydrocollator pack for 10 minutes before massaging an area. Then, while that area is being massaged, apply it to the part of the body that will be massaged next.

CONTRAST TREATMENT FOR SENSORY STIMULATION

Cross-Reference
See Chapter 6.

Duration and Frequency
12 minutes. Perform during a massage session.

Procedure
1. Apply a moist hot pack, a compress (washcloth wrung out in very hot water), or a hydrocollator pack to an area for 10 minutes.

2. Place an ice pack or a washcloth wrung out in cold water over the same area.
3. Leave the cold application on the area for 2 minutes before removing it.
4. Begin massage over the area.

COLD WATER IMMERSION AND EXERCISE FOR WEAK OR SPASTIC MUSCLES

For this treatment, after the cold immersion, have the client perform strengthening exercises or even contract muscles while you provide resistance. The client must have an incomplete lesion that leaves some function and sensation intact below the level of the injury.

Cross-Reference
See Chapter 7.

Duration and Frequency
5 to 10 minutes. Perform during a massage session, and repeat during the session if desired.

Special Instructions
A body part can also be wrapped in very cold towels (crushed ice wrapped in wet towels) if it cannot be immersed.

Procedure
1. Massage the weak or spastic part for 2 to 5 minutes.
2. Fill a large container with water and ice in order to chill the water to 35° to 40°F. (Check to make sure that the client is comfortably warm before beginning the cold water immersion.)
3. Warn the client that the part will be dipped in cold water.
4. Immerse the part in the water for 3 seconds.
5. Take the part out of the water and have the client perform exercises for 30 seconds. If he or she becomes fatigued, stop the exercises until after the next cold water immersion.
6. Repeat steps 4 and 5 twice more for a total of three rounds of cold immersion followed by exercises.
7. Massage the weak or spastic part for 2 to 5 minutes.

SPRAINS

A **sprain,** or ligament tear, occurs when a joint is wrenched or twisted past its normal range of motion. Minute tears occur in one or more of the ligaments that normally stabilize the joint, blood and fluid leak into the tissues around the joint, and trigger points in the ligaments and joint capsules may be activated immediately. Ligaments, like other soft tissues, respond to tensile strain and are more likely to tear if they are too short. For example, in the case of ankle ligaments, if one pronates while walking, the ligaments on the outside of the ankle tend to became shorter and the ones on the inside of the ankle stretch more and more. According to podiatrist Gary Null, "Under these conditions, all it takes is a moment of sudden pressure for the too-taut ligaments to rip."(13)

Sprains are classified by the amount of ligament fibers that are torn. First-degree tears, involving only a few fibers of a ligament, are characterized by slight swelling, pain, and loss of function. Second-degree tears involve many more fibers of a ligament and are characterized by modest swelling, diffuse tenderness, and loss of function. Third-degree tears are actual ruptures, where the ligament tears completely through and is no longer attached to the bone. A tear of this severity involves extensive bleeding, severe pain, and greater instability. Muscles spasms often occur near the sprained joint and are an indication that the person should rest the injured area; often there are spasms farther away as well. (Joint separations are also a type of ligament sprain.)

The specific treatment for sprains depends on their severity, but no matter how mild or severe the sprain is, the ligaments must be supported and protected during their healing process. For many years, first-degree sprains have been treated with ice, additional support such as braces or taping, compression, and elevation. Second-degree sprains have been treated with additional support, crutches, and isometric exercises. Third-degree sprains have been treated with a rigid cast and surgery to reattach the ligament in its proper place, followed by strengthening and stretching exercises once the cast is removed. As many as one-third of ankle sprains do not heal completely, and so proper care is very important.

Massage therapists should treat new sprains only after the client's injury has been diagnosed by a physician and massage has been recommended. Ice is applied during the first 24 to 48 hours, followed by contrast treatments to reduce joint swelling and pain. While ice applications can relieve muscle spasm, applications of ice also depress the circulation and so are useful primarily in acute stages, when bleeding is a concern. For sprains of the shoulder and spine, you can perform contrast treatment in the form of hot packs followed by ice massage. Mild sprains without swelling are sometimes treated by a heating compress that is left on overnight. For old, poorly healed ankle sprains, the deep heat of a paraffin bath may be used to ease joint stiffness, particularly before massage.

In the acute phase, massage may be performed proximal to the sprained joint but not on it. Massage is helpful for sprains in the subacute phase: circulatory, deep friction, and/or trigger point massage can reduce pain and swelling, which impair healing, and can relieve muscle tightness and spasm, which hamper movement and prevent or reduce adhesions. Massage of the area can also help prevent chronic muscular guarding caused by

trauma and pain. (See Box 13-1, second section, for presents an example of how musculoskeletal pain can lead to this problem.)

TREATMENT

ICE PACK OVER A SPRAINED JOINT IN THE ACUTE PHASE

Cross-Reference
See Chapter 6.

Duration and Frequency
20 minutes on, 20 minutes off, repeated every 2 hours for the first 24 to 48 hours

Cautions: Do not overuse ice. Injuries have occurred from ice being applied to acute injuries for too long.

LOCAL EPSOM SALT BATH

A local bath with Epsom salt can be used for subacute sprains to enhance local circulation and reduce edema. Gentle range-of-motion exercises may be performed during the bath.

Cross-Reference
See Chapter 7.

Duration and Frequency
20 minutes. Perform before a massage session, or the client may perform this as a home treatment three or four times daily.

Special Instructions
1. The water should be well over the sprained joint, so that even for a foot sprain, the water should be up to mid-calf level.
2. Gentle, painless movements performed while the part is in the water will further increase local circulation.

Procedure
1. Add 1 cup of Epsom salt per gallon to a container of water at 98° to 104°F.
2. Have the client soak the sprained part (e.g., hand and wrist, foot and ankle) in the tub for 15 to 20 minutes.
3. Dry the part and begin massage.

HEAT-TRAPPING COMPRESS

Heat-trapping compresses may be used for subacute sprains of the foot, ankle, knee, elbow, wrist, or hand to provide a mild prolonged warmth.

Cross-Reference
See Box 6-2.

Duration and Frequency
1 to 8 hours. This can be used daily in the subacute stages of healing. The client can apply the compress at bedtime and remove it in the morning.

Special Instructions

At the end of a massage session, the massage therapist may assist the client in applying a heat-trapping compress to keep the sprained joint warm for a few hours or overnight.

CONTRAST BATH FOR THE ANKLE JOINT

This treatment may be done on any joint, but because the most commonly sprained joint is the ankle, we use a contrast treatment for the ankle as an example.

Cross-Reference

See Chapter 7.

Duration and Frequency

15 minutes. Perform before or during a massage session. As a home treatment it can be performed two or three times daily.

Special Instructions

Gentle, painless movements performed while the part is in the water will further increase local circulation.

Procedure

1. Fill two deep buckets or washtubs with water, one at 110°F and the other at 50°F.
2. Put both feet in the hot water for 3 minutes. Water should reach mid-calf level.
3. Put both feet in the cold water for 30 seconds.
4. Repeat steps 2 and 3 three more times for a total of four rounds of hot followed by cold.
5. If prescribed by the client's physician, an adhesive bandage can now be applied to the sprained ankle.

PARAFFIN BATH FOR OLD, POORLY HEALED SPRAINS

We use the ankle as an example, but other joints may benefit from paraffin as well.

Cross-Reference

See Chapter 7.

Special Instructions

For joints that cannot be dipped, paraffin can be painted directly over the joint.

Duration and Frequency

10 to 15 minutes. Perform before a massage session, or the client may obtain a paraffin bath and perform this daily as a home treatment.

Procedure

1. Soak the client's foot and ankle in warm or hot water (98°–110°F) for 1 minute or longer.
2. Dip the foot and ankle at least six times in hot paraffin.
3. Wrap the foot to keep it warm and leave the paraffin on for at least 10 minutes before massage and range-of-motion exercises or stretching.

TENDONITIS

Tendonitis, or inflammation in a tendon, usually occurs when a muscle has been under extreme stress. Vigorous athletic training can create such conditions as biceps tendonitis (pitching), quadriceps tendonitis (dancing, basketball), rotator cuff tendonitis (tennis), or Achilles tendonitis (long-distance running), but tendonitis can also occur as the result of repetitive strain. Massage therapists are prone to this injury because their work involves the repetitive use of a few muscles for long periods, often while applying much force. Tears in the collagen of the tendon can cause pain, inflammation, and possibly a buildup of scar tissue as the tendon partly heals and then tears again. Tendon injuries take a longer time to heal than muscle injuries because they do not have as great a blood supply as muscles.

Standard medical treatment for tendonitis is rest, ice, and anti-inflammatory medications. These may include either steroidal or nonsteroidal anti-inflammatory types. A brace or wrapping may be used as well. Stretching and/or strengthening exercises are often prescribed. As their symptoms resolve, many clients gradually return to the aggravating sport or activity, although for some this may not be possible.

During the acute phase of tendonitis, contrast treatments, ice massage, and lymphatic drainage techniques may be used to increase local circulation and decrease inflammation.

In the subacute phase, contrast treatments continue to be appropriate for promoting healing, and both cross-fiber friction and techniques that treat muscle tension in the entire muscle (not just the tendon) are helpful to prevent scar tissue buildup.

Although the recommended treatments that follow may be used on any tendon, we show how to use them on the elbow for epicondylitis, a type of tendonitis caused by repetitive strain. There are two common types of epicondylitis. **Medial epicondylitis**—inflammation of the wrist flexor tendons at their insertion on the medical epicondyle—can be caused by repeated and forceful bending of the wrist, such as swinging a golf club, or in other activities that involve gripping or grasping and then turning the hand with a great deal of force. **Lateral epicondylitis**—inflammation of the wrist extensor tendons at their insertion on the lateral epicondyle, also known as tennis elbow or typing elbow—is far more common. It can be caused by many activities that are performed using repeated forceful contractions of the wrist extensors in a pronated position, such as during backhand strokes in tennis, pitching, and performing repetitive work with a hammer or screwdriver.

In both conditions, the treatment is basically the same. In the acute phase, the arm is rested and may even be splinted in a position that relieves tension on the tendons. Strengthening exercises may be begun after a week of rest so strength and flexibility are not lost. Contrast treatments may be used two or three times daily to relieve inflammation, as may ice massage or paraffin dips. Lymphatic drainage and gentle transverse friction techniques are appropriate for acute tendonitis. Local salt glows followed by castor oil and a heating compress may be applied during a massage session or used by the client at night. The client's doctor may also prescribe anti-inflammatory medication. In the subacute phase, this therapy may continue, except circulatory massage and deep transverse friction techniques are now appropriate. Massage therapists should not treat tendonitis until it has been diagnosed by a physician and massage has been approved.

TREATMENT
CONTRAST BATH TREATMENT OF INFLAMED TENDONS AT THE ELBOW

Cross-Reference
See Chapter 7.

Duration and Frequency
15 minutes. Perform before or during a massage session, or the client may perform this as a home treatment two or three times daily.

Special Instructions
1. The tendon and an area at least 6 inches around it should be covered by the water.
2. Gentle, painless movements performed while the elbow is in the water will further increase local circulation.
3. Contrast immersion baths are used here, but hydrocollator packs and ice massage can be used instead.

Procedure
1. Fill two deep buckets or washtubs with water, one at 110°F and the other at 50°F.
2. Put the elbow with the inflamed tendon in the hot water for 3 minutes.
3. Put that elbow in the cold water for 30 seconds.
4. Repeat steps 2 and 3 three more times for a total of four rounds of hot followed by cold.
5. Remove the elbow from the water and dry it thoroughly.

ICE MASSAGE OF ACUTELY INFLAMED TENDONS AT THE ELBOW

Cross-Reference
See Chapter 6.

Duration and Frequency
8 to 10 minutes

Special Instructions
Perform the ice massage on the tendon and 6 inches all around it.

LOCAL SALT GLOW FOLLOWED BY APPLICATION OF CASTOR OIL AND A HEAT-TRAPPING COMPRESS, SUITABLE FOR ACUTELY OR SUBACUTELY INFLAMED TENDONS AT THE ELBOW

Apply at the beginning of a massage session, remove after 30 minutes, and then perform massage over and around the inflamed tendon.

Cross-Reference
See Chapters 5, 6, and 11.

Duration and Frequency
45 minutes

Caution
Do not wrap the joint so tightly that you cut off circulation.

Special Instructions
If the client is using this as a home treatment, he or she may leave the heating pad on for up to 2 hours, then remove the heating pad and leave the compress on overnight.

Procedure
1. Perform a local salt glow over the muscle and tendon and about 6 inches around it, using Epsom salt.
2. Rub a liberal amount of castor oil over and around the tendon.
3. Cover the castor oil–coated skin with a piece of cellophane, then apply a heating compress over it.
4. Cover with a heating pad set on low and leave in place for 30 minutes or more. If the client is using this as a home treatment, he or she may leave the heating pad on for up to 2 hours, then remove the heating pad, go to bed, and remove the compress in the morning.
5. Remove the heating compress and wash the oil off using hot water and baking soda, then finish with a brief friction rub with very cold water.

PARAFFIN DIP BEFORE MASSAGE FOR SUBACUTELY INFLAMED TENDONS AT THE ELBOW

Cross-Reference
See Chapter 7.

Duration and Frequency
15 minutes. Apply before beginning a massage session.

Procedure
1. Immerse the elbow, especially the tendon, in the paraffin bath and wrap it well.

2. After unwrapping the area, either give the client's arm a cold mitten friction or have the client dip the elbow in cold water for a few seconds.
3. Begin massage.

TIRED FEET

Muscular fatigue in the feet often affects clients who have been walking or running long distances or who have been competing in sports that involve a great deal of running, such as basketball and soccer. It is also common in clients who have poor alignment, poorly fitting shoes, or structural problems in the feet. Along with hydrotherapy treatments, massage can address this type of simple muscular fatigue. Hydrotherapy is used frequently by competitive runners to ease muscular fatigue and rejuvenate muscles, and massage can bring great relief for feet that ache from or are fatigued by vigorous exercise. An athlete can receive these treatments and massage during a rest break and then go back on the field rejuvenated; using massage after a vigorous workout can reduce muscular fatigue more effectively than resting quietly.(11)

TREATMENT
CONTRAST FOOTBATH

Cross-Reference
See Chapter 7.

Duration and Frequency
10 minutes. Perform before or during a massage session. As a home treatment, it can be performed two or three times daily.

Special Instructions
Gentle, painless movements performed while the feet are in the water will further increase local circulation. Many runners find a simple cold footbath very refreshing and more practical. Simply follow the procedure that follows, but use only one footbath of water as cold as can be tolerated and have the client soak for 10 minutes. Another option is to have the client sit in a half-bath of cold water for 10 minutes.

Procedure
1. Fill two deep buckets or washtubs with water, one at 110°F and the other at 50°F.
2. Put both feet in the hot water for 3 minutes.
3. Put both feet in the cold water for 30 seconds.
4. Repeat steps 2 and 3 twice more, for a total of three rounds of hot followed by cold.

LOCAL SALT GLOW AND WARM FOOTBATH

Cross-Reference
See Chapters 7 and 11.

Duration and Frequency
5 to 10 minutes

Special Instructions
This technique may be performed with the client supine. In this case, put a towel at the foot end of the table, place the footbath on it, and tell the client to bend the knees and keep and feet in the warm water.

Procedure
1. Place a large towel on the floor.
2. Have the client sit in a chair.
3. Place a container of warm water (98°–105°F) on top of the towel.
4. Have the client soak the feet in the footbath for 2 minutes.
5. Take one of the client's feet out of the footbath.
6. Using a small amount of Epsom salt, perform a salt glow on one foot. Either hold the client's foot over the footbath while you do this, or lay her foot on the towel next to it.
7. Place the client's foot back in the warm footbath.
8. Repeat with the client's second foot.
9. Pour clean water over both feet and then move the footbath off the towel entirely, so there is room for the both feet on the towel.
10. Dry the feet and cover them with the towel, so they do not become chilled. Massage of the feet and lower legs may now be performed. The client may remain sitting in the chair or move to massage table.
11. Cover the feet with socks when massage is completed.

WHIPLASH

The head and neck can be snapped violently forward and back (Fig. 13-6) during a fall, a head-on collision in an athletic event, or a rear-end collision in a motor vehicle. This snapping action can cause what is known as a **whiplash** injury, that is, damage to many of the structures of the neck. Strain of the neck muscles, sprain of the neck ligaments, fractures of cervical vertebrae, herniation of cervical discs, and/or injury to the spinal cord itself can occur. Depending upon the severity of the whiplash, the result can be an accumulation of excessive scar tissue, ongoing muscle spasms in neck muscles that attempt to splint unstable joints (a job normally performed by the ligaments which now are weakened), trigger points, and possibly cranial bones being out of alignment. Muscles around the cervical spine, including the sternocleidomastoid, scalenes, and splenius cervicis, may be injured in a whiplash. The amount of damage to these muscles may be greater if they were very tight previously. Spinal ligaments may be sprained so severely that they will not hold the spinal column together tightly enough and the vertebrae are unstable. Clients may feel almost nothing at the scene of a car accident, be cleared by an emergency department doctor, and in the ensuing days have

Hyperextension
phase

Hyperflexion
phase

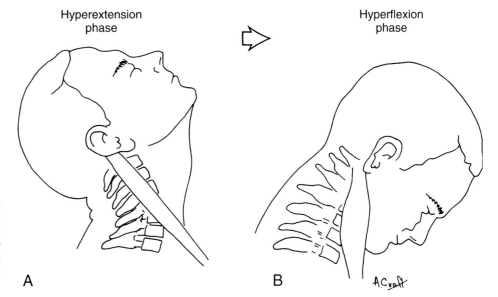

FIGURE 13-6 ■ Hyperextension and hyperflexion of the head and neck, or whiplash. (Reprinted with permission from Werner R. *Massage Therapists Guide to Pathology.* 2nd ed. Baltimore: Lippincott Williams & Wilkins, 2002: Fig. 3-9.)

A   B

increasing stiffness and pain. Whiplash injuries, even when they do not show up on radiography, are often serious and long-lasting, and they require a doctor's ongoing care.

During the subacute stage of whiplash, hydrotherapy treatments can reduce pain and inflammation, increase local circulation, and help relax muscles before massage. Many types of massage can help heal whiplash injuries, from trigger point to deep friction and craniosacral techniques. Because of the variety of injuries that can occur when the neck is forced into hyperextension and then hyperflexion, massage therapists should not work with clients with whiplash injuries until they have been diagnosed by a physician and massage has been approved.

TREATMENT

NECK EXERCISE PERFORMED IN A HOT SHOWER

This will gently warm and relax the neck muscle tension and improve local circulation. For subacute whiplash only

Cross-Reference
See Chapter 9.

Duration and Frequency
5 to 10 minutes. Perform at the beginning of a massage session, or if used as a home treatment, two or three times daily.

Special Instructions
Remind the client, if necessary, that this is a gentle limbering exercise and should not cause any pain or discomfort.

Procedure
1. Have the client step into a hot shower and let the water beat on the neck for at least 3 minutes to thoroughly warm the cervical muscles.

2. Have the client very slowly, and with no pain or straining, while the hot water continues to beat on the neck muscles, draw the letters of the alphabet with the nose one by one.
3. Have the client towel off and dress quickly to avoid chilling
4. The client may now lie down for a rest or a massage session, if planned.

CONTRAST TREATMENT FOR THE NECK

Cross-Reference
See Chapter 6.

Duration and Frequency
5 to 10 minutes. Perform at the beginning of a massage session, or if used as a home treatment, two or three times daily.

Special Instructions
A contrast treatment may be performed in the shower using a handheld shower attachment and the same intervals of hot and cold.

Procedure
1. Have the client lie prone upon the massage table.
2. Apply a moist heating pad or hydrocollator pack to the back of the neck for 3 minutes. Wrap it around to the front of the neck as far as possible but do not cover the carotid arteries.
3. Wring out a washcloth in ice water and rub the area that was under the moist heat for 30 seconds, or perform ice massage on the area for 1 minute.
4. Repeat hot and cold two more times for a total of three rounds.
5. Dry the client's skin and begin hands-on massage.

Hydrotherapy and Massage for Subacute Whiplash Injury

Background

Dimitri Hall was a 32-year-old landscaper who was in excellent health and who had no history of back or neck injuries. Recently, as he sat at a stoplight with his head turned to the right, his car was struck from behind by a car traveling 30 miles per hour. Within 2 hours after the accident, Dimitri's neck began to hurt. His neck pain gradually increased and he began to feel tingling and numbness in his right arm and right leg. After being examined at a hospital emergency department, where radiographs showed no cervical fractures, Dimitri received a cervical collar and was prescribed muscle relaxant, anti-inflammatory, and pain medications.

He later visited his family doctor, who examined him and found that his paraspinal muscles from T10 to C1 were hypersensitive to light touch and hurt far more on the injured side. He also found that Dimitri's neck range of motion was very limited and that even light pressure on suboccipital and scalene muscle trigger points caused severe referred pain up into his head. The doctor told Dimitri that he had soft-tissue damage and inflammation in his neck and prescribed physical therapy and massage therapy twice a week for 4 weeks. He advised Dimitri to wear a cervical collar for all but 2 or 3 hours out of every 24 and to avoid moving his neck when it was off.

Treatment

Session 1. On the seventh day after the accident, Dimitri entered the massage therapist's office wearing a cervical collar and having the moderate to severe neck pain, hypersensitivity to touch, highly active trigger points, and limited neck range of motion noted by his doctor. The session began with Dimitri lying prone on the massage table while hot compresses alternated with ice massage were applied to the back of his neck and his upper back. Dimitri stated that this made his neck feel better. He was then treated with gentle fingertip kneading and pétrissage on his neck, entire back, and chest. At the end of the session, the massage therapist explained how to perform contrast treatments to the upper back and neck in the shower, using a handheld shower attachment. Hot water could be used for 2 minutes, followed by cold for 30 seconds to 1 minute, and three to five rounds could be performed. Dimitri was told he could perform this treatment as many as four times daily.

Sessions 2 to 7 were similar to the first. Dimitri continued to have neck pain, although it was never as extreme as during the first few days, and his neck continued to hurt when he looked down. However, his pain very gradually began to decrease. He continued to wear his cervical collar almost all the time. He performed contrast treatments in the shower every day and found that they relieved his pain for 1 to 2 hours.

Dimitri's massage treatments were similar to what the therapist performed at the first visit but were always adjusted to the amount of pressure he could tolerate. Each session, before massage was performed on any part of his back or neck, he received 10 minutes of heat followed by a short ice massage of the area. First, a small towel wrung out in hot water was placed on his upper back and the back of his neck, then the towel was covered with a thin sheet of plastic and a heating pad set on medium. Massage was performed on the Dimitri's arms for 10 minutes. Then 1 minute of ice massage was performed on his upper back and the back of his neck. The massage therapist then placed the heat on Dimitri's lower back while she performed hands-on massage on his upper back and the back of his neck. After 10 minutes of hands-on massage, she removed the heat from his lower back and performed ice massage for 1 minute. She again placed the heat on the upper back while she performed hands-on massage on Dimitri's lower back. She then repeated this entire sequence and finished treating his back with 1 minute of ice massage on Dimitri's entire spine. He said this made his back feel great. He then turned to the supine position and massage was performed on the his neck, shoulders, and chest.

As time went on, Dimitri's situation began to improve. He received twice-weekly massage and physical therapy and continued contrast treatments in the shower for pain relief and relaxation. Although he had occasional setbacks caused by forgetting to wear his cervical collar or practicing his physical therapy exercises too vigorously, his neck pain began to decrease. Gradually, the muscles in his back and neck became noticeably less hypertonic and less swollen and he was able to tolerate more pressure during massage. At his eighth and last massage session, Dimitri entered with little or no pain and an improved range of motion in his neck. He was noticeably less sensitive to pressure on his entire back and shoulders, his upper back muscles were noticeably less hypertonic and swollen than they were at the beginning of massage therapy, and pressure on trigger points produced much less pain. Dimitri would continue to receive physical therapy for some time and planned to continue contrast treatments at home for residual pain and stiffness in his neck.

Discussion Questions

1. Why did the massage therapist recommend shower contrast treatments at home rather than hot showers or cold showers alone?
2. Why did the massage therapist use heat followed by hands-on massage followed by heat again?

FULL HOT BATH

Cross-Reference
See Chapter 7.

Duration and Frequency
15 to 20 minutes. Perform before a massage session.

Caution
This treatment should not be taken by those with high blood pressure or heart problems.

Special Instructions
A 10-minute hot application followed by a short cold rub may also be used directly on the back of the neck as soon the client leaves the tub and lies down on the massage table, to ensure complete relaxation of the neck muscles.

Procedure
1. Fill the bathtub with hot water (102°–110°F).
2. Place a cold compress on the forehead and a rolled-up towel or bath pillow behind the client's neck so the neck is in a comfortable position.
3. Have the client remain in the tub for 15 minutes or longer, depending upon tolerance.
4. Have the client sit on the side of the bathtub.
5. Perform a cold mitten friction while the client is sitting on the side of the bathtub. If lightheaded, the client should continue sitting on the side of the tub until thoroughly cooled off and no longer light-headed.
6. Have the client dry off and go directly to the massage table for treatment.

CHAPTER SUMMARY

In this chapter, you have learned some of the most common injuries you may see in your clients and their causes. You have also learned how hydrotherapy may be used in conjunction with massage to safely treat these injuries. Because massage therapists so often see clients with common musculoskeletal injuries such as muscle strains and joint sprains, the information in this chapter will prove invaluable in your practice.

REVIEW QUESTIONS

Fill in the Blanks

1. Mustard plasters provide intense local heat and can be used for _____ and _____ and _____.

2. Muscle soreness after exercise can be treated using _____ baths.

3. A cold leg bath relieves muscle fatigue by shifting blood flow from _____ to _____.

4. Sprains are injuries to _____, while strains are injuries to _____.

5. A cold-water immersion bath is given to someone with a spinal cord injury to stimulate _____.

Multiple Choice

6. All but one of the following are inflammatory conditions:
   a. Bursitis
   b. Epicondylitis
   c. Exhaustion after exercise
   d. Plantar fasciitis

7. All but one of the following can benefit from contrast treatments:
   a. Sprains
   b. Scar tissue
   c. Amputation
   d. Plantar fasciitis

8. All but one of these treatments is appropriate for acute bursitis:
   a. Upper half-body pack
   b. Paraffin bath
   c. Contrast treatment
   d. Ice massage

9. When scar tissue is formed improperly, one of the following results:
   a. Arthritis
   b. Swelling
   c. Hematoma
   d. Adhesions

10. All but one are signs of inflammation:
    a. Redness
    b. Cool skin
    c. Swelling
    d. Pain

REFERENCES

1. www.cdc.gov/national center for health statistics/faststats/injury/html. Accessed December 2005.
2. Simon R, Aleskovsky R. *Repetitive Strain Injury Handbook.* New York: Henry Holt, 2000, p 5.
3. Thrash A. *Home Remedies: Hydrotherapy, Massage, Charcoal and Other Simple Treatments.* Seale, AL: Thrash, 1981, p 60.
4. On AY, Colakoglu Z, Hepguler S, Aksit R. Local heat effect on sympathetic skin responses after pain of electrical stimulus. *Arch Phys Med Rehabil* 1997;78:1196.
5. Harden M. A new look at heat treatment for pain disorders. *Am Pain Soc Bull* 2005;15, No. 1, winter 2005.
6. www.caringmedical.com/ice-why we do not recommend it. Ross Hauser, MD. Accessed December 2005.
7. www.diabetes.niddk.nih.gov/dm/pubs/statistics/index.htm. Diabetes statistics. Accessed January 4, 2007.

8. www.aputee-coalition.org/fact-sheets/amp_stats_cause.html. Amputation fact sheet. Accessed January 4, 2007.

9. Simon R, Aleskovsky R. *The Repetitive Strain Injury Handbook.* New York: Henry Holt, 2000, p 65.

10. Aftimos S. Myofascial pain in children. *N Z Med J* 1989; 02:440.

11. Earr T et al. The effects of therapeutic massage on delayed onset muscle soreness and muscle function following downhill walking. *J Sci Med Sport* 2002;5:297.

12. Howatson G, Van Someren KA. Ice massage. Effects on exercise-induced muscle damage. *J Sports Med Fitness* 2003; 43:500.

13. Null G, Robins T. In *How to Keep Your Feet and Legs Healthy for a Lifetime.* New York: 4 Walls, 8 Windows, 2000, p 75.

14. Kesiktas N et al. The use of hydrotherapy for the management of spasticity. *Neurorehabil Neural Repair* 2004;18:268.

RECOMMENDED RESOURCES

Benjamin B. *Listen to Your Pain: The Active Person's Guide to Understanding, Identifying, and Treating Pain and Injury.* New York: Penguin, 1984.

Buchman D. *The Complete Book of Water Healing.* New York: Instant Improvement, 1994.

Clark G, Wilgis E, Aiello B, et al., eds. *Hand Rehabilitation: A Practical Guide,* 2nd ed. New York: Churchill Livingstone, 1997.

Finnerty G, Corbitt T. *Hydrotherapy.* New York: Frederick Ungar, 1960.

Gates S, Mooar P, eds. *Orthopedics and Sports Medicine for Nurses.* Baltimore: Williams & Wilkins, 1989.

Hauser H. *Prolo Your Pain Away,* 2nd ed. Oak Park, IL: Beulah Land, 2004.

Horay P, Harp D. *Hot Water Therapy.* Oakland, CA: New Harbinger, 1991.

Michlovitz S. *Thermal Agents in Rehabilitation.* Philadelphia: F.A. Davis, 1996.

Moor FB, Peterson SC, Manwell EM, et al. *Manual of Hydrotherapy and Massage.* Hagerstown, MD: Review and Herald, 1964.

Packman H. *Ice Therapy, Understanding its Application.* Flushing, NY: Author, 1987.

Simon R, Aleskovsky R. *The Repetitive Strain Injury Handbook.* New York: Henry Holt, 2000.

Thomas C. *Simple Water Treatments for the Home.* Loma Linda, CA: Loma Linda University School of Health, 1977.

Tierra M. *The Way of Herbs.* New York: Simon & Schuster, 1990.

HYDROTHERAPY AND MASSAGE FOR NONINJURY CONDITIONS

14

Most people view pain as an enemy. Yet, as my leprosy patients prove, it forces us to pay attention to threats against our bodies . . . Who would ever visit a physician apart from pain's warnings?. . . Virtually every response of our bodies that we view with irritation or disgust—blister, callus, swelling, fever, sneeze, cough, vomiting, and especially pain—demonstrates a reflex towards health. In all these things normally considered enemies, we can find a reason to be grateful.

—Paul Brand, MD, quoted in Soul Survivor: How Thirteen Unlikely Mentors Helped My Faith Survive the Church

Chapter Objectives

After completing this chapter, the student will be able to:

- Describe the most common types of chronic pain.
- Explain how hydrotherapy can relieve pain with either heat or cold.
- Explain the rationale for using four hydrotherapy treatments with conditions presented in this chapter.
- Describe the specific treatment with hydrotherapy for three painful conditions presented in this chapter.
- List three conditions that do not involve pain and describe their treatment with hydrotherapy.

In this chapter you will learn about hydrotherapy treatments you can combine with your massage techniques in order to help clients with a variety of problems and conditions. Since massage therapists are often consulted for help with both acute and chronic musculoskeletal conditions, special attention is devoted to them. Musculoskeletal pain, in particular, is surprisingly widespread; when surveyed, one-fifth to one-third of all American adults say they have chronic pain. Arthritis, rheumatism, chronic headaches, and spine and back problems head the list of these long-term pain problems.(1) Even higher percentages of elders, three-quarters or more, have chronic pain that affects the quality of their lives and their ability to function normally. Osteoarthritis is their single most common painful condition.(2)

Hydrotherapy treatments can help relieve much musculoskeletal pain and make massage sessions more effective and enjoyable. For example, for pain in an extremity,

fomentations applied on both the front and the back can relax muscles, relieve pain, and allow the client to tolerate massage better. Or, in areas of chronic tension, various forms of moist heat can be used to warm and loosen the client's muscles and fascia before massage. Ice massage can numb painful areas, especially sharp local pain, and relieve sciatica and muscle spasm. Heat-trapping compresses over joints are effective for joint pain. Paraffin baths can reduce joint stiffness. Neutral baths are excellent for almost any condition that causes general pain, such as severe arthritis, chronic low back pain, stroke, muscle spasticity, cerebral palsy, spinal cord injury, or postpolio pain. Clients with these conditions may experience joint pain after being active, and contrast treatments are an excellent way to boost local circulation and relieve their pain. When clients experience these treatments during sessions and use them at home, they will also see the effects of massage sessions last longer. Regularly exercising in warm water or receiving regular **Watsu** sessions

BOX 14-1 | *Point of Interest*

WATER MAKES AN IMPACT: TWO TREATMENTS THAT USE WATER STIMULATION ON THE SKIN TO TREAT CHRONIC CONDITIONS

The two hydrotherapy treatments described here are not practical for today's massage therapist, as they necessitate specialized equipment and, in the case of the continuous bath, much time. However, it is interesting to see that when water impacts the skin in specialized ways, it may benefit people with some specific problems.

The first treatment we discuss is the continuous bath, which is an ingenious extension of the soothing and pain-relieving abilities of neutral, warm, or hot baths. The patient is placed on a hammock suspended in a bathtub, then covered with a canvas sheet that has a hole for the head. A series of valves and temperature gauges allow the bath water to be kept at a constant temperature, and water runs for many hours or even for days. Water running over the skin creates a constant gentle barrage of nerve impulses, which reflexively produces a calming effect similar to the effect of the gentle, steady, and rhythmic rocking used by practitioners of the Trager method. For this reason, continuous neutral baths, sometimes of many hours' duration, were widely used in the late nineteenth and early twentieth centuries to calm restless, agitated, or combative patients at mental hospitals, to relieve the pain, spasm, burning sensation, and tremors of Parkinson's disease, to lower high blood pressure, and to treat chronic musculoskeletal pain, such as that of advanced arthritis. Continuous baths were safe and had no contraindications except skin rashes or other conditions that could be irritated by moisture.

The second treatment we discuss is the percussion douche, a spray of water at high pressure directed against some portion of the body. Much more like a very vigorous compression massage than a relaxing, gentle stimulation, the percussion douche is used for radically different purposes than the continuous bath. A percussion douche stimulates circulation and other local functions, decreases local congestion, and can relieve local pain. It was widely used in the days of the water cure to relieve such painful conditions as neuralgia, painful rheumatic joints, sciatica, chronic low back pain, and migraine headaches. For sciatica, the high-pressure stream of water would be used to spray along the path of the sciatic nerve from the heel up to the lumbar area and then back down to the heel again. For chronic low back pain, the spray would begin at the heel and move up the back of the leg to the lower back and then on to that side of the middle back, upper back, and neck. Often the client was sprayed with hot water followed by cold. Massage was often given after this procedure was finished.

References

1. Thrash A, Thrash C. *Home Remedies: Hydrotherapy, Massage, Charcoal and Other Simple Treatments*. Seale, AL: Thrash, 1981, pp 102, 120.
2. Kellogg JH. *Rational Hydrotherapy*. Battle Creek, MI: Modern Medicine, 1923, p 432.

---

will also benefit many chronic conditions by increasing joint range of motion, stimulating circulation, and relieving pain. The treatments presented in this chapter only begin to give an idea of the potential of treating chronic conditions with water. (For an example of other water treatments that were not included, see Box 14-1.) Research is badly needed on the use of more of these safe and effective ways to treat chronic pain and other conditions not related to injury.

ADHESIVE CAPSULITIS OF THE SHOULDER (FROZEN SHOULDER)

Adhesive capsulitis of the shoulder, also known as frozen shoulder, is a gradually progressive and quite painful restriction of joint motion. Rotator cuff tendonitis, cervical radiculopathy, bursitis, postmastectomy pain, prolonged immobilization of a minor shoulder injury, or even a muscle imbalance caused by inactivity can lead to this condition. Trauma to the joint such as a shoulder dislocation, shoulder fracture, or a tear in the rotator cuff muscles can also cause frozen shoulder. Adhesive capsulitis begins when someone's shoulder hurts whenever it is moved, so the person avoids moving it. Over time this leads to weakness in the muscles around the shoulder joint, which in turn leads to even less joint movement. As a result, adhesions develop between the

head of the humerus and the synovial joint capsule, and eventually the superior part of the joint capsule can adhere to the bicipital tendon and the head of the humerus. Some ligaments may become frozen in a shortened position, which severely limits the person's range of motion. The end result is decreased internal and external rotation, abduction and flexion, and general shoulder pain with active movement. Even passive movement will be decreased, compared to the opposite shoulder. Simple movements, such as those used in dressing, bathing, and combing the hair, may be impossible.

In most cases, with rest and careful rehabilitation—including massage and range of motion, stretching, and strengthening exercises—the frozen shoulder can be reversed, and the person can regain normal, pain-free motion. Otherwise, manipulation under anesthesia (to tear the joint capsule loose from the head of the humerus) or surgery may be performed. However, even with resolution of the frozen shoulder, there may be a permanent loss of range of motion at the shoulder. Many people who had frozen shoulder at one time still have a limitation in their shoulder range of motion or some residual reluctance to move their shoulder or arm.

Deep friction, trigger point massage, and myofascial release techniques are all appropriate techniques for adhesive capsulitis. Deep heat from hot packs or mustard plasters can be applied to the shoulder before massage and/or stretching in order to relax surrounding muscles and make scar tissue easier to stretch. Ice massage may be used to numb the shoulder so that gentle range-of-motion exercises can be performed.

TREATMENT

ICE MASSAGE AROUND THE SHOULDER JOINT OR ICE PACK APPLICATION TO THE SHOULDER

Cross-Reference
See Chapter 6.

Duration and Frequency
5 to 8 minutes for ice massage on the shoulder and 10 minutes for ice pack on the shoulder. Perform during a massage session.

Procedure
1. Perform ice massage around the shoulder joint for 5 to 8 minutes, or apply an ice pack for 10 minutes.
2. The client may now perform gentle range of motion exercises as long as they do not cause any pain.

MOIST HEAT APPLICATION TO THE SHOULDER

Cross-Reference
See Chapter 5.

Duration and Frequency
20 minutes. Perform during a massage session, or as a home treatment before stretching exercises, two or three times daily.

Special Instructions
Hot compresses may be substituted for fomentations, but an external heating device will be required to keep them hot. A hydrocollator pack may be used on the top of the shoulder but not on the underside.

Procedure
1. Apply two fomentations, one on the underside of the arm and one on the top surface of the arm, so that the shoulder joint is sandwiched between them. Monitor carefully for burning.
2. Wait 20 minutes, then remove the fomentations and begin massage, range-of-motion exercises, and/or stretching.

MUSTARD PLASTER APPLICATION

Cross-Reference
See Chapter 5.

Duration and Frequency
20 minutes. Perform during a massage session, or as a home treatment before stretching exercises, two or three times daily.

Procedure
Apply the mustard plaster over the top of the shoulder and tuck it around to the back. Monitor carefully for burning. Wait 20 minutes, then remove the plaster and begin massage, range-of-motion exercises, and/or stretching.

ARTHRITIS

Arthritis, or joint inflammation, is one of the most common causes of musculoskeletal pain and one of the most common reasons that people seek massage therapy. For this reason, both osteoarthritis (overuse arthritis) and rheumatoid (autoimmune arthritis) are discussed at length in this section. Usually, clients with these two types of arthritis already have discovered that applications of hot water, such as hot baths and showers, are a great way to relieve their pain, and many also use heating pads for this purpose.

OSTEOARTHRITIS

Osteoarthritis, which is also known as degenerative joint disease, is the most common form of arthritis. It affects most people over 55 years old and becomes even more common as people age.(3) The arthritic process begins when the cartilage covering joint surfaces begins to break down; then rough bony surfaces rub together, which causes stiff, painful, and hard-to-move joints (Fig. 14-1A). The most common joints to develop this condition are the fingers and weight-bearing joints such as the spine, knee, and hip. Factors that can contribute to the development of osteoarthritis include repetitive stress, aging, nutritional deficiencies, heredity, chronically loose joints (ligamentous laxity), muscle weaknesses, and traumatic injuries. Osteoarthritis in individual joints is most prevalent in individuals who performed heavy work using that joint for at least 15 years and in athletes whose sport stressed that particular joint or who injured it while playing.(4,5) Traumatic injuries are responsible for approximately 12% of osteoarthritis of the hip, knee, or ankle (Fig. 14-1B).(6)

Most chronic arthritis sufferers experience stiffness in their joints as well as dull, sometimes disabling pain. They may also experience discomfort in their joints before or during a change in weather. Bony lumps on the finger joints are common. Standard medical treatment for osteoarthritis includes medication to reduce pain and inflammation; low-impact exercise to keep joints flexible without stressing them; and warm baths, hot or cold compresses, and cold packs. Clients who have severe pain and who cannot exercise due to muscle weakness or imbalance benefit from gentle movement therapies such as

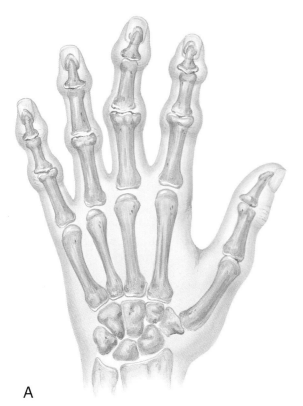
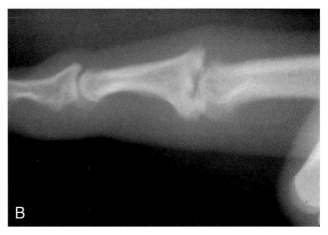

FIGURE 14-1 ■ Osteoarthritis. **A.** Osteoarthritis of the hand. (Asset provided by Anatomical Chart Co.)
B. Osteoarthritis caused by injury. A year after a traumatic injury, the middle phalanx of this index finger has developed significant osteoarthritis. (Reprinted with permission from Strickland JW, Graham TJ. *Master Techniques in Orthopedic Surgery: The Hand.* 2nd ed. Philadelphia: Lippincott Williams & Wilkins, 2005: Fig. 5-5.)

Feldenkrais and Alexander techniques, warm water exercise, and soft tissue massage. **Prolotherapy,** the injection of natural substances at the exact site of a ligament injury to repair damage, may also be an effective treatment for osteoarthritis. Corticosteroid injections and surgery are last-resort treatments.

Many patients with arthritis prefer to avoid medications with their many side effects, and regular hydrotherapy may help them do this. Many massage and hydrotherapy treatments give short-lived pain relief, but when they are performed regularly, the pain relief can last much longer. Massage techniques that address muscle tension and increase local circulation are very helpful for reducing the joint pain, stiffness, and restricted range of motion caused by osteoarthritis.(7) Before a massage session, a hydrotherapy treatment will ready the person's tissues by increasing circulation, making tissue more stretchable, and relaxing the muscles. Applications of heat are particularly effective in relieving muscle spasm, although for some people, cold works better. (You and your clients may need to experiment with both heat and cold to find out which works better for them.) Cold may be effective for clients with sharp and penetrating pain, rather than the dull pain that is more common. Contrast treatments can temporarily relieve pain and increase joint flexibility.

Whole-Body Treatments for Osteoarthritis in Multiple Areas

For a client who has a great deal of pain, try 15- to 20-minute hot tub baths, saunas, or steam baths followed by a full body massage. Do three sessions the first week, two the second week, and one the third week. Then skip a week, do one session the following week, skip 2 weeks, and do one session the next week. Thus you can gradually decrease the frequency to one session. As a follow-up between sessions, clients may take a hot sea salt bath two or three times a week, or if they have access to a hot tub, a 15- to 20-minute soak several times a week. They should perform gentle exercises while in the warm water.

Partial-Body Treatments for Osteoarthritis in Specific Areas

Many hydrotherapy treatments may be applied to specific arthritic joints. Hot applications are soothing, as well as an excellent preparation for hands-on massage. A mustard plaster, for example, can be put over a painful joint at the beginning of a session and removed after 15 to 30 minutes for massage on that area. A paraffin bath may be used at the beginning of a session and the paraffin removed 20 minutes later, immediately before massage of the painful part. A local salt glow and castor oil pack followed by a heat-trapping compress can be performed at the beginning of a session, followed by massage after 45 minutes. Hot packs of various types may be applied over joints for 20 minutes before massage. Between sessions clients can use one of these forms of heat along with gentle exercise.

TREATMENT
MUSTARD PLASTER OVER A JOINT

Cross-Reference
See Chapter 7.

Duration and Frequency
15 to 30 minutes. Perform during a massage session.

Procedure
1. Apply mustard plaster over painful joint. Monitor carefully for burning.
2. Wait 15 to 30 minutes, then remove plaster and begin massage.

CONTRAST BATH TREATMENT OF A PAINFUL JOINT

Cross-Reference
See Chapter 7.

Special Instructions
1. Gentle, painless movements performed while the joint is in the water will further increase local circulation and improve range of motion.
2. If possible, immerse the corresponding joint on the opposite side in the bath as well; that is, if the right hand is the painful one, place both hands in the water.

Duration and Frequency
15 minutes. Perform during a massage session, or the client may do this as a home treatment two or three times daily.

Procedure
1. Fill two buckets or washtubs with enough water to immerse the painful joint, one at 110°F and the other at 50°F.
2. Have the client put the painful joint in the hot water for 3 minutes.
3. Have the client put the painful joint in the cold water for 30 seconds.
4. Repeat steps 2 and 3 three times for a total of four rounds of hot followed by cold.
5. Remove the joint from the water and dry it thoroughly.
6. Begin massage.

LOCAL SALT GLOW FOLLOWED BY APPLICATION OF CASTOR OIL AND A HEAT-TRAPPING COMPRESS

Cross-Reference
See Chapters 5 and 11.

Duration and Frequency
45 minutes. Perform before a massage session, or the client may perform this as a nightly home treatment, leaving the compress on overnight.

Procedure
1. Perform a salt glow on and around the painful joint, then rinse off salt water.
2. Thoroughly dry the area.
3. Apply a generous amount of castor oil over and around the painful joint.
4. Cover the area with plastic wrap.
5. Wring out a cotton cloth in cold tap water and wrap it around the painful joint.
6. Cover the cold compress with the dry cloth, making sure the wet cloth is well covered, and pin it in place.
7. Wait 45 minutes, remove dry cloth and compress underneath, rub the area briskly, then begin massage.

MOIST HEAT TO LARGER JOINTS, SUCH AS THE KNEE

Cross-Reference
See Chapter 5.

Duration and Frequency
20 minutes. Perform before a massage session, or the client may perform this two or three times daily as a home treatment.

Procedure
1. Wring out a towel in warm water and wrap it around the joint.
2. Cover that with a thin sheet of plastic or two layers of plastic wrap.
3. Place a heating pad set on low over the plastic-wrapped joint.
4. Wait 20 minutes, then remove the entire compress and begin massage.

PARAFFIN BATH FOR PAINFUL OR STIFF JOINTS IN THE WRISTS AND HANDS OR IN THE ANKLES AND FEET

Cross-Reference
See Chapter 7.

Duration and Frequency
20 minutes. Perform before or during a massage session, and the client may perform this as a home treatment once daily.

Procedure
1. Briefly immerse the joint in a hot local bath, then dry the area.
2. Dip the joint area in paraffin six times. (Dip the entire hand up to the wrist, or the entire foot up to the ankle.)

3. Encase the area in a plastic bag or cellophane wrap, cover with a dry towel, or for the feet or hands, use socks or gloves. If desired, apply a heating pad on a low setting over the paraffin-wrapped joint.
4. Leave the paraffin on for about 10 minutes, then remove the covering and the paraffin, and begin massage.

COLD APPLICATIONS FOR SHARP LOCALIZED PAIN

Cross-Reference
See Chapter 6.

Duration and Frequency
5 to 8 minutes for ice massage on and around a painful joint, 10 minutes for an ice pack on the painful joint, or 20 minutes using a cold compress around the painful joint. Perform during a massage session.

Procedure
1. Perform ice massage around the joint for 5 to 8 minutes, apply an ice pack for 10 minutes, or apply a cold compress for 20 minutes.
2. Dry the area and begin massage.

RHEUMATOID ARTHRITIS

Rheumatoid arthritis is an autoimmune disease that primarily affects connective tissue. The synovial membranes that normally protect and lubricate the joints become inflamed, leading to arthritis that involves many joints, especially those of the hands and feet. Sufferers experience pain, swelling, and stiffness in these joints, as well as a loss of range of motion and eventually deformity of the joints (Fig. 14-2). Pronounced morning stiffness, fatigue, and malaise are also common. Standard medical treatment for rheumatoid arthritis usually consists of medications to relieve pain and swelling, physical therapy, medications that affect the immune system, and even corticosteroid injections. A last option is surgery to rebuild damaged tendons, remove portions of affected synovial membranes, or replace the entire joint. Severe sensitivities to allergens such as corn and wheat may also affect the course of this disease.

Many patients with rheumatoid arthritis prefer to avoid medications with their many side effects, and regular hydrotherapy may help them do this. In one study, researchers found that sufferers who took saunas on a regular basis had less pain and easier movement than controls.(8) One-time hydrotherapy treatments offer temporary relief of pain, and for this reason alone massage therapists may wish to combine them with massage. For example, a massage therapist could have clients with rheumatoid arthritis take a sauna before their massage session. Since massage techniques targeted to relieve pain and improve joint mobility are more effective when an area is relaxed and has extra blood circulating through it, hydrotherapy treatments can also increase the effectiveness of massage sessions. As a follow-up between sessions, clients can take regular whole-body heating treatments or use local treatments over painful joints as desired. Clients with rheumatoid arthritis may also benefit from gentle movement therapies such as the Feldenkrais and Alexander techniques and warm water exercise.

Whole-Body Treatments for Rheumatoid Arthritis in Multiple Areas

For a client who has pain in more than one area of the body, a whole-body heating treatment can help relieve pain and prepare his or her tissues for massage, and as a home treatment it can relieve morning stiffness. Simply help the client into a warm or hot tub bath, shower, sauna, or steam bath, and after 20 minutes help him or her out and onto the massage table and begin massage. As a follow-up between sessions, clients may take a daily hot bath or shower and perform gentle exercises while in the water. For full instructions for and contraindications to full-body heating treatments, see the sections on each one in Chapters 7 to 9.

Partial-Body Treatments for Rheumatoid Arthritis in Specific Areas

Rather than treating the whole body, the following treatments target specific joints. They can be performed in your office before or during massage.

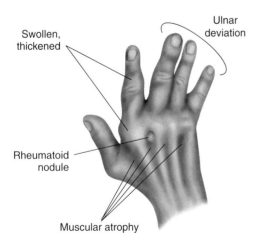

Swollen, thickened

Ulnar deviation

Rheumatoid nodule

Muscular atrophy

FIGURE 14-2 ■ Rheumatoid arthritis. (Reprinted with permission from Bickley LS, Szilagyi P. *Bates Guide to Physical Examination and History Taking.* 8th ed. Philadelphia: Lippincott Williams & Wilkins, 2003: Fig. 15-6.3.)

TREATMENT

PARAFFIN BATH FOR PAINFUL OR STIFF JOINTS

Cross-Reference
See Chapter 7.

Duration and Frequency

20 minutes. Perform before or during a massage session, and the client may perform this as a home treatment once daily.

Procedure

1. Immerse the joint in a hot local bath, then dry the area.
2. Dip the joint area in paraffin six times.
3. Encase the area in a plastic bag or cellophane wrap, cover with dry towel, or for the feet or hands, use socks or gloves. If desired, apply a heating pad on low setting over the paraffin-wrapped joint.
4. Leave the paraffin on for about 10 minutes, then remove the covering, bag or cellophane, and paraffin, and begin massage.

MOIST HEAT COMPRESS ON A SPECIFIC JOINT

Cross-Reference

See Chapter 5.

Duration and Frequency

20 minutes. Perform before a massage session, or the client may perform this two or three times daily as a home treatment.

Special Instructions

More than one joint may be wrapped at the same time. Fomentations may also be used.

Procedure

1. Wring out a large or small towel, depending upon the size of the joint, in warm water and wrap it around the joint.
2. Cover the towel with a thin sheet of plastic or two layers of plastic wrap.
3. Place a heating pad set on low over the plastic-wrapped joint.
4. Wait 20 minutes, then remove the entire compress and begin massage.

CONTRAST BATH TREATMENT OF A PAINFUL JOINT

Cross-Reference

See Chapter 7.

Special Instructions

1. Gentle, painless movements performed while the joint is in the water will further increase local circulation and improve range of motion.
2. If possible, immerse the corresponding joint on the opposite side in the bath as well; that is, if the right hand is the painful one, place both hands in the water.

Duration and Frequency

15 minutes. Perform during a massage session, or the client may perform this as a home treatment two or three times daily.

Procedure

1. Fill two buckets or washtubs with enough water to immerse the painful joint, one at 99° to 110°F and the other at 50° to 65°F.
2. Have the client put the painful joint in the hot water for 3 minutes.
3. Have the client put the painful joint in the cold water for 30 seconds.
4. Repeat steps 2 and 3 three times for a total of four rounds of hot followed by cold.
5. Remove the joint from the water and dry it thoroughly.

ICE MASSAGE TO RELIEVE PAIN IN A SPECIFIC JOINT

Cross-Reference

See Chapter 6.

Duration and Frequency

20 minutes. Perform during a massage session.

Procedure

1. Perform ice massage around the joint for 5 minutes.
2. Use hands-on massage techniques around the painful area or elsewhere in the body for 5 minutes.
3. Repeat steps 1 and 2 three more times, for a total of 20 minutes of ice massage.
4. Dry the area and begin massage.

CHRONIC TENSION IN SPECIFIC BODY AREAS

Helping clients deal with specific areas in their body that are chronically tense is a critical aspect of most massage therapists' work. Massage techniques targeted to specific areas can help clients release muscles that have been tense for years. Using hydrotherapy treatments before actually massaging an area can help release surface tension, give the client an enjoyable sensation in the tight area, make tissues more pliable, and make deeper work more tolerable. Following are three examples of areas of chronic tension that can be treated with moist heat before hands-on techniques, but there are many other areas of the body where these treatments can be applied.

CHRONIC TENSION IN THE FACIAL MUSCLES

Chronic tension in the facial muscles can be caused by habits such as:

1. Tensing the muscles around the eyes and forehead because of visual difficulties, injury, eyestrain, or emotional stress

CASE HISTORY 14-1

Releasing Muscle Tension With a Simple Treatment

Background

Steve was an 84-year-old massage client who had faced many major challenges in recent years. He underwent quadruple bypass surgery, received serious injuries in a motor vehicle accident, was diagnosed with macular degeneration, and then his wife of many years died. He exercised three times a week at the cardiac rehabilitation center at a local hospital, took a wide variety of supplements, and came in for a whole-body Swedish massage session once every 2 weeks. For Steve, massage sessions were used to help ease his many musculoskeletal aches and pains, stimulate his circulation, and help meet his need for touch. Because of his macular degeneration, Steve experienced a great deal of eyestrain. He squinted constantly because he was light sensitive, and continually tensed the muscles of his eyes and forehead as he strained to see, and so his upper face and scalp were extremely tight.

Treatment

The massage therapist closed the curtains in the therapy room to eliminate the outside light, which bothered Steve's eyes. For the first time, she tried adding moist heat to Steve's massage session (with his physician's permission). Using hot water from a slow cooker on a counter, she soaked a washcloth, wrung it out, and gently laid it over his eyes. She checked with him to be sure the cloth was not too hot, since elderly people have thin skin and can be burned easily. She then proceeded to massage Steve's neck and shoulders, applying a new hot cloth every 2 minutes. Normally Steve enjoyed chatting with the therapist during the entire massage time, but this time something different occurred. He stopped talking and settled down completely after only a minute or so, and after the fifth hot cloth was applied, he let out a deep sigh and said, "My eyes haven't felt this relaxed in years."

After another minute, the therapist removed the now-lukewarm cloth, wrung out a washcloth in cold water and laid that over his eyes for 30 seconds, then gently dried the area. As the therapist began to massage his forehead and around his eyes, she could see that his skin was pink and could feel that the tissues under her fingers were warmer and more elastic than usual. The top layer of tension that normally required some minutes of massage to release was already gone.

Discussion Questions

1. Name three reasons that the application of a cloth over the eyes was helpful.
2. Why did the therapist finish the session with a cold washcloth?

2. Tensing the muscles around the nose because of sinus problems, injury, or emotional stress
3. Tensing the muscles of the jaw because of poor alignment of teeth, dental pain, injury, or emotional stress
4. Tensing the muscles of the throat because of discomfort from overusing the voice, swallowing difficulties, injury, frequent sore throats, or emotional stress

Massage is an effective way to release tension in the facial muscles, and moist heat can also warm and relax them. An ideal way to integrate moist heat into a treatment is to apply the moist heat, then massage another part of the client's body for 10 minutes, then remove the moist heat and begin massage. A container of hot water, such as a slow cooker, may be used to obtain hot water for compresses. Other small heat applications include warm gel packs over a moist cloth and miniature hydrocollator packs. A hot towel cabinet that contains warm moist washcloths or small towels is also very convenient for this treatment. For an example of using moist heat and massage for tension in the facial muscles, see Case History 14-1.

TREATMENT

MOIST HEAT ON THE FACIAL MUSCLES

Cross-Reference
See Chapter 5.

Duration and Frequency
10 minutes

Caution
Facial skin is thinner than skin on many other parts of the body and should be monitored carefully for burning.

Procedure
1. Apply moist heat (hot water compress, warm gel pack over moist washcloth, miniature hydrocollator pack) over the area for 2 minutes. Massage elsewhere on the client's body at this time.

2. Apply a new warm cloth and leave it on for 2 minutes.
3. Repeat steps 1 and 2, for a total of 8 minutes of heat over the area.
4. Apply cold for 30 seconds, applying a cloth wrung out in ice water, or perform ice massage.
5. Begin massage of the facial muscles.

CHRONIC TENSION IN THE ABDOMINAL MUSCLES

Chronic tension in the abdominal muscles is very common. A pattern of carrying tension in these muscles can begin with abdominal injuries, with pain from internal organ problems, or as a sequela of abdominal surgery. Holding emotional stress in the abdominal muscles is not only common but this habit can begin early in life. One-third to one-half of those who have stress-related abdominal pain as children continue to experience it when they are adults.(9) Because tension in this area is often emotionally-based, many clients who know that they are tense in these muscles still feel tentative and vulnerable about local massage. As an introduction to massage of the abdominal muscles, a few minutes of relaxing moist heat over the abdomen can remove superficial tension, make muscles more pliable, and provide a very soothing sensation. Here we use a moist heating pad because it is lightweight, which generally feels more comfortable on the abdomen, and because it drapes well over body curves.

TREATMENT

MOIST HEATING PAD FOLLOWED BY MASSAGE

Cross-Reference
See Chapter 5.

Duration and Frequency
10 to 15 minutes. Perform during a massage session.

Special Instructions
A flat plastic hot water bottle or fomentation may be substituted for the moist heating pad.

Procedure
1. With the client lying supine, apply a moist heating pad on a medium setting while massaging another part of the body. Monitor carefully for burning.
2. After 10 minutes, remove the heat and perform massage of the abdomen.

CHRONIC TENSION IN THE RESPIRATORY MUSCLES

Chronic respiratory problems, such as emphysema or lung cancer, can cause a great deal of tension in the muscles of respiration. Years of difficult breathing may cause extreme tension in not only the intercostal muscles but many muscles of the back and rib cage, along with reduced mobility in the rib cage, diaphragm, and spine. Breathing may become chronically shallow, the chest cavity may narrow, the shoulders may become rounded, and the posture of the neck and upper back can be distorted. Struggling for breath during asthma attacks can be frightening and emotionally traumatic and can also lead to chronic tension in the respiratory muscles. Emotional stress can also cause chronic tension.

Massage is an effective way to release tension in the respiratory muscles, and moist heat can improve local circulation, deepen the respiration, and warm and loosen both the anterior and posterior fascia and muscles. An ideal way to integrate moist heat during a session is to apply it to the chest, then massage another part of the client's supine body for 10 minutes, and then massage the chest. Then repeat the procedure on the posterior side of the rib cage with the client prone. Contrast treatments of the chest can be performed to increase local circulation even further and to give the client a more stimulating treatment.

TREATMENT

FOMENTATION OR HYDROCOLLATOR PACK TO THE CHEST AND UPPER BACK, FOLLOWED BY MASSAGE

Cross-Reference
See Chapter 5.

Duration and Frequency
20 minutes. Perform during a massage session.

Special Instructions
Hot compresses may be substituted for fomentations, but an external heating device will be required to keep them hot.

Procedure
1. With the client lying supine, apply a hot fomentation or hydrocollator pack to the chest while massaging another part of the body. Monitor carefully for burning.
2. After 10 minutes, remove the heat and perform massage of the chest.
3. Have the client lie prone and apply moist heat to the upper back.
4. After 10 minutes, remove the heat and perform massage of the entire back, emphasizing the upper back and the intercostal muscles.

CONTRAST TREATMENT OF THE CHEST AND UPPER BACK

Cross-Reference
See Chapters 5 and 11.

Duration and Frequency
10 minutes. Perform before or during a massage session.

Caution

Do not allow anyone receiving this treatment to become chilled during or after the treatment.

Procedure

1. Place a flat plastic hot water bottle on the massage table, cover it with a cloth, and have the client lie supine so that the heat is directly on the upper and middle back.
2. Place a fomentation or hydrocollator pack on the chest.
3. After 3 minutes, remove the hydrocollator pack and give a 30-minute cold mitten friction.
4. Repeat steps 1 and 2 twice for a total of three rounds of hot followed by cold.
5. Have the client sit up, and give a 30-second cold mitten friction to the middle and upper back.
6. Remove the flat plastic hot water bottle from the massage table, and have the client lie prone.
7. Begin massage of the chest and upper back.

CONSTIPATION, CHRONIC

Constipation, a condition in which bowel movements are reduced or difficult, can occur from a variety of medical conditions or by less complicated factors. Chronic dehydration, a lack of dietary fiber, and poor muscle tone in the abdominal area from a lack of exercise may contribute to chronic constipation as well. Bed-ridden, sedentary, and wheelchair-riding clients are prone to constipation.

Massage therapists do not treat constipation per se, but it is often the case that abdominal massage stimulates peristalsis and elimination. If a client has constipation and no underlying pathologies, massage and contrast treatments that relax the abdomen and stimulate circulation there may help relieve it.

TREATMENT

CONTRAST TREATMENT TO THE ABDOMEN

Cross-Reference

See Chapters 5 and 11.

Duration and Frequency

12 minutes. Perform before or during a massage session.

Procedure

1. Apply a hot fomentation or a hot compress covered with plastic and a heating pad to the client's abdomen.
2. After 3 minutes, remove the fomentation or compress and give a cold mitten friction for 30 seconds to the abdomen, using ice water if the client can tolerate it.
3. Repeat steps 1 and 2 for a total of three rounds of hot followed by cold.
4. Begin massage.

DIABETES

Diabetes is a common and often devastating metabolic disorder characterized by glucose intolerance, excessive discharge of urine containing glucose, and disturbances in the metabolism of fat, protein, and carbohydrates. Many factors can contribute to diabetes, including a diet that is high in saturated fats, obesity, lack of exercise, and aging. Because diabetes is becoming far more frequent in the United States, it is likely that every massage therapist will be treating some individuals with this disease. Massage is appropriate for clients with diabetes, provided that they do not have very advanced diabetes, arteriosclerosis, or kidney failure. Hydrotherapy, too, can be useful but should be applied with caution.

Diabetes often causes arterial disease, with a reduction in blood flow to the extremities. We know that the application of local heat, such as a hot footbath, will increase the metabolism of the warmed tissues; however, because in diabetes the skin blood vessels do not dilate well, less oxygen is available to nourish the tissues than would be the case in a person without diabetes. As a result, the increased metabolic needs of the warmed tissues can very quickly exhaust the nutrients and oxygen available from the blood, and the cells can actually die of lack of oxygen. This is why hot footbaths are contraindicated for diabetics. Nerve degeneration in the feet, called **peripheral neuropathy,** is another common complication of diabetes. This degeneration makes the affected body region (usually the feet) much less sensitive to all stimuli—in some cases almost numb. In this scenario, a client who receives a hot footbath may not be able to sense that the feet are getting too hot, and burning the feet is a real danger. Therefore, do not apply heat to the feet with hot water bottles, moist heat such as fomentations or hydrocollator packs, or even paraffin dips. Steam cabinets in which the steam is coming up from the floor of the cabinet should also be avoided.

Many people with diabetes do not handle heat well, and in your medical history, be sure to ask the client how he or she responds to heat, including hot showers or baths. If the client dislikes being warm, this is even more of a reason to avoid heating applications. Mild treatments using warm water are appropriate, such as warm whole-body baths, warm footbaths (no hotter than 102°F), salt glows, and body wraps. Also appropriate are treatments using cold, such as heat-trapping compresses and cold mitten frictions. Contrast foot-baths using water no hotter than 102°F help increase circulation without excess heat, although the increase in blood flow will be 50% less than that of clients without diabetes. All of these treatments may be performed before or during massage sessions.

Endocrinologist and diabetes specialist Phil Hooper, MD, who conducted a small study of the safety of hot tubs for diabetics,(10) believes that regular hot tubs at no more than 102°F can be beneficial for patients with diabetes, in part because they can stimulate blood flow to the extremities (Hooper PL, personal communication with author, August 10, 2006). However, to ensure that no one with diabetes is burned by hot water, you or the client should always use a water thermometer to check temperature before the client enters a bathtub or hot tub.

DRY SKIN

Many hydrotherapy treatments effectively treat dry skin; below are just a few traditional ones that are appropriate to use before a massage. In itself, massage is an excellent treatment for very dry skin because not only are massage emollients absorbed by the skin, preventing it from drying out, massage stimulates the sebaceous glands as well.

WHOLE-BODY TREATMENTS FOR DRY SKIN

The treatments that follow benefit the skin over the entire body.

TREATMENT
WHOLE-BODY OIL APPLICATION AFTER A WARM OR HOT SHOWER

Cross-Reference
See Chapter 9.

Duration and Frequency
10 to 15 minutes. Perform before or after a massage and as a daily home treatment.

Procedure
1. Have the client take a warm or hot shower.
2. After the shower, when the skin will have absorbed some moisture and is still wet, the client should put 5 drops of vegetable oil on the palms and rub them over the entire skin surface, so the oil is well mixed with the water on the skin.
3. Now have the client dry the skin, leaving a very fine film of vegetable oil on it.

WHOLE-BODY HONEY WRAP

Cross-Reference
See Chapter 10.

Duration and Frequency
20 minutes. Perform before a massage session.

Special Instructions
This treatment is a great deal easier to perform using a wet room table.

Caution
Contraindicated for diabetics.

Procedure
1. Have the client take a short shower, sauna, or steam bath and blot the skin so it is mostly dry.
2. Have the client lie down on a wet table (or a table covered with towels).
3. Pour $\frac{1}{4}$ cup of warmed honey onto your hands and apply it onto the client's still-moist skin, or mix the honey with $\frac{1}{4}$ cup of water and paint it onto the client's body. If honey is applied to the feet, they should be carefully encased in plastic bags so that the client does not track honey anywhere.
4. Wrap the patient in a dry sheet and have him or her go into a steam bath or sauna for 15 minutes. After that time, the honey should be completely absorbed into the skin. If it is not, have the client take a shower.
5. Begin massage.

MOISTURIZING WRAP WITH SHEA BUTTER OR A THICK OIL, SUCH AS WHEAT GERM OIL

Cross-Reference
See Chapter 10.

Duration and Frequency
20 minutes. Perform before a massage session.

Procedure
1. Apply a liberal amount of warmed shea butter or thick oil to the skin and gently massage in.
2. Wrap the client as for a full body wrap, using a dry sheet.
3. Wait 20 minutes, during which time the face may be massaged.
4. Unwrap the client and proceed with massage on the rest of the body. The shea butter or thick oil may be sufficient for massage; if not, more may be added.

PARTIAL-BODY TREATMENTS FOR DRY SKIN

Dry, cracked skin on the feet and hands can benefit greatly from applications of paraffin or honey before massage. However, do not massage skin that is so dry and cracked that it is open, due to the risk of infection.

Paraffin or honey wraps may be given to the hands or feet even if the client does not receive any massage in those areas during a massage session.

TREATMENT
PARAFFIN APPLICATIONS ON THE HANDS AND FEET

Cross-Reference
See Chapter 7.

Duration and Frequency
10 minutes. Perform before a massage session or as a daily home treatment.

Procedure
1. Briefly soak the client's hands or feet in warm water to clean them.
2. Apply a thick layer of emollient cream on the client's hands or feet.
3. Dip the hands or feet in paraffin, wrap them in a plastic bag and then wrap them in a cloth covering such as terry cloth gloves for the hands or socks for the feet.
4. After 10 minutes, remove the coverings and paraffin and begin massage.

LOCAL HONEY WRAP

Cross-Reference
See section on whole-body honey wrap treatment in this chapter.

Duration and Frequency
10 minutes. Perform before a massage session or as a daily home treatment.

Procedure
1. Briefly soak the client's hands or feet in warm water to clean them.
2. Pour about 2 tbsp of warmed honey onto your hands and apply it to the client's still moist hands or feet, then clean your hands.
3. Wrap the client's hands or feet in plastic bags and add a cloth covering such as gloves for the hands or socks for the feet.
4. After 10 minutes, remove the coverings and clean off the honey with warm, wet towels or a brief warm soak.
5. Dry the hands or feet and begin massage.

DYSMENORRHEA

Women who have **dysmenorrhea**, significant pain before or during their menstrual periods, may find the pain severe enough to interfere with their activities. Pain medication is often used for dysmenorrhea. For centuries, women have found that after their period begins, local heat on the abdomen is relieving, and they have used many types of heat, including animal bladders filled with hot oil, burning moxa, warm bricks wrapped in flannel, hot sitz baths, hot half-baths, hot compresses, heating pads, and hot water bottles. Although clients generally do not seek out massage therapists for relief of menstrual cramps, they sometimes arrive for a massage session while they are experiencing them. To relieve cramps, the massage therapist may apply local heat, such as a hot-water bottle, during the session. Massage of the abdomen is contraindicated at this time, but techniques that employ pressure points in other areas, such as shiatsu on the lower back, are appropriate. Clients who have no pelvic pathologies are good candidates for tonic treatments between their menstrual periods and local applications when pain is present.

TONIC TREATMENTS BETWEEN MENSTRUAL CYCLES

Discontinue these treatments 12 hours before the period is expected to start.

TREATMENT
DAILY CONTRAST PELVIC SHOWER

Cross-Reference
See Chapter 9.

Duration and Frequency
10 minutes

Special Instructions
Contrast sitz baths may also be used.

Procedure
1. Using a hand shower attachment, spray the pelvic area with water as hot as can be tolerated for 2 minutes.
2. Spray the pelvic area with water as cold as can be tolerated for 1 minute.
3. Repeat steps 1 and 2 twice for a total of three rounds.

WEEKLY CONTRAST TREATMENT

Cross-Reference
See Chapters 5 and 11.

Caution
Monitor the client's posterior body carefully for burning.

Duration and Frequency
45 minutes. Perform during a massage session once a week.

Procedure
1. Place two hot fomentations or flat plastic water bottles filled with hot water on the massage table and have the client lie supine on them, so that they

are in contact with her body from her scapula to the top of her thighs.

2. Cover her abdominal and pubic areas with another hot fomentation or moist cloth and heating pad.
3. Leave the heat on for 15 minutes, during which time massage may be performed upon another part of the body.
4. Remove the heat on the abdomen.
5. Have the client roll onto one side.
6. Give a 30-second cold mitten friction, with water as cold as can be tolerated, where the heat was applied, that is, on the abdomen and the posterior of the body from the top of the thighs to mid scapula.
7. Have the client roll onto her back and place heat back on her abdominal and pubic area.
8. Leave the heat on for 15 minutes.
9. Repeat steps 5 and 6, the cold mitten friction in side-lying position.
10. Repeat steps 7 to 9 for a total of three rounds of hot followed by cold.
11. Begin massage of the abdominal area.

TREATMENTS FOR PAIN RELIEF DURING MENSTRUAL PERIOD

TREATMENT
MOIST HEAT APPLICATIONS

Cross-Reference
See Chapter 5.

Duration and Frequency
20 minutes. Use during a massage session.

Procedure
Have the client lie prone with a flat plastic hot water bottle or rubber hot water bottle contacting the low back and another lightweight warm application (flat plastic hot water bottle, moist heating pad set on medium, moist cloth covered by a heating pad, or hot fomentation) over the lower abdomen. Leave on for no more than 20 minutes.

ECZEMA

Eczema is a generic term for a number of noncontagious inflammatory skin conditions which appear in the form of a skin rash. Eczema is very common and is believed to be linked to a number of factors, mostly genetic, that cause an overactive immune response to irritating substances. Emotional stress can contribute to outbreaks of eczema, even in infancy.(11) Eczema is often helped by avoiding irritating substances, taking supplements with essential fatty acids, reducing stress, and taking baths with soothing

substances. Massage is contraindicated over the area of eczema if the skin is puffy, weepy, open, or contains blisters, but massage is appropriate in other areas of the body to help the client relax.

TREATMENT
OATMEAL BATH

Cross-Reference
See Chapter 7.

Duration and Frequency
20 minutes. Perform before or after a massage session, or may be used twice daily as a home treatment during a flare-up.

Procedure
1. Add oatmeal to bath water as the tub begins filling.
2. Have the client remain in the tub for 20 minutes.

SODIUM BICARBONATE, OR BAKING SODA, BATH

Cross-Reference
See Chapter 7.

Duration and Frequency
20 minutes. Perform before or after a massage session, or may be used twice daily as a home treatment during a flare-up.

Procedure
Add baking soda to bath water while the tub is filling. Have the client remain in the tub for 20 minutes.

EYESTRAIN

Eyestrain is a feeling of discomfort and pain in and around the eyes. It is commonly caused by activities that require extended periods of near-vision tasks, such as reading, sewing, or using a computer. Other factors that encourage eyestrain include emotional stress, incorrect prescriptions for corrective lenses, squinting due to light sensitivity or poor vision, or looking into the sun for long periods. People with chronic eyestrain may become so accustomed to it that they are no longer aware how much tension and discomfort they are holding. Often, however, they find hydrotherapy applications and massage tremendously relaxing.

Hydrotherapy and massage can increase circulation and ease muscle tension in and around the eyes. Heat applications over the eyes are soothing and increase circulation, while cold applications can relieve pain and promote healing in the eyes. Contrast applications cause a dramatic increase in the blood flow to the eyes. (See Chapter 12 for eye tonic treatments.) The goals of massage are to relieve muscle tension and to improve circulation for the eyes and the area around them. Because eyestrain may cause tension not only in the eyes but in other parts of the body as well, a massage for eyestrain includes techniques for the face, especially around the eyes, and techniques for the neck and upper trapezius.

TREATMENT

HOT APPLICATIONS COMBINED WITH ICE MASSAGE FOR EYESTRAIN

Cross-Reference
See Chapters 5 and 6.

Duration and Frequency
10 minutes. Perform during a massage session or as a home treatment once or twice daily.

Caution
This treatment is not to be used with anyone with eye pathologies, such as macular degeneration, without a physician's permission.

Procedure
1. Soak and wring out a cloth in water as hot as the client can tolerate (it will cool rather quickly) and apply it over the client's closed eyes. Because the skin over the eyes is very thin, be careful not to use too much heat: be sure to check with the client.
2. While the cloth is over the eyes, perform ice massage around the heated area for about 2 minutes. Use a dry washcloth to catch any drips.
3. Repeat steps 1 and 2 twice for a total of three rounds.
4. Dry the client's face.
5. Begin massage.

CONTRAST COMPRESSES FOR EYESTRAIN

Cross-Reference
See Chapters 5 and 6.

Duration and Frequency
10 minutes. Perform during a massage session or as a home treatment once or twice daily.

Special Instructions
Hot and cold eye gel packs may be used instead of hot and cold cloths.

Procedure
1. Soak and wring out a cloth in water as hot as the client can tolerate (it will cool rather quickly) and apply it over the client's closed eyes. Because the skin over the eyes is very thin, be careful not to use too much heat: be sure to check with the client.
2. After 2 minutes, soak and wring out a cloth in water as cold as the client can tolerate and apply it over the client's closed eyes.
3. Leave the cold compress on for 1 minute.

4. Repeat steps 1, 2, and 3 twice more, for a total of three rounds of hot followed by cold.
5. Dry the client's face.
6. Begin massage.

FIBROMYALGIA

Fibromyalgia is a musculoskeletal pain and fatigue disorder that primarily affects women. The word *fibromyalgia* itself means *pain in the muscles, tendons, and ligaments*. Although its exact cause is unknown, triggers include physical trauma, viral infections such as the flu, and depression. Fibromyalgia is characterized by chronic pain in the muscles and soft tissue surrounding joints, tenderness to pressure at specific sites in the body, stiffness after rest, low pain tolerance, sensitivity to cold, sleep that is not restful, constipation, and chronic fatigue. Symptoms may wax and wane, and some persons with fibromyalgia have more extreme symptoms than others. Standard medical treatment consists of regular physical therapy, medication to improve sleep and reduce pain, and emotional support.

Hydrotherapy can help fibromyalgia patients feel better and move more comfortably during the day and can make a massage session more effective. Hot baths and showers are helpful for morning stiffness and pain, and pool therapy in a 91° to 94°F pool can decrease pain and fatigue and improve muscle function. During a massage session, moist heat applications, such as hydrocollator packs or fomentations, can help relieve pain, and ice massage may also be used to deactivate trigger points. Many massage techniques are effective for someone with fibromyalgia, although overtreating is always a hazard. Too much or too deep massage can cause a flare-up of pain, and massage must be carefully adjusted to how much a client with fibromyalgia can tolerate.

TREATMENT

ICE MASSAGE TO DEACTIVATE TRIGGER POINTS, FOLLOWED BY LOCAL HEAT

Cross-Reference
See Chapter 6.

Duration and Frequency
About 1 minute. Apply during a massage session.

Procedure
1. Gently stretch the muscle to the greatest extent possible without overstretching.
2. Maintaining the muscle stretch, stroke the entire length of the muscle three times with the ice, which is wrapped in plastic.
3. Gently stretch the muscle to the greatest extent possible without overstretching.

4. If the muscle is still not capable of fully lengthening without pain, try applying direct pressure to the trigger point for 10 to 30 seconds, then gently stretch the muscle again. Or have the client contract the antagonist muscle for 30 seconds and relax completely as you gently stretch the muscle again.
5. Repeat steps 4 to 6 until the muscle is pain free when completely stretched.
6. Gently return muscle to a comfortable position and massage the area further if desired.
7. Apply a heating pad or moist hot pack to the muscle for 5 minutes or more.

GOUT

Gout is a type of arthritis typically caused by an overproduction of uric acid or an inability to excrete it. Excess uric acid crystals are deposited in the joints of the knees, ankles, and big toes, causing not only swelling but excruciating pain. Nine in ten of those with gout are men. Standard medical treatment focuses on medications for inflammation and pain medications to decrease the production of uric acid or increase its excretion, occasional aspiration of fluid from affected joints, and a diet high in fluid intake and low in purines.

Hydrotherapy may be helpful in temporarily easing pain and inflammation in clients with gout. Either hot or cold applications may relieve pain, whereas contrast applications can relieve swelling. (Baths may be the best treatment, as some clients cannot tolerate even the slight weight of a cloth.) Herbs have been used in footbaths for generations. Contrast baths may also force blood flow into hard-to-reach joints and break up crystalline deposits of uric acid. Massage is contraindicated for gouty areas but may be helpful for general relaxation. Acute attacks of gout are very painful, and a client who has had one may welcome relaxing touch.

TREATMENT

COLD APPLICATIONS (COLD COMPRESS OR ICE PACK)

Cross-Reference
See Chapter 6.

Duration and Frequency
20 minutes. Apply during a massage session.

Procedure
Apply a cold wet compress or an ice pack covered with a thin cloth, and leave on for 20 minutes.

HOT FOOTBATH

Cross-Reference
See Chapter 7.

Duration and Frequency
20 minutes. Perform during a massage session.

Procedure
1. Rest the client's feet in the hot footbath with the client either seated or supine on the massage table.
2. Massage of other parts of the body that can be done with the client in this position may proceed.
3. After 20 minutes, remove the client's feet, dry them gently, and continue massage on other parts of the body.

CONTRAST FOOTBATH

Cross-Reference
See Chapter 7.

Duration and Frequency
10 minutes

Procedure
1. Fill two deep buckets or washtubs with water, one at 110° and the other at 50°F.
2. Put both feet in the hot water for 3 minutes.
3. Put both feet in the cold water for 30 seconds.
4. Repeat steps 2 and 3 at least twice more for at total of three rounds, or more if desired.

HEADACHES

MIGRAINE HEADACHE

Migraine headaches are severely painful, usually limited to one side of the head, and often accompanied by vertigo, nausea, hypersensitivity to light, a perception of flashing lights, or other visual disorders. They begin with an extreme constriction of the blood vessels of the brain on the affected side of the head. During this phase, the client may have feelings of dread, blurred vision, or other sensations that warn that a migraine is imminent. After 2 to 4 hours the vasoconstriction phase ends and the next phase, extreme dilation of the blood vessels of the brain, begins. This vasodilation causes the actual pain of the migraine. Because the brain is encased in the bones of the skull, the dilated blood vessels have no space to expand, and consequently there is increased pressure on the brain itself. This pressure causes not only the pain but also the neurological symptoms, both of which typically last for several hours.

Migraines have many known triggers, including emotional stress; dehydration; eating an allergenic food; altitude changes; fatigue; fluctuations in hormone levels related to menstruation; low blood sugar; trigger points in the temporalis, occipitalis, sternocleidomastoid, and posterior cervical muscles; and possibly malalignment of the cranial bones. Before diagnosing migraine, physicians rule out brain tumors, hemangiomas, carotid aneurysms,

Ménière's disease, and seizure disorders. Once diagnosed, the standard medical treatment for migraine consists of medication and avoidance of aggravating foods. Some relaxation methods and biofeedback can also be effective.

Although it is unlikely that a client will seek out a massage therapist for treatment of a migraine headache, sometimes it happens that the client thinks he or she may have a tension headache at first, then realizes that it is a migraine headache, or that the headache began after the massage session was scheduled. In this case, the classic hydrotherapy treatment for a migraine headache, a hot footbath, can be performed. Immersing the feet in hot water dilates the blood vessels of the feet and reduces blood flow into congested areas. The hands may be immersed in hot water at the same time. An ice pack on the back of the neck will stimulate constriction of blood vessels to the brain. Be careful not to apply heat alone to the client's head. A client of the author's, who has had migraine headaches for 30 years, inadvertently showed the vasodilating effect of heat to the head: she applied heat to her head when she had her first migraine headache and ended up with the most painful and longest-lasting migraine of her life.

Although some therapists have reported success in relieving migraine headaches with deep tissue massage or craniosacral therapy, in general, once a migraine headache has begun, massage treatment cannot always relieve it, and the longer the migraine has gone on, the less likely it is that massage will help. The author has had the greatest success with abolishing full-blown migraines by combining massage with heat to the feet and cold to the head.

TREATMENT

All hydrotherapy treatments should be begun as soon as possible after the headache or any warning signs of a headache begin.

APPLICATION OF COLD RUNNING WATER TO THE BACK OF THE NECK AND SCALP

Cross-Reference
See Chapter 6 for effects of cold.

Duration and Frequency
3 minutes. Perform at the beginning of a massage session or as a home treatment at the first sign of a headache.

Procedure
1. Run water in the sink as cold as the client can tolerate it.
2. Have the client place the head under the faucet for 3 minutes, being careful to keep the nostrils out of the water so as to breathe comfortably.

3. Let the cold water run over the back of the client's head with as much force as is tolerable. Include the occipital area.
4. Dry the client's hair.
5. Begin massage.

HOT FOOTBATH COMBINED WITH ICE PACK ON THE BACK OF THE NECK

Cross-Reference
See Chapters 6 and 7.

Duration and Frequency
20 minutes. Perform before or during a massage session.

Special Instructions
1. The water in the footbath must be kept at 110°F for the entire treatment. This means that as the water cools, more hot water must be added. The fresh hot water should be added carefully, so that it is not poured directly on the client's feet.
2. The footbath may be given with the client supine upon the massage table.
3. Massage can be given on other areas of the body during the footbath, and then massage can be given directly to the head and upper body during the rest period afterward.

Procedure
1. Give the client a footbath at 110°F, combined with a cold compress to the forehead and an ice pack to the back of the neck. If desired, add 1 tbsp of mustard powder per 1 to 2 gal of water in the footbath.
2. Change the cold compress every 3 minutes. Another cold compress may also be placed on the top of the client's head.
3. After 20 minutes, remove the ice pack and the cold compress.
4. Pour cold water over the client's feet, dry them off, and then have the client lie down and rest for 20 minutes.

HOT FOOTBATH COMBINED WITH CONTRAST TREATMENT FOR THE HEAD AND CERVICAL SPINE

Cross-Reference
See Chapters 6 and 7.

Duration and Frequency
20 minutes. Perform before or during a massage session.

Procedure
1. Give the client a 20-minute footbath at 110°F. (See step 1 of the previous hot footbath treatment for further details.)

2. After the client's feet are in the footbath, apply a hot water bottle, hot compress, or hot miniature fomentation to the base of the neck and the cervical spine. At the same time apply ice water compresses or a cloth and then cold miniature gel packs to the upper face (forehead, eyes, temples, and ears).
3. Wait 3 minutes, then switch the hot and cold applications on the head, so that now you apply ice-water compresses where the heat was on the base of the neck and cervical spine and hot water compresses to the face, temples, ears and forehead.
4. After 3 minutes, repeat steps 2 and 3 twice more for a total of three rounds.
5. Remove all hot and cold applications from the head.
6. Remove the client's feet from the hot foot soak and dry them well.
7. Begin massage.

HOT HALF BATH

Cross-Reference
See Chapter 7.

Duration and Frequency
15 minutes. Perform before or during a massage session.

Special Instructions
This should be taken as soon as possible after the client senses the beginning of a migraine.

Procedure
1. Fill tub to waist level with 104°F water.
2. Have the client enter the tub, wearing a dry shirt or sheet to keep the upper body warm if desired.
3. After 15 minutes, have the client leave the tub, dry off vigorously, and lie down for rest or massage.

MUSCLE CONTRACTION HEADACHE

A muscle contraction headache (also known as a tension headache) is caused by muscle contraction, spasm or irritation, or active trigger points in the face, head, neck, or upper back. Tension in the neck and shoulder muscles can have many causes, including eyestrain, poorly aligned teeth or cranial bones, poorly healed injuries, poor posture, and emotional stress.

Hydrotherapy treatments can increase circulation to the muscles of the neck and head and relax them. Moist heat can decrease muscle spasm. Massage techniques to relieve muscle tension are generally effective for muscle contraction headaches; however, they will be more effective if the client is already relaxed and the circulation to neck and shoulder muscles has been increased. In addition, treatments that are soothing may address the stress component of the tension headache.

TREATMENT

APPLICATION OF COLD RUNNING WATER TO THE BACK OF THE NECK AND SCALP

Cross-Reference
See Chapter 6 for effects of cold.

Duration and Frequency
3 minutes. Perform at the beginning of a massage session, or as a home treatment at the first sign of a headache.

Procedure
1. Run water in the sink as cold as the client can tolerate.
2. Have the client place the head under the faucet for 3 minutes, being careful to keep the nostrils out of the water so as to breathe comfortably.
3. Let the cold water run over the back of the client's head with as much force as is tolerable. Include the occipital area.
4. Dry the client's hair.
5. Begin massage.

ICE PACK APPLICATION

Cross-Reference
See Chapter 6.

Duration and Frequency
15 minutes. Perform during a massage session, or as a home treatment at the beginning of a headache.

Procedure
Apply an ice pack on the back of the client's neck for 15 minutes. Remove the ice pack and begin massage.

MOIST HEAT APPLICATION

Cross-Reference
See Chapter 5.

Duration and Frequency
15 minutes. Perform before or during a massage session.

Procedure
1. Place a hot water bottle, moist heating pad, hot gel pad, fomentation, or hydrocollator pack on the upper back and neck for 15 minutes.
2. Remove the hot application and begin massage.

CONTRAST TREATMENT TO THE UPPER BACK AND NECK

Cross-Reference
See Chapters 5 and 6.

Procedure
1. With the client prone, place a hot water bottle, moist heating pad, fomentation, hot gel pack, or hydrocollator pack on the upper back and the back of the neck for 3 minutes.

2. Remove the hot application and place an ice pack, cold gel pack, or ice water compress on the upper back and the back of the neck for 1 minute. Make sure the client is warm, so the ice pack does not cause chilling.
3. Repeat steps 1 and 2 twice for a total of three rounds of hot followed by cold.
4. Remove the cold application and begin massage.

POSTCONCUSSION HEADACHE

When a person has a brain **concussion** (an injury to a soft structure caused by force or violent shaking), a *postconcussion headache* may result. Brain concussions most commonly occur from being hit on the head, car accidents, sports-related injuries, and slips and falls. The cause of the postconcussion headache is not always clear because while brain inflammation and bleeding can produce pressure inside the head, musculoskeletal injuries, such as skull fractures and injuries to vertebrae, discs, and myofascia in the upper cervical area may have occurred as well. Muscle spasm in involved muscles, such as the upper trapezius and semispinalis capitis, often follows. Many but not all postconcussion headaches can be successfully treated with migraine headache medication, indicating that pressure inside the head is a problem. However, other types of headaches such as tension or cluster headaches are also common. Most postconcussion headaches take place in the initial weeks after an injury and resolve within a few months.

When a client with postconcussion headaches sees you for massage therapy, make sure that he or she is under a physician's care for the headaches. Then, a hot foot soak combined with an ice pack to the back of the neck to relieve the headache can be performed before or during a massage session. Unfortunately, no research has been done on using this hydrotherapy treatment for postconcussion headaches. However, some people claim to have found relief this way. and because it is safe and easy to use a hot footbath, there is certainly no harm in offering one to a client with a postconcussion headache.

SINUS HEADACHE CAUSED BY NONINFECTIOUS SINUSITIS

Sinus headaches, often caused by chronic sinus inflammation from allergies, may develop during hay fever season. Although massage therapists do not treat the common cold or sinus infections, which sometimes develop after a cold, a client who has chronic sinusitis may find sinus contrast treatments and massage very invigorating and relieving.

TREATMENT

STEAM INHALATION ON THE MASSAGE TABLE

Cross-Reference
See Chapter 8.

Duration and Frequency
15 minutes. Perform before or during a massage session.

Procedure
1. Place a small steam unit on the table underneath the face cradle and place a face towel over the face cradle.
2. Have the client lie prone upon the table so her face is touching the face towel.
3. After 15 minutes of steam inhalation, have the client sit up and dry her face with the face towel.
4. Begin massage of the face.

SINUS CONTRAST TREATMENT

Cross-Reference
See Chapters 5 and 6.

Duration and Frequency
10 minutes. Perform before or during a massage session.

Caution
Do not use when the client has a sinus infection except with physician's permission.

Procedure
1. Dip a washcloth in 110°F water and wring it out.
2. Place it across the nose, leaving the nostrils exposed. Fold down the ends 90° from the central point so they lie alongside the nose.
3. After 2 minutes, replace the first washcloth with a second washcloth or small bath towel that has been wrung out in ice water, and leave it on for 1 minute.
4. Repeat steps 1 and 2 twice for a total of three rounds.
5. Begin massage.

LIFE STRESS

High levels of stress affect all aspects of a client's life—emotional, physical, and mental. Clients may experience great muscle tension, muscular aches and pains, stiffness, insomnia, and a host of other symptoms. Hydrotherapy and massage are both classic treatments for this problem; the soothing effects of relaxation massage are even more effective when combined with relaxing water treatments.

When working with someone who is seeking massage for life stress, your choice of treatment will vary depending upon what is most soothing for your client. Perhaps some prefer a steam bath, tub bath, or sauna that is quite hot. Others may prefer lying on a bed of fomentations; still others, taking a neutral bath. Treatments with ice or

---

CASE HISTORY 14-2

Noninfectious Sinus Headache Treated by Hot Footbath and Sinus Contrast Treatment

Background

Terry was a 45-year-old librarian who had no health problems but received a massage once a month to help relax her very tense neck and shoulder muscles. One month in the spring, however, she began having severe headaches and sinus congestion, which her family physician diagnosed as allergy related. She arrived for her massage session with a headache and a feeling of congestion in her upper face and was unsure that she would be comfortable lying prone for this reason. The massage therapist asked her if she would like to try a hot foot soak for her headache and a contrast treatment over her sinus area to make her more comfortable. She agreed to try this.

Treatment

With Terry lying supine, the massage therapist placed her feet directly in a hot footbath and began massage of her head, neck, and shoulders. Within 10 minutes Terry said her sinus area felt more open and her headache was gone. The therapist then removed the footbath, dried Terry's feet, and continued the massage. During the massage, the therapist also performed a contrast treatment to Terry's upper face using hot and cold compresses, finishing with a cold compress. Terry then lay prone and was pleasantly surprised to find that her face was not uncomfortable in this position. After the session, her headache was still gone, her sinuses felt more open, and she was as relaxed as usual after a session.

---

cold water are not as conducive to relaxation. They require more effort for many people to tolerate them at all and are more invigorating than soothing. Neutral baths, with their ability to reduce stimulation, can be very effective for nervous tension. Historically, many herbs and essential oils have also been added to bath waters to enhance their relaxing effect, such as chamomile and lavender. Numerous studies have found that body heating, using hot footbaths or warm full-body baths 30 minutes before bedtime, causes a person to fall asleep sooner and sleep more deeply.(12–17)

How would you combine hydrotherapy treatments with massage for clients in your practice who are experiencing problems with high levels of stress? To give just one example, for a client who is having trouble sleeping, an evening massage session in your office could be followed by a hot bath there, or you can send the client home after the massage session to take a neutral or hot bath and then go directly to bed. You might also suggest a nightly warm bath as a regular self-care treatment. Another treatment that relaxes and enhances sleep is hot fomentations to the spine during an evening massage. Clients find these treatments nurturing and relaxing as well.

TREATMENT
NEUTRAL BATH

Cross-Reference
See Chapter 7.

Duration and Frequency
20 to 30 minutes. Perform after a massage session.

Special Instructions
The client may also take a neutral bath at home after a massage session and then go directly to bed.

Procedure
1. Help the client into the bath.
2. Maintain water temperature at 98°F so the client will not become chilled.
3. After 20 to 30 minutes, have the client dry off gently, dress, and go home to go directly to bed.

HOT FOMENTATIONS TO THE BACK AND THIGHS PRIOR TO MASSAGE, FOLLOWED BY OPTIONAL SALT GLOW

Cross-Reference
See Chapters 5 and 11.

Special Instructions
Flat plastic hot water bottles may be substituted for the fomentations.

Duration and Frequency
30 minutes

Procedure
1. Prepare and heat the fomentations.
2. Place a plastic tub under the massage table.
3. Lay one fomentation on the massage table where the client's back will be and one where each thigh

will be. It is important to cover them very carefully so the client will not be burned and to check the skin frequently.

4. Have the client lie supine on the fomentations for 30 minutes during massage on the front of the body.
5. Have the client turn over, removing the fomentations as he or she does so. Place them in the plastic tub under the table.
6. Dry the skin if there is any sweat on it, and cover the client to prevent chilling.
7. If desired, give a salt glow to the client's back and the back of the legs. If you plan to do this, add a towel under the fomentations before the client gets on the table so that it will be there after you remove them. It will protect the sheets when you give the salt glow.
8. Begin massage.

LOW BACK PAIN

Lower back pain is such a common complaint that it is one of the top 10 reasons that patients in the United States visit their physicians. In a 2006 survey of massage therapists in two states, chronic back pain was the reason for 12% of all visits.(18) Lower back pain—the source of one third of all disability costs in the United States—can have many causes, including disease processes such as osteoporosis, connective tissue disease, fibromyalgia, cancerous tumors, even infections in the spine. Mechanical causes of back pain include traumatic injuries to the structures of the back—muscles, ligaments, discs, bones, and joints—as well as osteoarthritis and spinal stenosis. Inactivity and weak abdominal muscles can worsen lower back pain. Improperly healed injuries, such as muscle strains and ligament sprains, may cause back pain for the rest of the person's life. And finally, one very important cause of lower back pain is emotional stress. For more on this topic, see the section on lower back muscle spasm in this chapter.

Lower back pain is classified as either acute (lasting 6 weeks or less), subacute (lasting 6–12 weeks), or chronic (lasting 12 weeks or more). Standard medical treatment of acute lower back pain involves medications for pain, inflammation, and muscle spasm, as well as heat to the back rather than ice. After a month or two, if low back pain is not resolved, physicians generally begin to perform diagnostic tests to find other causes. If nonmechanical causes, such as a disease, are found, they are treated. If no specific cause can be found, standard medical treatment may include physical therapy, other medications, and as a last resort, surgery.

Although most lower back pain is either mechanical or stress related, since diseases can also cause back pain, it is vital that the client with lower back pain be evaluated by a physician before receiving massage. How disastrous it would be if a client with bone cancer was treated with massage rather than receiving the medical treatment he or she needed!

ACUTE LOWER BACK PAIN

Hydrotherapy and massage not only can relieve much lower back pain but, by increasing local circulation and reducing muscle tension, can also promote healing. If the client's pain is linked to emotional stress, the nurturing and relaxing qualities of these modalities can also assist healing. For acute pain, hydrotherapy using heat is generally recommended. Hot applications can vary from a hot bath, which will heat the entire back, to local applications such as moist heat (fomentations) or mustard plasters. When the client's tissues are thoroughly warmed and relaxed, massage can be far more effective. For some clients, however, ice massage may help numb the area and give more relief.

TREATMENT
MOIST HEAT APPLICATION

Cross-Reference
See Chapter 5.

Duration and Frequency
20 minutes. Perform before or during a massage session.

Procedure
1. Apply moist heat over the lower back, using a hydrocollator pack, fomentation, moist heating pad, or flat plastic hot water bottle (Fig 14-3, A and B). The application should stay hot; if it cools off, reheat it or replace it.
2. After 20 minutes, remove moist heat, give a brief cold mitten friction (Fig 14-3C), dry the skin briskly, and begin massage.

FULL HOT BATH FOLLOWED BY LOCAL MOIST HEAT APPLICATION

Cross-Reference
See Chapters 5 and 7.

Duration and Frequency
45 minutes. Give the bath before the massage session, and begin the massage session with the moist heat application in place on the lower back.

Procedure
1. Help the client into a hot bath (103°–110°F).
2. After 25 to 30 minutes, help the client out of the bath. Watch for signs of lightheadedness. Have the client dry off.

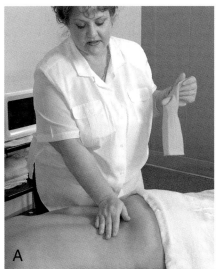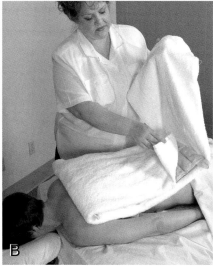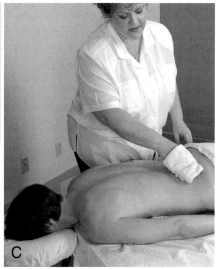

FIGURE 14-3 ■ Moist heat application followed by cold mitten friction for acute lower back pain. **A.** Checking the area visually. **B.** Placing large silica gel pack on lower back. **C.** Performing brief cold mitten friction to the lower back.

3. Have the client lie prone on the massage table, and apply moist heat to the lower back. Begin massage on another part of the body.
4. After 20 minutes, remove the moist heat over the lower back and perform a brief cold mitten friction over the area.
5. Dry the area briskly and begin back massage.

MUSTARD PLASTER APPLICATION

Cross-Reference
See Chapter 5.

Duration and Frequency
20 minutes. Perform during a massage session or as a home treatment before stretching exercises two or three times daily.

Procedure
Apply the mustard plaster over the entire lower back. Monitor carefully for burning. Begin massage on another part of the body. Wait 20 minutes, then remove the plaster and begin massage.

ICE MASSAGE

Cross-Reference
See Chapter 6.

Duration and Frequency
8 to 10 minutes. Perform before massage of the lower back or as a home treatment ice massage two or three times daily.

Procedure
1. Perform ice massage on the entire lower back for 8 to 10 minutes, until the area is thoroughly numb.

2. Dry the skin briskly.
3. Begin massage.

CHRONIC LOWER BACK PAIN

As with acute lower back pain, it is vital that the client has been evaluated by a physician and approved for massage treatment. Perpetuating factors are very important in this condition. Hydrotherapy and massage can help with symptoms, but such factors as leg-length inequality, emotional stress, postural distortion, muscular imbalance, and poorly healed injuries can all perpetuate low back pain and must be addressed for real relief. Someone who has been hurting for a long time may also be experiencing a high level of stress from the back problem and feel worried, discouraged, and worn down by pain. In this sense, treating someone with chronic back pain can be quite different from treating someone with acute back pain.

Both hydrotherapy treatments and massage are relaxing and nurturing. They enhance circulation, ease muscle tension, and may be the best nondrug approach to this problem. Any massage techniques that relieve muscle tension, including circulatory, myofascial, and trigger point, may help relieve pain as well. Of course, if there is an underlying perpetuating factor, the best approach is to address the cause. But even as a symptomatic treatment, massage can be tremendously comforting, and hydrotherapy treatments can make massage more effective. Salt glows, contrast showers, and ice massage may all help relieve pain and enhance massage. Patients who have severe chronic lower back pain are likely to fare better with ice massage and exercise than with hot packs and exercise. For some clients, both heat and ice may have to be tried to determine which relieves their pain the best.

TREATMENT

MOIST HEAT APPLICATION FOLLOWED BY SALT GLOW OF THE ENTIRE BACK

Both the moist heat and the salt glow increase circulation to the back.

Cross-Reference
See Chapters 5 and 11.

Duration and Frequency
25 to 30 minutes. Perform during a massage session.

Procedure
1. Place a towel on the massage table.
2. With the client prone, apply moist heat in the form of a hydrocollator pack, fomentation, moist heating pad, or flat plastic hot-water bottle. Keep it hot for the entire treatment time. If a hot pack cools off, replace it with another one.
3. After 20 minutes, remove the moist heat and give a brief cold mitten friction.
4. Inform the client that he or she will feel warm water on the back.
5. Gently wash the back with warm water.
6. Apply about 2 tbsp of moistened salt to the client's back. Rub the entire back for about 3 minutes, especially in the lower back area.
7. Gently wash the salt off with a wet washcloth and then dry the skin briskly with a dry washcloth.
8. Remove the towel from underneath the client.
9. Begin massage.

CONTRAST SHOWER

This is a modified version of an old treatment, the hot and cold percussion douche to the back, using the spray from a full-body shower.

Cross-Reference
See Chapter 9.

Duration and Frequency
About 11 minutes. Perform before a massage session, or as a home treatment as often as once an hour.

Procedure
1. Have the client enter a hot shower (up to 110°F) and remain for 5 minutes, so that the body is thoroughly warm. Use the strongest spray that can be tolerated directly on the lower back.
2. Change the water temperature to cold for 30 seconds, and target the lower back as much as possible.
3. Change the water temperature to hot for 2 minutes.
4. Change the water temperature to cold for 30 seconds.
5. Repeat steps 3 and 4.
6. Have the client dry off and lie down for a rest or a massage session.

ICE MASSAGE

Cross-Reference
See Chapter 5.

Duration and Frequency
8 to 10 minutes. Perform before massage of the back or as a home treatment up to five times daily.

Procedure
1. Perform ice massage on the lower back for 8 to 10 minutes, until the area is thoroughly numb.
2. Dry the skin briskly.
3. Begin massage.

MULTIPLE SCLEROSIS

Multiple sclerosis is a progressive autoimmune disease in which the body attacks the myelin of the brain and spinal cord, which leads to degeneration of the myelin sheaths that surround the sensory and motor neurons. Symptoms may include muscle weakness, stiffness, spasticity, bladder problems, and the loss of both sensation and motor control. The cause of multiple sclerosis is unknown; although it is thought to be an autoimmune disease, it is may be triggered by environmental factors. The standard medical treatment for this disorder consists of medication to reduce symptoms and mild exercise to maintain strength and function. Although patients are warned not to become overheated—an increase in core temperature of as little as 1°F may cause extreme fatigue—some old-time hydrotherapists used fever treatments to address the underlying immune system dysfunction.(19) (For more information on this type of therapy, see Appendix C.) Pool therapy can help patients with multiple sclerosis, but care must be taken that they not become overheated. When overheating does occur, patients become very weak and are likely to fall. (Alternating 10 minutes of exercise in an 80°F cold pool with 5 to 10 minutes of exercise in a 94°F neutral pool avoids this problem.)

Hydrotherapy and massage may both be used to alleviate the symptoms of multiple sclerosis, especially muscle spasticity, poor circulation caused by that spasticity, and muscle stiffness. Keeping the tissue of a wheelchair-bound or bedridden person healthy and mobile not only reduces the person's subjective feelings of discomfort but may help him or her to be more active. Someone who has stiff extremities and difficulty moving often feels a great deal better after hydrotherapy treatments and massage. If desired, exercises prescribed by a patient's physical therapist may be incorporated into a massage session after the application of cold has temporarily decreased spasticity and muscle weakness. In this case, ice water compresses or cold water immersion are used prior to massage. For a case history of hydrotherapy treatments for a client with multiple sclerosis, see Chapter 7.

TREATMENT
WHOLE-BODY SALT GLOW

Cross-Reference
See Chapter 11.

For someone who cannot exercise, a whole-body salt glow is an excellent way to stimulate the circulation without using heat. It may be done in a bathtub, with the client sitting on a bath chair, on a therapy table, or for a bedridden client, on the client's bed. For house calls to bedridden clients' homes, simply spread a tarp or plastic sheet over the bed, cover that with a cloth sheet, and perform the salt glow there. With the client rolled first to one side and then to the other, the sheet and tarp can be removed and the bed underneath will be dry.

ICE WATER COMPRESS

Cross-Reference
See Chapter 6.

Duration and Frequency
8 minutes. Perform during a massage session.

Procedure
1. Prepare a compress by wringing out a towel of the appropriate size in a container of half ice and half cold water or by wrapping crushed ice in wet towels and applying that to an entire extremity.
2. Apply the towel to the spastic muscles for 4 minutes.
3. Wring out towel in the ice water and reapply it, leaving it on for 4 more minutes.
4. Dry the area well.
5. Perform stretching or strengthening exercises, then finish with massage.

COLD WATER IMMERSION FOLLOWED BY EXERCISE

Cross-Reference
See Chapter 5.

Duration and Frequency
1 to 5 minutes. Perform before or during a massage session.

Procedure
1. Begin with a large bowl or bucket of water at 35° to 40°F. Ice cubes will be needed to achieve this temperature. Check to make sure that the client is comfortably warm before beginning the cold-water immersion.
2. Immerse the body part in the water for 3 seconds.
3. Take the body part out of the water and have the client do isometric contractions or contractions against resistance for 30 seconds. If the client becomes fatigued, stop the exercises until after the next cold-water immersion.
4. Repeat steps 2 and 3 two to five times.

MUSCLE CRAMPS AND SPASMS

Both **muscle cramps** and **muscle spasms** are involuntary contractions of skeletal muscles. Muscle cramps are generally sudden, strong, and short-lived, which is fortunate, since they can be very painful. Muscle spasms, on the other hand, are not as strong of a contraction, but they last much longer. Muscle spasms can be very uncomfortable and so are a common reason to seek massage therapy. Many factors contribute to muscle cramps and spasms, including tightness of the affected muscle, poor local circulation, vitamin and mineral deficiencies, sudden movement or chilling of a tight muscle, inactivity, dehydration, and some medical conditions. Acute muscle cramps can also occur when a person has been sitting or sleeping in a cramped position or overstretches a muscle that is not properly warmed up before exercising. Hand cramps sometimes occur from overuse of the hand muscles, such as from playing a musical instrument, sewing, typing, massaging, carpentry, tennis, writing, or gardening.

MUSCLE CRAMPS

Some clients, particularly elderly people whose local circulation is poor, are prone to calf or foot cramps when receiving massage therapy. Should their calf or foot muscles cramp, immediately apply moist heat or put the part in a hot-water bath. Often this helps relieve the cramp immediately, but if it is not successful, ice should be tried next. A contrast treatment may also be effective. Sometimes all that is needed is to have the person contract the antagonist muscles, causing the contraction of the cramping muscle to cease, as it automatically relaxes. Following are instructions for moist heat, ice massage, and contrast treatments.

TREATMENT
MOIST HEAT APPLICATION ON AN ACUTELY CRAMPING CALF MUSCLE

Cross-Reference
See Chapter 5.

Duration and Frequency
30 seconds to a few minutes, until the cramp has gone away. Perform during a massage session immediately when a muscle cramp begins.

Special Instructions
The application must be hot, not warm, to be effective.

Procedure
1. Apply a hot fomentation, moist heating pad, or hot compress to the cramping calf muscle. Leave it on until the cramp has gone away.
2. Begin massage of the calf muscles.

CASE HISTORY 14-3

Spasmodic Muscle Contraction Treated by a Combination of Ice Massage and Manual Massage

Background

Rose was a woman in her early sixties who suffered from a twitch in the muscles around her right eye that could continue for hours at a time and sometimes even woke her from sleep. She was referred to a massage therapist by her ophthalmologist, who approved the use of both ice cube massage and manual massage.

Treatment

The massage therapist began the by performing ice massage along the path of the right facial nerve. Using an ice cube, he began at the front of the earlobe, moved upward to the temple, down along the underside of the eye socket, and finally downward along the jaw. The area was treated with ice massage 5 minutes on, 5 minutes off, and this sequence was repeated three more times. After a total of 20 minutes of ice massage, Rose rested for 15 minutes. Then the massage therapist treated the entire right side of her face with Swedish massage. This concluded her session. Rose was treated three times a week for 2 weeks, twice a week for 2 weeks, and once a week for 2 weeks, for a total of 12 sessions. At the end of this time, her muscle twitch was gone and her treatment concluded. She experienced no muscle twitching at all for 2 years. Since then she occasionally feels muscle twitches and has noticed that they occur only during times of great emotional stress.(20)

Discussion Questions

1. Why was ice applied to the facial nerve?
2. Why was the combination of ice massage and manual massage better than manual massage alone?

ICE MASSAGE ON AN ACUTELY CRAMPING MUSCLE IN THE ARCH OF THE FOOT

Cross-Reference
See Chapter 6.

Duration and Frequency
30 seconds to a few minutes, until the cramp has gone away. Perform during a massage session immediately when a muscle cramp begins.

Procedure
1. Using an ice cup or ice cube, massage directly over the cramping muscle, and continue until the cramp has gone away.

CONTRAST COMPRESS FOR ANY ACUTELY CRAMPING MUSCLE

Cross-Reference
See Chapter 6.

Duration and Frequency
4 minutes

Procedure
1. Apply a hot compress to the cramping muscle for 3 minutes.
2. Apply ice water compress to the cramping muscle for 1 minute.
3. Repeat steps 1 and 2 until the muscle stops cramping.

TREATMENT

HOT HAND BATH WITH STRETCHING FOR ACUTE SPASMS IN THE HAND MUSCLES

Cross-Reference
See Chapter 7.

Duration and Frequency
15 minutes. Perform during a massage session. Use the hand bath for self-care if the hands spasm after giving massages.

Procedure
Have the client soak the hands in hot water (about 110°F), wiggling the fingers and stretching the hand muscles while soaking. After 15 minutes, dry the hands and begin massage

ACUTE SPASM OF LOWER BACK MUSCLES

Acute spasms of the lower back muscles are extremely common and can have a variety of causes, including muscle strain such as can occur with heavy lifting, structural and postural problems, poor healing of previous back injuries, and emotional stress. As professionals who deal with muscle tension, massage therapists are often called when a person's lower back muscles have gone into spasm.

Of all of the factors that can cause acute spasm of lower back muscles and pain, emotional factors are one of the most common and the least understood. Suppressed emotions, particularly anxiety and anger, can cause a person to tighten up the musculature of the back, resulting in not only muscle tension but muscle spasm and a drastically reduced blood supply to the back muscles.(21) During more than 20 years as a massage therapist, the author has asked each client with acute lower back muscle spasm about his or her life stress, and almost without exception, clients have said that their stress levels were very high. Some representative events that happened just before clients experienced acute lower back spasm: a college student just finished her last final examination, a young mother was taking care of a baby with severe asthma attacks, an elderly woman was packing up and moving out of her home of 40 years, a 30-year-old man was leaving to be the best man at a wedding he desperately did not want to attend, and a 50-year-old woman was caring for a severely mentally ill child. These were all situations in which the spasm was triggered by the client bending over and in which the physician was not able to find any organic problem. A typical comment from clients was: "I just reached over to pick up something [often as light as a speck of dust] and then I couldn't even straighten back up." A simple movement that results in spasm of back muscles is often simply the final straw for a treacherously tense body.

When a person experiences acute low back spasm accompanied by pain, the first step should be a thorough examination by his or her physician. The standard protocol for this situation is to first rule out serious injuries and disease. Then anti-inflammatories and/or muscle relaxants are usually prescribed, and the patient is advised to rest in bed for at least a few days. Massage therapists may work with clients as soon as they have been evaluated by a physician and massage has been approved.

Hydrotherapy treatments can relieve pain, deeply relax the muscles of the lower back, and increase circulation to them as well. Ice massage can dull pain. Many experienced hydrotherapists favor deep heating of acute muscle spasms to relax them, but occasionally a spasm will respond better to cold, such as ice massage or an ice water compress. Any type of massage that addresses muscle tension will be helpful and can also help the client with stress.

TREATMENT

MOIST HEAT APPLICATION TO THE LOWER BACK

Cross-Reference
See Chapter 5.

Duration and Frequency
30 minutes. Perform during a massage session or as a home treatment two or three times daily.

Procedure
1. Apply a hot fomentation, moist heating pad, or hot compress to the lower back for 30 minutes.
2. Remove the heat, and give a 1-minute ice application (ice massage or cold mitten friction with ice water).
3. Begin massage of the lower back.

FULL HOT BATH FOLLOWED BY LOCAL MOIST HEAT APPLICATION

Cross-Reference
See Chapters 5 and 7.

Duration and Frequency
45 minutes. The bath may be given before a massage session, and the moist heat application can be put on at the beginning of the massage session.

Procedure
1. Help the client into a hot bath (103°–110°F).
2. After 25 to 30 minutes, help the client out of the bath. Watch for signs of lightheadedness. Have the client dry off.
3. Have the client lie prone on the massage table, and apply moist heat to the lower back. Another part of the body may be massaged at this time.
4. After 20 minutes, remove the moist heat over the lower back and perform a brief cold mitten friction over the area.
5. Dry the area briskly and begin massage.

ICE MASSAGE OF THE LOWER BACK

Cross-Reference
See Chapter 6.

Duration and Frequency
About 8 minutes, until the painful area is numb. Perform during a massage session or as a home treatment three or more times daily.

Special Instructions
As an alternative, an ice pack may be applied for 20 minutes.

Procedure
With the client supine, use an ice cup or ice cube to massage the painful area and about a 4-inch margin on all sides. Then begin hands-on massage.

ACUTE SPASM OF NECK MUSCLES

This condition, which clients may refer to as a "crick in the neck," is usually caused by a severe spasm of the sternocleidomastoid muscle, although the levator scapulae and trapezius muscles may also be involved.(22) As with spasm of the low back muscles, many factors, including muscle strain, emotional stress, poor work posture, structural and postural problems, and poor healing of previous injuries may combine to render the client vulnerable to a "neck attack." On rare occasions, mechanical problems such as herniated discs may also cause neck spasm. This condition may be precipitated when an already tight muscle becomes chilled (for example, by sleeping under an air conditioning vent or next to an open window in the dead of winter), when life stress increases to a high level, or when the client has had an upper respiratory infection. The first step in dealing with this condition should be a thorough examination by his or her physician to rule out diseases or other problems.

Usually a client with this problem enters with an extremely stiff neck—he or she may have to turn the entire body to look directly at you—and some degree of neck pain. The client's neck muscles may be extremely sensitive to the touch as well. A common scenario is the person who "slept wrong" and woke up in the morning with a stiff neck. Most likely this person had tight neck muscles and possibly weakened or injured neck ligaments as well; sleeping in an awkward position can stretch those ligaments. The muscles in that area then spasm to protect the joint, causing pain and stiffness.

Hot applications increase lymphatic drainage and blood circulation to muscles in spasm and bring relief to the client. Ice applications will relieve pain and muscle spasm and can also be used after trigger point treatment to assist in stretching the muscle in spasm to its full length again. Hands-on massage—using Swedish, myofascial, trigger point release, or other techniques—can be very effective in relieving the spasm of the sternocleidomastoid and related muscles and works beautifully in conjunction with these hot and cold applications. However, if a ligament injury is causing the person's problems, treatment of the ligament is what the client most needs in the long run. Likewise, if emotional stress is a big factor, only dealing with the stress will address the heart of the problem.

TREATMENT

ICE STROKING (INTERMITTENT COLD WITH STRETCH) OF THE STERNOCLEIDOMASTOID MUSCLE

Cross-Reference
See Chapter 6.

Duration and Frequency
5 minutes. Perform during a massage session after trigger point release of the muscle.

Special Instructions
In acute spasm of the neck muscles, the sternocleidomastoid muscle on both sides of the neck should be treated, along with any associated trigger points in the levator scapulae, trapezius, splenius cervicis, and other posterior neck muscles.

Procedure
1. Treat trigger points in the sternocleidomastoid with trigger point pressure release (Fig. 14-4).
2. Gently stretch the muscle to the greatest extent possible without overstretching. While you maintain the muscle stretch, stroke the entire length of the muscle three times with the plastic-wrapped ice.
3. Again gently stretch the muscle to the greatest extent possible without overstretching.
4. If the muscle still cannot fully lengthen without pain, try applying direct pressure to the trigger point, then gently stretching the muscle again or have the client contract the antagonist muscle for 30 seconds and relax completely as you gently stretch the muscle again.
5. Repeat steps 2 to 4 until the muscle is pain free when completely stretched.
6. Apply a heating pad or moist hot pack to the muscle for 5 minutes or more to eliminate posttreatment soreness.
7. Have the client gently move the head back and forth from the fully lengthened to the fully shortened position three times for each division of the muscle.

HOT MOIST APPLICATION TO THE NECK

Cross-Reference
See Chapters 6 and 11.

Duration and Frequency
30 minutes. Perform during a massage session or as a home treatment two or three times daily.

Procedure
1. Apply a hot fomentation, moist heating pad, or hot compresses to the neck for 30 minutes.
2. Finish with a 1-minute ice application (ice massage or cold mitten friction using ice water) to the client's neck.
3. Begin massage of the neck muscles.

For full instructions and contraindications, see sections on hot moist applications, Chapter 6.

FULL HOT BATH FOLLOWED BY LOCAL MOIST HEAT APPLICATION

Cross-Reference
See Chapters 5 and 7.

Duration and Frequency
40 minutes. Have the client take the hot bath before the massage session; then apply the local heat to the neck at the beginning of the session.

Procedure
1. Help the client into a hot bath (103°–110°F)

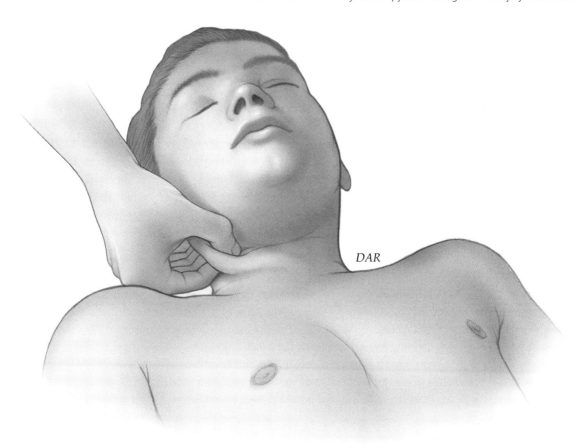

FIGURE 14-4 ■ Trigger point pressure release of the sternocleidomastoid muscle. (Reprinted with permission from Sinclair M. *Pediatric Massage Therapy*. 2nd ed. Baltimore: Lippincott Williams & Wilkins, 2004: Fig. 5-5.)

2. After 25 to 30 minutes, help the client out of the bath. Watch for signs of lightheadedness. Have the client dry off.
3. Have the client lie either supine or prone on the massage table and apply moist heat to the neck. Another part of the body may be massaged at this time.
4. After 20 minutes, remove the moist heat over the neck and perform a brief cold mitten friction over the area.
5. Dry the area briskly and begin massage of the neck muscles.

ICE MASSAGE OF THE NECK MUSCLES

Cross-Reference
See Chapter 6.

Duration and Frequency
5 to 10 minutes. Perform during a massage session or as a home treatment three times daily.

Caution
To avoid pressure on the carotid arteries, do not massage the anterior neck medial to the sternocleidomastoid muscles.

Procedure
Perform ice massage gently on the posterior and lateral neck muscles and continue around to the sternocleidomastoid muscle. Continue ice massage for 5 to 10 minutes.

MUSCLE SPASTICITY

Muscle spasticity is an extreme degree of muscle tone even when a person is at rest. It can occur after a stroke, spinal cord injury, or other central nervous system injury, and it may be painful, interfere with easy movement, and lead to contractures. Although the process is not completely understood, it is believed that applications of cold to spastic muscles cools muscle spindles, whose job it is to maintain muscle tone, and this allows spastic muscles to relax.

> **CASE HISTORY 14-4**
>
> ### Treatment of an Acute Neck Spasm With Heat, Ice Massage, and Hands-on Massage
>
> **Background**
>
> Martin was a 32-year-old man who worked full time and took college classes at night. A cramped work space for his home computer meant that his body was in an awkward position as he did much of his homework. His head was often twisted far to the left as he read from a stack of papers as he typed. While working a school deadline, he put in almost an entire week-end at the computer with his head twisted to the left, but when he awoke the next morning he found he could not turn his head at all.
>
> **Treatment**
>
> First Martin took a hot shower, letting the hot water beat directly on the muscles on the front and sides of his neck, which loosened them. Then he consulted with his physician by telephone, who concurred that visiting his massage therapist was a sensible course of action. At the beginning of the session, his therapist applied very hot compresses to both sternocleidomastoid muscles for 20 minutes while massaging his upper back and shoulders. After 20 minutes, the therapist removed the compresses, performed ice massage for 1 minute, and then applied Swedish and trigger point techniques to the muscles, followed by gentle stretching. Martin left her office feeling much better, but it took 3 more days before he began to feel completely well again. On those days, he did no typing and twice a day he took a 20-minute hot shower or bath followed by 1 minute of ice massage on his sternocleidomastoid muscles and then gentle stretching. To avoid a recurrence of the same problem, Martin also began to rearrange his workspace to avoid twisting his head so much when he worked at his computer.

Massage techniques that increase circulation and decrease tension are useful to temporarily decrease muscle spasticity, but because spasticity is the result of an injury to the central nervous system, massage must be regular to be helpful. It can also help relieve stress, ease muscle pain, and help maintain joint range of motion. Warm water exercise can also be very helpful because it reduces spasticity and retains muscle strength and range of motion.

The following cold applications must be carefully used, with the awareness that the core temperature will drop if more than one-fifth of the body is covered with a cold compress or if one part is immersed in cold water long enough. Be sure the client is warm before you begin.

TREATMENT
ICE WATER COMPRESS

Cross-Reference
See Chapter 6.

Duration and Frequency
8 minutes. Perform during a massage session.

Procedure
1. Prepare a compress by wringing out a towel of the appropriate size in a container of that is half ice and half cold water. Crushed ice may be wrapped in wet towels and applied to an entire extremity.
2. Apply the towel to the spastic muscles for 4 minutes.
3. Wring out towel in the ice water and reapply it, leaving it on for 4 more minutes.
4. Dry the area well.
5. Perform stretching or strengthening exercises, then begin massage.

COLD WATER IMMERSION FOLLOWED BY EXERCISE

Cross-Reference
See Chapter 7.

Duration and Frequency
5 to 10 minutes. Perform during a massage session.

Procedure
1. Begin with a large bowl or bucket of ice cubes and water at 35° to 40°F. Check to make sure that the client is comfortably warm before beginning the cold-water immersion.
2. Immerse the body part in the water for 3 seconds.
3. Take the body part out of the water and have the client perform exercises for 30 seconds.
4. Repeat steps 2 and 3 five times, for a total of six cold water immersions.
5. Perform other stretching or strengthening exercises.
6. Begin massage.

MUSCLE WEAKNESS

Chronic muscle weakness can be caused by a variety of disabilities, including muscular dystrophy, spinal cord injury, postpolio syndrome, strokes, and some types of cerebral palsy. Muscle weakness not only makes many movements difficult or impossible but contributes to chronic tension. Constantly straining to move causes tension and, if the person uses a few stronger muscles to substitute for the weaker ones, those muscles become overdeveloped and tight.

Hydrotherapy can be used in a variety of ways to help clients with muscle weakness:

1. Cold water immersion can temporarily stimulate muscle strength so that muscles can be exercised. Then strengthening exercises that are recommended by the client's physical therapist can be incorporated into a massage session. (Massage can be used to help the client relax and reduce chronic muscle tension, but it can also be performed in a more stimulating manner if called for.) For example, exposure to cold can be used to stimulate the action of the extensor muscles. A weak or paralyzed hand or foot can be immersed in very cold water and then exercised while the strength of the muscles is stimulated. At the moment of immersion, a contraction will be noticed, even if it is weak or inhibited by spasticity. The first contraction will be the strongest, and the successive contractions, which will occur each time the body part is immersed in cold water, will be weaker. However, the extensors will be stimulated and the flexors inhibited for about 20 minutes following the treatment. Exercises and massage strokes can be combined; for example, when the client can only do a few contractions without becoming fatigued, this is a perfect time for using either relaxing or stimulating massage techniques.

2. Another way to combine massage and exercise that builds muscle strength is to combine warm water exercise with massage techniques. Massage therapist Meir Schneider's self-healing approach has documented success in improving muscle strength in patients with muscular dystrophy, using gentle massage techniques and repeated gentle exercise, especially in warm baths or pools.(23) Watsu water massage has been combined with exercise for this purpose as well.

3. For some movement problems deriving from brain dysfunction, such as strokes, heat and cold may be of benefit because of their brain-stimulating effect. In 2005 a research study with partially paralyzed stroke survivors used contrast applications to paralyzed hands and wrists (hot packs followed by cold packs) five times a day for 6 weeks. Compared to other stroke survivors whose rehabilitation was the same in every other way, the contrast application group improved far more in the ability to flex and extend their wrists. Researchers concluded that the contrast applications were effective because they helped stimulate and reorganize large areas in the brain.(24)

TREATMENT

COLD WATER IMMERSION FOLLOWED BY EXERCISE

Cross-Reference
See Chapter 5.

Duration and Frequency
1 to 5 minutes. Perform before or during a massage session.

Procedure
1. Begin with a large bowl or bucket of water at 35° to 40°F. Ice cubes will be needed to achieve this temperature. Check to make sure that the client is comfortably warm before beginning the cold water immersion.
2. Immerse the body part in the water for 3 seconds.
3. Take the body part out of the water and have the client do isometric contractions or contractions against resistance for 30 seconds. If he or she becomes fatigued, stop exercises until after the next cold water immersion.
4. Repeat steps 2 and 3 two to five times.

SCIATICA

Sciatica is a relatively common type of pain in the lower back and leg, which radiates from the lower back along the large sciatic nerve. True sciatica, a compression or inflammation of this nerve, can be caused by a disc herniation (usually at L5 or S1 level) which pinches or irritates the nerve root or by entrapment of the sciatic nerve in the gluteal area by the piriformis muscle (piriformis syndrome). Sciatic symptoms very similar to those caused by a herniated disc can also be caused by trigger points in the gluteus medius that refer pain down the back of the leg along the path of the nerve.

Sciatic pain can range from sharp to burning to tingling to shooting pain and can be mild, moderate, or severe. Weakness, numbness, and difficulty moving the affected leg or foot also may occur. Standard medical treatment for sciatica includes medications for inflammation and pain, physical therapy including manual manipulation, and surgery. However, patients with persistent sciatica from lumbar disc herniations have no better results with surgery than with physical therapy and exercise.(25)

Both hydrotherapy and massage can increase circulation to painful areas, decrease muscle spasm, and quiet trigger points. True sciatica caused by a disc herniation will not be healed by massage, and clients with such a condition should be treated by an orthopedic physician.

TREATMENT
HOT HALF-BATH

Cross-Reference
See Chapters 6 and 7.

Duration and Frequency
20 minutes. Perform before a massage session or as a home treatment two or three times daily.

Procedure
1. Have the client sit in a hot bath (102°–108°F).
2. After 20 minutes, finish the half-bath with a cold local shower to the area or have the client lie prone with a bag of crushed ice or a frozen cold compress over the lower back for 2 minutes.
3. Begin massage.

ICE MASSAGE FOR SCIATICA

Cross-Reference
See Chapter 6.

Duration and Frequency
20 minutes. Perform during a massage session.

Procedure
1. Using an ice cube or ice cup, perform ice massage over the gluteal muscles and down the back of the leg, following the path of the sciatic nerve. Continue ice massage for 5 minutes.
2. Allow the client to rest without the use of ice for 5 minutes. Massage may be performed on another part of the body at this time.
3. Repeat steps 1 and 2 three more times, for a total of 20 minutes of ice.

ICE MASSAGE FOR PIRIFORMIS SYNDROME

Cross-Reference
See Chapter 6.

Duration and Frequency
5 to 10 minutes. Perform during a massage session.

Procedure
1. Have the client lie with the painful side up.
2. Using an ice cube or ice cup, do ice massage over the piriformis and down the back of the leg for 5 to 10 minutes, until the area is thoroughly numb.
3. Begin hands-on massage.

CONTRAST TREATMENT WITH HOT FOMENTATIONS AND ICE PACKS

Cross-Reference
See Chapters 5 and 6.

Duration and Frequency
25 minutes. Perform during a massage session.

Procedure
1. With the client prone, apply moist heat over the gluteal muscles in the form of a hydrocollator pack, fomentation, moist heating pad, or a flat plastic hot water bottle. Hands-on massage may be done on another part of the body at this time.
2. After 10 minutes, remove moist heat and apply an ice pack for 2 minutes.
3. Apply the moist heat again.
4. After 5 minutes, remove moist heat and apply an ice pack for 2 minutes.
5. Repeat steps 3 and 4 for a total of three rounds of hot followed by cold.
6. Begin massage.

SPASTIC PARALYSIS

Spastic paralysis is the term used to describe a condition in which the nerves controlling muscles are hyperirritable and their impulses cause persistent spasms and exaggerated tendon reflexes. In this condition, muscles are contracted so hard and for so long that the person literally cannot move. Spastic paralysis is the result of damage to the motor nerves of the central nervous system, such as can be caused by a stroke or spinal cord injury. Cerebral palsy, which a person can be born with which or can develop after a brain injury, can also cause spastic paralysis. Muscle relaxants such as baclofen are the standard treatment of choice for this condition.

Hydrotherapy and massage cannot cure spastic paralysis but can relieve some of its discomfort and pain. Ice water compresses can relieve spasticity for short periods, so that muscles can be exercised or stretched. Neutral baths can be tremendously relaxing as the person is surrounded by water and floats free of gravity. Massage gives the person not only skin stimulation and relaxation of normal muscles but a great amount of sensory stimulation.

TREATMENT
ICE WATER COMPRESS

Cross-Reference
See previous section on muscle spasticity.

Duration and Frequency
8 minutes. Perform during a massage session.

NEUTRAL BATH

Cross-Reference
See Chapter 7.

Duration and Frequency
1 hour

Special Instructions
1. The client should have a family member or other caregiver present during this treatment.
2. Massage may be performed in the bath itself, using soap lather instead of oil or lotion. Or massage may be performed once the client is transferred out of the tub and onto a bed or therapy table.

Procedure
1. Assist the client into the bathtub, then fill it with neutral-temperature water. Depending upon the client's degree of paralysis, he or she may need to wear a flotation vest or other flotation device. Some clients benefit from sitting in a bath chair placed in the tub.
2. The client remains in the bathtub for 1 hour. The bath water must be carefully monitored so that the client does not become chilled, and someone must be with him or her at all times.

TEMPOROMANDIBULAR JOINT DISORDER

Temporomandibular joint disorder (TMD) is a painful condition of the jaw which may accompanied by stiff neck, stuffy nose, ringing in the ears, and pain in the face, temples, and ears. The client may have pain in the jaw joint, difficulty opening the mouth, and headaches or ear pain. Causes of TMD include improper alignment of the teeth, injury, and arthritis in the temporomandibular joint. Emotional stress can cause a person to tense the muscles around the temporomandibular joint, and this is perhaps the most common cause of TMD. This condition is generally treated with physical therapy (gentle stretching of involved muscles); anti-inflammatory, muscle relaxant, or pain medications; and for advanced cases, dental appliances or prolotherapy injections.

Hydrotherapy can be helpful with TMD. Ice packs to the side of the face and temple can be used to relieve muscle spasms, and moist heat may be used before stretching the jaw muscles. A hot pack applied to the masseter muscle can cause a significant increase in local blood flow and oxygen saturation.(26) Contrast treatments can be used to increase circulation, ease pain, and decrease inflammation. Massage techniques that decrease muscle tension in the jaw and facial muscles or address malalignment of cranial bones may relieve pain as well.

Massage therapists should not treat facial pain until the client has been diagnosed by a physician or dentist and massage has been approved.

TREATMENT

ICE PACK TO SIDE OF FACE AND TEMPLES TO RELIEVE SPASM

Cross-Reference
See Chapters 6 and 7.

Duration and Frequency
15 minutes

Procedure
1. With the client in side-lying position and the affected side up, place a thin cloth on the client's skin over the side of the face and the temples, and then place the ice pack on top.
2. Remove the ice pack after 10 minutes. Gentle stretching may be performed at this time.
3. After stretching, apply a warm compress to the muscles for 5 minutes to prevent muscle soreness.

MOIST HEAT APPLICATION TO REDUCE JAW MUSCLE TENSION

Cross-Reference
See Chapter 5.

Duration and Frequency
20 minutes. Perform during a massage session. Or as a home treatment, when the TMD pain is particularly strong, the client may use moist heat as much as once an hour during the day.

Procedure
Apply moist heat (hot water compress, hot gel pack, or miniature fomentation) over the painful area for 20 minutes. Follow with stretching and/or massage.

CONTRAST TREATMENT TO THE JAW MUSCLES

Cross-Reference
See Chapters 5 and 6.

Duration and Frequency
15 minutes. Perform during a massage session or as a home treatment three or four times during the day.

Procedure
1. Apply moist heat (hot water compress, hot gel pack, baby hot water bottle, miniature fomentation) over the area for 5 minutes.
2. Remove the moist heat and apply an ice water compress for 1 minute.
3. Apply the moist heat again.
4. After 3 minutes, remove the moist heat and apply an ice water compress for 1 minute.
5. Repeat steps 3 and 4 for a total of three rounds of hot followed by cold.
6. Begin massage.

TERMINAL ILLNESS

The client who is terminally ill, no matter what the age, is experiencing a constellation of unpleasant experiences. These may include feelings of general malaise, nausea, fatigue, difficulty breathing, or pain; fear of death; an awareness of the extra stress on the client's caregivers; unpleasant procedures; and side effects from medications. Many terminally ill people receive a great deal of touch from caregivers as they are propped up, rolled over, bathed, diapered, fed, and have oxygen or intravenous lines adjusted. However, the undemanding, supportive touch of massage is contact purely for the sake of comfort; it can relieve nervous tension as well as physical aches and pains, and it may indeed be the nicest, most enjoyable touch of the terminally ill person's day.

Massage therapists working under physicians' direction at hospices are finding that some forms of hydrotherapy may also be particularly helpful in specific cases because they can soothe, comfort, and relieve pain. These treatments may also be prescribed to avoid more medications when a client is already taking a lot of them. Local salt glows, warm compresses, and warm hand baths or footbaths gently promote circulation and are nurturing and relaxing. Moist heat applications can help relieve many types of pain, from gas pain to bone metastasis pain. Neutral or warm baths ease the pull of gravity and soothe pain. Simple hydrotherapy treatments may also prove invaluable when massage has been prescribed but the patient has never had a massage. As a gentle introduction, a warm hand bath or footbath and local salt glow can soothe and relax the patient in an unthreatening way. Below are some examples of specific clients and how hydrotherapy was used to help them, drawn directly from the author's experience with patients:

- An 82-year-old woman was living in a nursing home because she required 24-hour care. She had diabetes, dementia, and chronic urinary tract infections, was incontinent and barely conscious, and lay in a fetal position much of the time. Massage was relaxing to her but challenging to give due to her fetal position. Every few days, nursing assistants at the nursing home transported her in a bath gurney, a chaise lounge–like contraption, down the corridor to the tub room. There, she was lowered into a 100°F tub and given a bath, which lasted about 20 minutes. Nursing assistants reported that she not only relaxed in the water but clearly enjoyed being there, and when taken back to her bed, she slept longer and more deeply than usual. This routine was continued until barely a week before her death, when she became too fragile to move out of bed.
- A 14-year-old boy had advanced metastatic cancer that caused severe pain, seizures, vision loss, and very high levels of stress. His pain was well controlled by medications, but as a side effect of one medication, his skin

was extremely sensitive to the touch. Massage with this teenager was a challenge because of his skin sensitivity, but warm footbaths and arm baths, followed by very light Swedish massage or energetic techniques, was an effective and deeply enjoyed answer to this problem. At times the therapist would spend much time simply pouring water gently over his hands and feet. Another feature of this boy's case was severe eyestrain caused by his vision loss, and warm compresses over the eyes followed by gentle pressure on the acupuncture points around them relaxed him greatly.

- A 70-year-old woman had a neurological disorder that caused spasticity in some muscles and weakness in other muscles. She found relief with massage techniques and warm moist compresses. A particular problem for this patient was too-high muscle tone in her sternocleidomastoid muscles accompanied by muscle weakness in her hyoid muscles. The tightness in her sternocleidomastoids made it more difficult for her weak hyoid muscles to propel food down into her esophagus and made it more likely that she would aspirate the food into her lungs. Specific trigger point treatment of her sternocleidomastoids helped temporarily reduce their tension, but another approach to the overly weak and overly tight muscles was suggested by an occupational therapist who was part of the hospice team. At mealtimes, warm moist compresses applied directly over the sternocleidomastoids reduced their tone, while ice was applied to the outside of the patient's cheeks and inside her mouth to stimulate tone in her swallowing muscles.
- An 87-year-old man had dementia, myoclonus (chronic muscle twitching), and failure to thrive. This frail gentleman was generally awake most of the night and slept during much of the day. Only two interventions would help him to sleep all night. One was a massage at bedtime, and the other was a 10-minute warm shower. Staff would have him sit on a shower bench and use a hand sprayer with 110°F water. As he sat, they would clean him with soap lather, wash him off with the warm water, dry him, and put him to bed, where he would sleep all night.

TREATMENT

LOCAL SALT GLOW AND WARM FOOTBATH

Cross-Reference
See Chapters 7 and 11.

Duration and Frequency
5 to 10 minutes. Perform during a massage session.

Procedure
1. Have the client sit in a chair, with a towel on the floor under his or her feet. If the client cannot sit up, this technique may be performed with him or

her lying in bed. In this case, put a towel under the feet and tell the client he or she will have to bend the knees to keep the feet in the warm water.

2. Place a dishpan or other container of warm water (98°–102°F) on top of the towel.
3. Place the client's feet in the footbath.
4. Take one foot out of the footbath, and using a small amount of Epsom salt, perform a salt glow on one foot. Either hold the client's foot over the footbath while you do this or lay the foot on the towel next to it.
5. Place the client's foot back in the warm footbath.
6. Repeat steps 4 and 5 with the client's other foot.
7. Holding the client's first foot above the footbath, pour clean water over it and then move the footbath slightly so the client may put his or her foot on the towel.
8. Repeat step 7 with the other foot. After pouring water over the second foot, move the footbath off the towel entirely so there is room for the second foot on the towel.
9. Dry the feet and cover them with the towel so they do not become chilled.
10. Massage of the feet and lower legs may be done at this point. The client may remain sitting in the chair or move to a therapy table.
11. Cover the feet with socks when the massage is over.

CHAPTER SUMMARY

In this chapter you have learned how to apply hydrotherapy techniques to a variety of specific conditions. Hydrotherapy can be applied in numerous ways to help the massage therapist meet the special needs of the client, whether he or she needs pain relief, easing of nervous tension, release of a muscle spasm, or stimulation of the skin and nervous system. The treatments detailed here will make massage more effective, feel good to your clients, leave them with an increased sense of well-being, and make your sessions far more versatile.

REVIEW QUESTIONS

Short Answer

1. Explain how hydrotherapy can relieve pain with either heat or cold.

2. Name three types of chronic pain and discuss their treatment with hydrotherapy.

3. Name three conditions that involve difficult movement and discuss their treatment with hydrotherapy.

4. Describe three options for a hydrotherapy treatment of a client with acute low back pain who has been referred by a physician 1 day after his pain began.

5. Name three conditions for which contrast baths may be used.

Fill in the Blank

6. Acutely cramping muscles can be treated with _____.

7. Three conditions for which contrast baths may be used are _____, _____, and _____.

8. Full hot baths can be useful for _____, _____, and _____, but not for patients with _____.

9. Muscle cramps are _____ and _____, while muscle spasms are _____ and _____.

10. Pool therapy is recommended for patients with _____, _____, and _____.

Matching

11.
___ 1. Continuous bath   **a.** Fibromyalgia
___ 2. Mustard plaster   **b.** Muscle weakness
___ 3. Moist heat   **c.** Parkinson's disease
___ 4. Ice water immersion   **d.** Rotator cuff tear

12.
___ 1. Contrast compress   **a.** Migraine headache
___ 2. Ice water immersion   **b.** Low back spasm
___ 3. Full hot bath   **c.** Eyestrain
___ 4. Hot footbath   **d.** Muscle spasticity

13.
___ 1. Moist heat to abdomen   **a.** Diabetes
___ 2. Baths less than 103°F   **b.** Terminal illness

____ **3.** Contrast treatment over the eyes

c. Chronic tension in abdominal muscles

____ **4.** Local salt glow and footbath

d. Eyestrain

14.

____ **1.** Diabetes

a. No core temperature over 99. 6°F

____ **2.** Multiple sclerosis

b. No ice pack to the abdomen

____ **3.** Constipation

c. No paraffin foot dip

____ **4.** Scar tissue

d. No ice massage

15.

____ **1.** Eczema

a. Oatmeal bath

____ **2.** Dry skin

b. Heat to abdomen and lower back

____ **3.** Osteoarthritis

c. Heat trapping compress

____ **4.** Menstrual cramps

d. Moisturizing wrap

REFERENCES

1. www. niams. nih. gov/mel. reports. Lappin, D. Arthritis— What We Know Today. Accessed January 2007.
2. Gloth FM 3rd. Pain management in older adults: prevention and treatment. *J Am Geriatr Soc* 2001;49:188.
3. D'Ambrosia RD. Epidemiology of osteoarthritis. *Orthopedics* 2005;28(2 Suppl):5201.
4. Kujala UM et al. Knee osteoarthritis in former runners, soccer players, weight lifters, and shooters. *Arthritis Rheum* 1995;38:539.
5. Roach KE et al. Biomechanical aspects of occupation and osteoarthritis of the hip: A case control study. *J Rheumatol* 1994;21:2334.
6. Brown TD et al. Posttraumatic osteoarthritis: A first estimate of incidence, prevalence, and burden of disease. *J Orthop Trauma* 2006;20:739.
7. Perlman A, Sabina A, et al. Massage therapy for osteoarthritis of the knee: A randomized controlled trial. *Arch Intern Med* 2006;166:2533.
8. Matvelkov GP, Marushchak YV. An evaluation of the effect of the sauna on the clinical, laboratory and psychological indices in rheumatoid arthritis. *Ter Arkh* 1993;65:48.
9. Wasserman P et al. Psychogenic basis for abdominal pain in children and adolescents. *J Am Acad Child Adolesc Psychiatry* 1988;27:179.
10. Hooper PL. Hot-tub therapy for type 2 diabetes mellitus. *N Engl J Med* 1999;341:924.
11. Rosenthal M. Psychosomatic study of infantile eczema. *Pediatrics* 1952;10:581.
12. Sung E, Tochihara Y. Effects of bathing and hot foot bath on sleep in winter. *J Physiol Anthropol Appl Human Sci* 2000;19:21.
13. Kanda K, Tochihara Y, Ohnaka T. Bathing before sleep in the young and in the elderly. *Eur J Appl Physiol Occup Physiol* 1999;80:71.
14. Liao WC. Effects of passive body heating on body temperature and sleep regulation in the elderly: A systematic review. *Int J Nurs Stud* 2002;39:803.
15. Karuchi K, Cajochen C, Werth E, Wirz-Justice A. Warm feet promote the rapid onset of sleep. *Nature* 1999;401:36.
16. Ebben MR, Spielman AJ. The effects of distal limb warming on sleep latency. *Int J Behav Med* 2006;13:221.
17. Raymann RJ, Swaab DF, Van Someren EJ. Cutaneous warming promotes sleep onset. *Am J Physiol Regul Integ Comp Physiol* 2005;288:R1589. Epub 2005 Jan 27.
18. Sherman K et al. The diagnosis and treatment of chronic back pain by acupuncturists, chiropractors, and massage therapists. *Clin J Pain* 2006;22:227.
19. Doub L. *Hydrotherapy.* Fresno, CA: Author, 1971, p 70.
20. Packman H. *Ice Therapy, Understanding its Application.* Flushing, NY: Author, 1987, p 16.
21. Sarno J. *Healing Back Pain: the Mind-Body Connection.* New York: Warner, 1991.
22. Travell J, Simons D. *Myofascial Pain and Dysfunction: The Triggerpoint Manual,* 2nd ed., vol 1. Baltimore: Williams & Wilkins, 1999, p 322.
23. Schneider M, Larkin M. *Handbook of Self-Healing.* New York: Arcana, 1994.
24. Chet J, Liang C, Shaw F. Facilitation of sensory and motor recovery by thermal intervention for the hemiplegic upper limb in acute stroke patients. *Stroke* 2005;36:2665.
25. Weinstein J. Herniated discs improve with either surgical or nonsurgical treatment. *JAMA* 2006;296:2441.
26. Okada K, Yamaguchi, T, Minowa, K, Inque, N. The influence of hot pack therapy on the blood flow in masseter muscles. *J Oral Rehabil* 2005;32:480.

RECOMMENDED RESOURCES

1. Boyle W, Saine A. *Lectures in Naturopathic Hydrotherapy,* Sandy, OR: Eclectic Medical, 1988.
2. Buchman D. *The Complete Book of Water Healing.* New York: Instant Improvement, 1994.
3. Finnerty G, Corbitt T. *Hydrotherapy.* New York: Frederick Ungar, 1960.
4. Michlovitz S. *Thermal Agents in Rehabilitation.* Philadelphia: FA Davis, 1996.
5. Moor FB, Peterson SC, Manwell EM, et al. *Manual of Hydrotherapy and Massage.* Hagerstown, MD: Review and Herald, 1964.
6. Packman H. *Ice Therapy, Understanding its Application.* Flushing, NY: Author, 1987.
7. Skole G, Greenberg S, Gaszi M. *Self-Care Anywhere.* East Canaan, CT: New Century, 2000.
8. Thomas C. *Simple Water Treatments for the Home.* Loma Linda, CA: Loma Linda University School of Health, 1977.
9. Thrash A, Thrash C. *Home Remedies: Hydrotherapy, Massage, Charcoal and Other Simple Treatments.* Seale, AL: Thrash, 1981.

SIMPLE HYDROTHERAPY RECORD AND SELF-TREATMENT HANDOUTS

The following pages contain handouts for your clients. A simple chart allows them to track their self-treatments and the results, and individual self-treatments are briefly described. Space is also left for you to give them special tips or directions.

1. Your Home Hydrotherapy Record
2. Warm Epsom Salt Bath
3. Neck-Limbering Exercises in a Hot Shower
4. Contrast Treatment with Handheld Sprayer
5. Ice Massage
6. Whole-Body Contrast Shower

YOUR HOME HYDROTHERAPY RECORD

Name of treatment: _____

How often: _____

Day of the Week	Time of Day Treatment Completed	Time of Day Treatment Completed	Time of Day Treatment Completed	How I Felt Afterward
Monday				
Tuesday				
Wednesday				
Thursday				
Friday				
Saturday				
Sunday				

WARM EPSOM SALT BATH

Your massage therapist may have recommended an Epsom salt bath for bruises, sprains in the subacute stage, soreness after exercise or after massage, nervous tension, arthritis pain, or as a general tonic. Do not take a warm bath if you have any of the following conditions: seizure disorder, loss of sensation (lack of feeling), multiple sclerosis, inability to tolerate heat, recent ingestion of alcohol or drugs, or obesity. Do not eat at least 1 hour before you take a bath.

You will need a water thermometer, a bath towel, a bath mat, and 1 cup Epsom salt for a child or 2 to 4 cups of Epsom salt for an adult.

PROCEDURE

1. Pour the Epsom salt directly under the spigot as soon as the tub begins filling with warm water, to make sure it dissolves completely.
2. Get carefully into the tub when it is half full. Use a grab bar if you have one.
3. Adjust the temperature to your tolerance as the bath finishes filling. Check with a thermometer to make sure it is 98° to 102°F.
4. Stay in for 15 to 20 minutes.
5. At the end of your bath, thoroughly wash off the Epsom salt residue.
6. Get out of the tub carefully so that you do not slip.
7. Apply a moisturizing lotion or oil to your skin and then dress.
8. Lie down and rest for 20 minutes or more.

SPECIAL TIPS OR INSTRUCTIONS

_____

_____

_____

_____

_____

NECK-LIMBERING EXERCISES IN A HOT SHOWER

Your massage therapist may have recommended a hot shower and neck-limbering exercises for tightness in the neck caused by chronically tight muscles, stress, injury, soreness after exercise, muscle spasms, or arthritis pain.

Do not stay in a long hot shower if you have any of the following conditions: cardiovascular problems, diabetes, hepatitis, lymphedema, multiple sclerosis, seizure disorder, hypothyroid condition, loss of sensation (lack of feeling), any condition that might make you unsteady on your feet, inability to tolerate heat, or recent ingestion of alcohol or drugs. If you do have any of these conditions, you may take a short hot shower of about 5 minutes.

You will need a water thermometer, bath towel, and bath mat.

PROCEDURE

1. Turn on your shower, let the water run until it is warm, and get carefully into the shower.
2. Adjust the temperature so that it is comfortably hot (about 105°–115°F).
3. Let the water beat upon your neck for at least 3 minutes. Then, very slowly and with no pain or straining, continue to stand with the hot water beating on the neck muscles while drawing the letters of the alphabet with your nose. This will gently release muscle tension and improve range of motion.
4. Stay in for about 10 minutes.
5. Get out of the shower carefully so that you do not slip.

SPECIAL TIPS OR INSTRUCTIONS

_____

_____

_____

_____

_____

CONTRAST TREATMENT WITH HANDHELD SPRAYER

Your massage therapist may have recommended a contrast shower over one part of the body with a handheld sprayer for soreness after exercise, muscle spasm, muscle fatigue, arthritis pain, tendonitis, poor local circulation, or joint swelling from a sprain or after the removal of a cast. Do not take a contrast shower if you are cold or if you have any of the following conditions: peripheral vascular disease such as diabetes, Buerger's disease, arteriosclerosis of the lower extremities, Raynaud's syndrome, or loss of sensation (lack of feeling).

Never spray water over implanted devices such as cardiac pacemakers, ports, defibrillators, or pumps.

You will need a handheld sprayer, a bath towel, and a bath mat.

PROCEDURE

1. Step carefully into the shower stall or bathtub. If you are going to spray the legs or feet, you may sit on the side of the bathtub.
2. Spray the area with water as hot as you can comfortably tolerate for 2 minutes.
3. Spray the area with water as cold as you can comfortably tolerate for 30 seconds.
4. Repeat steps 2 and 3 twice for a total of three rounds.
5. Get out of the shower carefully so that you do not slip.
6. Dry the area off and dress quickly to avoid chilling.

SPECIAL TIPS OR INSTRUCTIONS

_____

_____

_____

_____

_____

ICE MASSAGE

Your massage therapist may have recommended ice massage after a muscle strain, joint sprain, or bruise, or for acute muscle spasm, arthritis pain, stiff or spastic muscles, bursitis, or muscle weakness. Do not perform ice massage if you really dislike cold or if you have Raynaud's syndrome, Buerger's disease, a prior history of frostbite, peripheral vascular disease, a lack of feeling (impaired sensation), marked hypertension, arteriosclerosis, or diminished circulation.

Use a chunk of ice made by freezing a paper cup full of water. Perform ice massage for about 5 to 10 minutes, until the area is numb.

PROCEDURE

1. Drape towels around the area to be iced if necessary.
2. Hold the cup of ice in one hand and gently rub it in a circular motion over the area you are treating and a few inches above and below the area as well.
3. Continue until the area is numb, about 5 to 10 minutes. Generally you will first feel a sensation of cold; second, a burning or pricking feeling; third, an aching sensation; and fourth, numbness. These sensations are a good sign that the ice is doing its work. Take the ice away as soon as the area is truly numb.
4. Remove the ice, dry the skin, and cover it.
5. If your massage therapist has given you exercises to do, perform them now.

SPECIAL TIPS OR INSTRUCTIONS

_____

_____

_____

_____

_____

WHOLE-BODY CONTRAST SHOWER

Your massage therapist may have recommended a contrast shower to increase your general wellness, relieve postexercise soreness, or help you tolerate cold better. Do not take contrast showers if you really dislike cold; if you have Raynaud's syndrome, cardiovascular problems, diabetes, hepatitis, lymphedema, advanced kidney disease, multiple sclerosis, a seizure disorder, hyperthyroid condition, or lack of feeling (loss of sensation); if you are cold, very tired, or pregnant; or if you have just eaten a meal.

If you are not accustomed to very hot or cold temperatures, try a warm shower alternated with a cool shower at first to be sure you can tolerate them.

PROCEDURE

1. Carefully get into the shower.
2. Adjust the water so it is as hot as you can comfortably tolerate.
3. Stay under the water for 2 to 5 minutes.
4. Change the water temperature to as cold as you can comfortably tolerate for 30 seconds to 1 minute.
5. Change the water temperature back to hot for 2 minutes.
6. Change the water temperature to cold for 30 seconds to 1 minute.
7. Repeat steps 5 and 6.
8. Get out of the shower carefully so that you do not slip.
9. Towel off and dress quickly to avoid chilling.

SPECIAL TIPS OR INSTRUCTIONS

_____

_____

_____

_____

_____

POOL THERAPY

Pool therapy can be a great way for your clients to experience the therapeutic effects of water immersion. When a body is wholly or partially immersed in a fluid, it experiences an upthrust that is equal in force to the weight of the fluid it displaces. This buoyant thrust temporarily takes away the pull of gravity, so that there is a dramatic decrease in the weight-bearing forces on all joints and intervertebral discs. When water's buoyancy is combined with its soothing feel on the skin and a specific temperature, it can be therapeutic in a number of ways.

Many approaches to working in a swimming pool for therapeutic purposes have been developed: these include the Bad Ragaz ring method, Watsu, the Halliwick method, and Cardiaquatics. Many community swimming pools now offer specific classes for children with special needs, elderly people with arthritis, and other special populations.

The temperature of the water in the pool is an important consideration, as it affects the comfort of the client and the benefit of the exercise. Most community swimming pools are heated to 80° to 84°F, which is comfortably cool and ideal for movement, since the client will become warmer when exercising. Therapeutic pools are heated to 86° to 90°F and are ideal for arthritis, chronic musculoskeletal problems, and postsurgical problems.

Below are some examples of the therapeutic effects of immersion in a pool.

MUSCULOSKELETAL EFFECTS: INCREASED RANGE OF MOTION, INCREASED STRENGTH, AND DECREASED PAIN

Clients who have difficulty moving or who have musculoskeletal pain may benefit greatly from exercising in a pool. Exercising in the water gives them increased range of motion, increased muscle strength, and relief of pain. Those with the following conditions can benefit:

- Moderate to severe chronic spasticity
- Multiple sclerosis
- Parkinson's disease
- Muscular dystrophy
- Cerebral palsy
- Hemiplegia
- Traumatic brain injury
- Rheumatoid arthritis
- Osteoarthritis

- Poliomyelitis
- Peripheral nerve injuries
- Acute and chronic low back strain
- Muscle contractures
- Recent injuries such as those received in motor vehicle accidents
- Postoperative follow-up for muscle and tendon transplants
- Dislocated hip
- Joint replacement
- Bone graft

Massage therapist Meir Schneider, whose self-healing technique has been effective for many people with chronic musculoskeletal problems, incorporates gentle exercises in a warm bathtub or pool with massage.(1) For pregnant women, exercising in a swimming pool reduces weight bearing, thus making exercise easier and more effective. This allows for greater ease of movement and deeper stretching than on land, thus helping prepare the woman's abdominal muscles for birth and speeding postpartum recovery.

IMPROVED CARDIAC AND RESPIRATORY FUNCTION DUE TO AEROBIC EXERCISE

Even people without musculoskeletal problems can benefit from working out in a pool if they are elderly, frail, obese, or find it difficult to exercise on land for other reasons. For example, middle-aged and elderly patients with emphysema or bronchial asthma typically find it very challenging to exercise. However, when a group of them participated in an aerobic exercise program in 100°F water for 2 months, their respiratory function and arterial blood gases (levels of oxygen in the blood) increased. These improvements were attributed to an increase in respiratory muscle strength and airway clearance.(2)

IMPROVEMENT IN SOME MEDICAL CONDITIONS DUE TO THE COMPRESSIVE EFFECT OF HYDROSTATIC PRESSURE

Hydrostatic pressure increases as a person goes deeper in the water, so the farther under the water he or she is, the more difficult it is to move. A person of average height who is standing immersed in water up to the neck will be under pressure at 1.74 lb per square inch. Greater hydrostatic pressure is on the lower body than on the upper, causing fluid to be squeezed upward. On average, 700 mL of blood moves from the limbs to the thorax. This alerts the blood pressure receptors that pressure is too high, which stimulates the bladder. This is why you are likely to feel the need to urinate when you are swimming in a pool.

Hemodilution (shown by a fall in the hemoglobin, packed cell volume, and red blood cell count) also occurs during the first hour a person is immersed, indicating that extracellular fluid enters the bloodstream. This returns to normal when the person gets out of the water.

The shift in blood from the legs to the thorax produces an increase in cardiac output and stroke volume (due to improved diastolic filling), but no change in heart rate. (If one is floating supine, this does not apply; the mechanical effect of the water is not much different from when the person is lying on dry ground.)

All these effects of hydrostatic pressure mean that deep-water immersion can be an effective treatment for edema, including lymphedema, ascites resulting from cirrhosis of the liver, some cases of high blood pressure, and some types of lead poisoning.(3) Scuba divers who have chronic lymphedema have found that the hydrostatic effect of water has a similar effect to that of compression bandaging.(4) Pregnant women in water exercise programs have found that in addition to enhancing exercise, the hydrostatic effect upon the body reduces varicose veins and swelling in their arms and legs, improving overall body circulation and stabilizing blood pressure.

Pool therapy has also been used by some doctors as an alternative to prescription medication for **preeclampsia.** In this condition, the pregnant woman retains salt; hence, arterial blood pressure rises rapidly, and body fluids build up at the expense of blood volume. The health and even life of both mother and baby may be at risk. Various diuretic drugs can be used to combat this fluid retention, but their effects on the fetus are not well established, and so a drugless treatment may be preferred.

Bathing neck-deep in a pool for a few hours has been found to effectively shift fluids from the limbs into the central body cavity, markedly increasing urination and excretion of salt.(5) Another medical use of this hydrostatic effect is to cool a dangerously overheated marathon runner: immersion of the athlete in a tub of ice water that is deep enough to submerge the trunk and limbs allows the hydrostatic pressure to squeeze blood back into the thorax, which helps to maintain normal blood pressure.(6)

SOOTHING EFFECTS

The soothing effect of water not only makes it popular for recreational soaking, bathing, and swimming, but it can also be put to use for many therapeutic purposes. For example, a mother who gives birth in a warm whirlpool tub is likely to have an easier birth, as the water's soothing and relaxing effect may ease the pain of uterine contractions, shorten labor, and help the woman enjoy greater freedom of movement. As of 2004, 250 U.S. hospitals offered water births as an option.(7) Fussy newborns often quiet remarkably when they are given a warm bath. Watsu aquatic bodywork has many of the benefits of massage therapy, but when a person is cradled in the arms of the therapist while floating in water, it greatly enhances the relaxing and nurturing effect of the massage techniques.(8)

SENSORY STIMULATION

People with disabilities can benefit from pool therapy for yet another reason: sensory stimulation. Children with conditions such as autism or tactile defensiveness benefit not only from being in water but from learning to tolerate the sensations of water on the skin, of buoyancy, and of hydrostatic pressure.

Aquatic therapists who work with these children over time see an increase in confidence, as they not only learn new skills and move better in water than they have ever done on dry land but become far more comfortable with tactile stimulation (Pam Davidson, PT and aquatic therapist, personal communication with author, February, 2005).

REFERENCES

1. Schneider M, Larkin M. *Handbook of Self-Healing*. New York: Arcana, 1994.
2. Kurabayashi H et al. Effective physical therapy for chronic obstructive pulmonary disease: Pilot study of exercise in hot spring water. *Am J Phys Med Rahabil* 1997;76:204.
3. Root-Bernstein R, Root-Bernstein M. *Honey, Mud, Maggots and Other Medical Marvels: the Science Behind Folk Remedies and Old Wives' Tales*. Boston: Houghton Mifflin, 1997, p 50.
4. Chikley B. *Silent Waves: The Theory and Practice of Lymph Drainage Therapy*. Scottsdale, AZ: IHH, 2001, p 27.
5. Harper, B. *Gentle Birth Choices*. Rochester, VT: Healing Arts Press, 2005.
6. Roberts W. Tub cooling for exertional heatstroke. *Physician Sports Med* 1998;26:1.
7. www.aqua-eez.com. Water birth site. Accessed December 2005.
8. www.waba.edu. Site of the World Aquatic Bodywork Association. Accessed December 2005.

PYROTHERAPY: USING ARTIFICIAL FEVER TO TREAT DISEASE

Fever is a complex physiologic reaction to an infectious organism such as a virus or bacterium. One important characteristic of a fever is the increase in core temperature. As a result of the body shunting blood from the skin surface to the interior to conserve heat, reducing sweating, and inducing shivering, core temperature begins to rise. At the same time, cellular messengers called **pyrogens** reset the anterior hypothalamus to a new, higher body temperature. Now producing more heat than it is losing, the body heats up, which stimulates the release of more white blood cells into the bloodstream and makes them more active against infection.(1,2)

One research study found that after healthy subjects were immersed in a 103°F water bath, their macrophages were more active and better able to respond to bacteria.(3) Higher core temperatures also damage or kill many viruses and bacteria, including those that cause HIV, the common cold, herpes, gonorrhea, polio, and syphilis. The HIV virus can be significantly inactivated by prolonged core temperatures of 102°F; gonorrhea bacterium dies at 104°F; and cancer cells are selectively destroyed at temperatures between 106° and 110°F.(4,5)

How was the connection between elevated body temperature and recovery from infectious illness discovered? Probably either a person with an infectious illness was accidentally warmed to a high body temperature and got better, or a person with an immune system illness such as syphilis or cancer ran a fever due to a second illness, and when that illness was over, was much improved. Observant folk may have noticed that someone who took regular saunas had less colds than other people. (In 1990, the first systematic study of this phenomenon confirmed that this was true.)(6) Or observation of sick animals may have been responsible: Wholistic veterinarian Martin Goldstein once treated an 8-year-old boxer dog with leukemia and lymph cancer who ran an untreated fever of 102–107°F for a week and was completely cured, as confirmed by blood tests and clinical findings.(7)

As discussed in Chapter 1, cultures around the world have treated infectious illnesses with body heating using hot baths, steam baths, sweat lodges, and other heating hydrotherapy treatments. In many cultures, at the onset of a cold or influenza, the person is encouraged to take hot baths or other heating treatments or eat heating foods such as hot peppers. The ancient Greeks treated syphilis and tuberculosis with heating treatments. Before the advent of Western medicine, Native Americans used the sweat lodge to treat many infectious illnesses. In the days of the water cure, whole-body heating treatments were used extensively for infectious illnesses. Father Sebastian Kneipp used steam baths for influenza, and wet sheet packs were widely used for pneumonia during the 1918 influenza epidemic (see Table 1-1). At Battle Creek Sanitarium, full hot baths or sweat packs were used for influenza, laryngitis, acute bronchitis, scarlet fever, and many other infectious illnesses. In the early part of the twentieth century, mainstream medicine used artificial fevers to treat gonorrhea, rheumatic fever, syphilis, and other conditions. Fevers were induced by giving patients other diseases (such as injecting patients with the blood of people with malaria or giving them megadoses of typhoid vaccine), or by using electric lights or hot baths to raise the body temperature. Such treatments were mainstream medicine until the introduction of penicillin in 1943.

Since the early twentieth century, however, only a few wholistically oriented physicians, principally naturopaths and Seventh Day Adventist medical doctors, have continued to use whole-body heating to strengthen the immune system and inactivate viruses and cancer cells.(5,8,9) Seventh Day Adventist nurse and chiropractor Louella Doub used artificial fever for over 30 years to stop the progression of diseases such as multiple sclerosis and rheumatoid arthritis. Doub employed Russian steam baths to raise core temperature to 103°F and held it there for 30 minutes or more.(10) Fever treatments for cancer and other immune system problems have been performed at other Adventist facilities as well. At Uchee Pines Institute in Seale, Alabama, a typical regimen for cancer patients is to give them full-body hot baths (which raise patients' core temperatures to 102°–104°F for 20 minutes) five times weekly for 3 weeks, followed by 3 weeks with no hot baths. The patient stays on this regimen indefinitely (C. Thrash, personal communication with author, July 1998).

More recently there has been a resurgence of interest in using pyrotherapy to treat immune system dysfunction, along with basic research on how heat affects the immune system. Work is being done to investigate pyrotherapy's effect on diseases such as cancer, AIDS, hepatitis, rheumatoid arthritis, chronic fatigue syndrome, multiple sclerosis, and other immune system conditions.(11,12) Many heating techniques, from the traditional full-body hot bath to hot wax, saunas, warming blankets, infrared lamps, and whole-body ultrasound, are now being used to raise patients' temperatures. A newer technique is to use a machine that extracts small amounts of blood from the bloodstream and warms it to nearly 108°F before returning it to the body. Pyrotherapy (also called therapeutic hyperthermia) is better known in Europe than in the United States, and some European hyperthermia centers treat patients with cancer and immune system conditions. As discussed in Chapter 10, whole-body heating in combination with chemotherapy is being researched at the Center for Hyperthermia Cancer Treatment at the University of Texas Medical School in Houston.

Case reports of dramatic improvement after pyrotherapy in patients with a variety of illnesses are available. For example, at Uchee Pines Institute in 1991, a male patient severely affected with multiple sclerosis received a series of 12 artificial fever treatments using hot baths and experienced a dramatic reduction in symptoms and a significant improvement in his general health (Wynn Horsley, MD, personal communication with author, December 16, 2005). Two patients with chronic fatigue syndrome experienced dramatic improvement in their illnesses after taking daily 140°F saunas for a month.(12) Research is needed to follow up on these anecdotal reports.

REFERENCES

1. Conti, C et al. Antiviral effects of hyperthermic treatment in rhinovirus infection. *Antimicrob Agents Chemother* 1999; 43:822. This study found that when a flask containing human cells and **rhinovirus** cells was immersed in a 113°F hot water bath, the heat suppressed the multiplication of the virus by 90%, but did not kill the human cells.
2. Bellin B, Shavit Y, Azuovsky, J, Wolloch, Y, et al. Effects on mild perioperative hypothermia on cellular immune responses. *Anesthesiology* 1998 Nov; 89(5):1133-40.
3. Zellner M et. al. Human monocyte stimulation by experimental whole body hyperthermia. *Wein Klin Wochenehr* 2002;114:73.
4. Standish L. *AIDS and Complementary Medicine*. London: Churchill Livingstone, 2002.
5. Thrash A, Thrash C. *Home Remedies: Hydrotherapy, Charcoal, and Other Simple Treatments*. Seale, AL: Thrash, 1981, p 106.
6. Ernst E, Pecho E, Wirz P, Saradeth T. Regular sauna bathing and the incidence of common colds. *Ann Med* 1990;22:225.
7. Goldstein M. *The Nature of Animal Healing*. Ballantine/Random House, 2000, p 41.
8. Boyle W, Saine A. *Lectures in Naturopathic Hydrotherapy*. Sandy, OR: Eclectic Medical, 1988, pp 53–62.
9. Weil A. *Spontaneous Healing: How to Discover and Embrace Your Body's Natural Ability to Maintain and Heal Itself*. New York: Ballantine, 2000, p 204.
10. Doub L. *Hydrotherapy*. Fresno, CA: Author, 1971.
11. Alonso K, Pontiaggia P, Sabato A, et al. Systemic hyperthermia in the treatment of HIV-related disseminated Kaposi's sarcoma: Long-term follow-up of patients treated with low-flow extracorporeal perfusion hyperthermia. *Am J Clin Oncol* 1994;17:353.
12. Masuda A, Kihara T, Shinsato T, et al. The effects of repeated thermal therapy for two patients with chronic fatigue syndrome. *J Psychosom Res* 2005; 58:383.

RECOMMENDED RESOURCES

1. *International Clinical Hyperthermia Society*. www.hyperthermia-ichs.org.
2. *International Journal of Hyperthermia*.
3. *Society for Thermal Medicine*, www.thermaltherapy.org.

WHERE TO BUY HYDROTHERAPY EQUIPMENT

1. Steam canopies
   - www.steamywonder.com; 1-800-417-6789
   - www.sacredstonehealing.com
2. Steam cabinets, steam generators
   - www.steamembrace.com; 1-800-231-7832
   - www.saunasteam.com
3. Thermophores (moist heating pads)
   - www.thermophore.com; 1-877-633-9464
4. Fomenteks
   - www.fomentek.com; 1-800-562-4328. This company manufactures three sizes of flat plastic hot water bottles.
5. Fomentations
   - www.wildwoodlsc.org (Wildwood Hospital, Wildwood, Georgia); 1-800-844-1099
6. Local arm and leg baths and other European hydrotherapy supplies
   - www.h-e-a-t.com; 1-800- 473-HEAT
   - www.torfspa.com; 1-877-811-1008
7. Specialty showers and hydrotherapy tubs
   - www.h-e-a-t.com; 1-800- 473-HEAT
   - www.torfspa.com; 1-877-811-1008
   - www.touchamerica.com; 1-800-678-6824
8. Hot tubs or spas
   - www.spaspecialist.com; 1-888-478-2224
   - www.keidel.com; 1-800-346-6536
   - www.plumbingworld.com
   - www.bainultra.com; 1-800-463-2187
9. Saunas
   - Finnleo sauna and steam, 1-800-275-0888
   - www.steamembrace.com; 1-800-231-7832
   - www.saunasteam.com
   - www.saunawarehouse.com
10. Specialty salts
    - www.sfbsc.com (San Francisco Bath Salt Company); 1-800-480-4540
    - www.saltworks.us
11. Water purifiers
    - Ingram C. *The Drinking Water Book*. Berkeley, CA: Celestial Arts, 2006. This book gives detailed information on selecting a water purifier, testing water for pollutants, drinking bottled water versus tap water, and improving the quality of tap water without special equipment.

ANSWERS TO CHAPTER REVIEW QUESTIONS

CHAPTER 1

SHORT ANSWER

Student answers may vary. Key elements follow.

1. Possible answers include the following:
   - Achieve same therapeutic goals as massage
   - Relaxing and stress reducing
   - Help adjust client's body temperature
   - Provide a variety of skin sensations
   - Help the therapist move into a spa setting
   - Reduce stress on the massage therapist's hands
   - Make the massage therapist more versatile
   - Provide home self-treatments for clients
   - Adjunct to massage and bodywork for rehabilitation
   - Part of a health-promoting regimen
2. Possible answers include the following:
   - Spiritual power of deity is in water, heals ailment
   - Water helps balance humors in the body
   - Applications of hot and cold strengthen body
   - Water is a chemical compound with scientific effects
3. The bather would first go to the tepidarium, then to the calidarium, then finally take a cold dip in the frigidarium.

MULTIPLE CHOICE

4. B; 5. D; 6. B; 7. A

TRUE/FALSE

8. true; 9. true; 10. false; 11. true

MATCHING

12. 1, D; 2, C; 3, A; 4, B
13. 1, E; 2, D; 3, C; 4, B; 5, A
14. 1, B; 2, C; 3, D; 4, A
15. 1, E; 2, D; 3, A; 4, C; 5, B
16. 1, E; 2, D; 3, C; 4, Λ; 5, B

CHAPTER 2

SHORT ANSWER

Student answers may vary. Key elements follow.

1. Possible answers include the following:
   - Abundant and affordable
   - Weight and hydrostatic pressure
   - Versatile
   - Easy to use
   - Provides a variety of tactile sensations
   - Buoyancy
   - Mind-body effects
   - Ability to dissolve many substances
   - Absorbs and holds heat or cold
   - Conducts both heat and cold
2. Convection is the giving off of heat by moving currents of liquid or gas. Conduction is the transfer of heat by direct contact of one heated or cooled substance with another. Condensation is the process which changes water vapor (a gas) into water (a liquid). Evaporation, the reverse of condensation, is the process of changing water, a liquid, into water vapor, a gas. Radiation is the transfer of heat through space, without two objects touching, through the emission of heat.
3. Water stores energy by absorbing heat or cold.
4. Every one of our vital organs needs water to carry out basic chemical reactions, such as to maintain body temperature at 98.6°F, digest food, process nutrients, and eliminate wastes.

MULTIPLE CHOICE

5. C; 6. D; 7. C

TRUE/FALSE

8. true; 9. false; 10. true; 11. true; 12. false

MATCHING

13. 1, D; 2, A; 3, C; 4, B
14. 1, C; 2, D; 3, A; 4, B
15. 1, D; 2, C; 3, B; 4, A
16. 1, C; 2, D; 3, B; 4, A

CHAPTER 3

SHORT ANSWER

Student answers may vary. Key elements follow.

1. Heat, cold, heat-pain, cold-pain, light touch, deep pressure, vibration, proprioception
2. See Tables 3-1 and 3-3.
3. See Tables 3-2 and 3-4.

FILL IN THE BLANK

4. Dilation, reflex areas
5. Metabolic, glucose
6. Stimulation

MULTIPLE CHOICE

7. D; 8. C; 9. D; 10. C

MATCHING

11. 1, C; 2, D; 3, E; 4, A; 5, B
12. 1, C; 2, E; 3, A; 4, D; 5, B
13. 1, B; 2, D; 3, C; 4, A

CHAPTER 4

SHORT ANSWER

Student answers may vary. Key elements follow.

1. Possible answers include the following: body composition, genetics, season, physical condition, skin temperature, core temperature, part of body treated, treatment temperature, abruptness of temperature, duration of temperature, proportion of the body exposed, use of friction or pressure, body temperature after the treatment, aversion to heat or cold.
2. See Figure 4-7.
3. The derivative effect caused by dilation of skin blood vessels shifts blood flow away from the brain and internal organs.

4. The goals of treatment, such as stress relief, treatment of injury, or nurturing touch

MULTIPLE CHOICE

6. D; 7. D; 8. D; 9. C; 10. B

TRUE/FALSE

11. true; 12. false; 13. true; 14. true; 15. true

MATCHING

16. 1, F; 2, D; 3, E; 4, B; 5, A; 6, C
17. 1, E; 2, G; 3, D; 4, C; 5, B; 6, A; 7, F
18. 1, C; 2, E; 3, D; 4, B; 5, A
19. 1, C; 2, D; 3, E; 4, A; 5, B
20. 1, D; 2, E; 3, C; 4, B; 5, A

CHAPTER 5

SHORT ANSWER

Student answers may vary. Key elements follow.

1. Burns to the skin
2. Possible answers include the following: diabetic neuropathy, spinal cord injury, implanted device, inflammation, malignancy, rashes, swelling, broken skin.
3. Possible answers include the following: muscle spasm, poor local circulation, musculoskeletal pain, muscle tightness, warming of tissue to make it more pliable and stretchable, post-massage soreness after deep massage, menstrual cramps, active trigger points, derivation, nervous tension, chilled local area.
4. First type of heat is dry. Second type of heat is wet.
5. Local heat makes myofascial trigger points less painful to pressure while they are treated, then reduces muscle soreness afterward.

MULTIPLE CHOICE

6. E; 7. E; 8. C; 9. C; 10. D

TRUE/FALSE

11. false; 12. true; 13. true; 14. true; 15. false

CHAPTER 6

MULTIPLE CHOICE

1. B; 2. A; 3. E; 4. A; 5. D

TRUE/FALSE

6. true; 7. false; 8. true; 9. true; 10. false

CHAPTER 7

SHORT ANSWER

Student answers may vary. Key elements follow.

1. Possible answers include the following: paraffin bath, continuous bath, hot local bath, Epsom salt bath.
2. Possible answers include the following: hot half-bath, hot footbath, hot sitz bath.
3. Baking soda neutralizes toxins, Epsom salt draws water and toxins and provides magnesium and sulfate needed for detoxification, sea salts draw water and toxins, and the warm water promotes a moderate amount of sweating.
4. Possible answers include the following: hot footbath, neutral bath, powdered mustard bath, hot full bath, warm full bath.
5. Water completely surrounds an area so its hot and cold can be conducted to all surfaces.

FILL IN THE BLANK

6. Burns, pressure sores
7. Hot footbaths
8. Poor
9. Irritation
10. Perform active movements

CHAPTER 8

SHORT ANSWER

1. Room air is dry in a sauna and wet in a steam bath.
2. Core temperature rises in both, but with steam the core temperature rises faster, and muscles become more relaxed.
3. Blood pressure rises briefly at the beginning of a sauna, then falls, and remains lower for at least an hour afterwards.

4. Steam inhalation liquefies nasal mucus and moistens, warms, and soothes the respiratory tract.
5. The lungs may not be able to process the water introduced by the steam.

MULTIPLE CHOICE

6. C; 7. B; 8. B; 9. C; 10. B

CHAPTER 9

SHORT ANSWER

Student answers may vary. Key elements follow.

1. By adding a friction treatment such as a salt glow.
2. It should be set as high as client can tolerate to desensitize the area but not so high that it causes pain or discomfort.
3. A hot shower causes generalized skin vasodilation, a cold shower causes generalized skin vasoconstriction, and a contrast shower combines vasodilation and vasoconstriction, ultimately increasing blood flow to the peripheral blood vessels even more than a hot shower.
4. The hot chest shower increases local blood flow and relaxes the chest muscles.
5. When cold is applied to the arms and hands, it can cause prolonged vasospasm.

TRUE/FALSE

6. false; 7. true; 8. true; 9. true; 10. false

CHAPTER 10

MULTIPLE CHOICE

1. A; 2. B; 3. B; 4. B; 5. C

FILL IN THE BLANK

6. Stimulate, cancer cells
7. Moist blanket, wet sheet
8. Tonic, muscle or joint
9. Cooling
10. Sedative

CHAPTER 11

SHORT ANSWER

Student answers may vary. Key elements follow.

1. Cold mitten friction
2. People who could not tolerate the application of cold could tolerate a salt glow because it uses warmer water.
3. Friction stimulates pressure receptors in the skin and cold stimulates cold receptors in the skin.
4. Use water of different temperatures or chemical additives such as essential oils.
5. Because it stimulates blood flow to all the blood vessels on the skin surface.

MULTIPLE CHOICE

6. A; 7. D; 8. B; 9. B; 10. C

CHAPTER 12

MULTIPLE CHOICE

1. C; 2. D; 3. C; 4. D; 5. C

FILL IN THE BLANK

6. Gently, pain
7. Faster and more forcefully
8. Muscles, trained
9. Retained, illness, poor
10. Cold, cuts, wounds

CHAPTER 13

SHORT ANSWER

1. Rotator cuff tears, muscle strains, and subacute bursitis
2. Contrast
3. Peripheral blood vessels, deeper vessels
4. Ligaments, muscles
5. Muscle contraction

MULTIPLE CHOICE

6. C; 7. B; 8. B; 9. A; 10. B

CHAPTER 14

SHORT ANSWER

Student answers may vary. Key elements follow.

1. Heat relieves muscle spasm; cold slows nerve conduction which numbs tissue.
2. Review treatments for three of these conditions: arthritis, fibromyalgia, migraine headache, low back pain.
3. Review treatments for three of these conditions: arthritis, fibromyalgia, muscle weakness, muscle spasticity, multiple sclerosis, spastic paralysis.
4. Hot, moist application to the lower back, full hot bath followed by local moist heat application, or ice massage of the lower back
5. Arthritis, constipation, dysmenorrhea, eyestrain, migraine headache, sinus headache, muscle spasms, sciatica, TMD

FILL IN THE BLANK

6. Contrast compresses
7. Arthritis, constipation, dysmenorrhea, eyestrain, migraine headache, sinus headache, muscle spasms, sciatica, TMD
8. Arthritis, fibromyalgia, low back pain, nervous tension; not for multiple sclerosis or diabetes
9. Short-lived and strong, longer-lasting and not as strong
10. Three of the following: Parkinson's disease, spinal cord injury, multiple sclerosis, arthritis, fibromyalgia

MATCHING

11. 1, C; 2, D; 3, A; 4, B
12. 1, C; 2, D; 3, B; 4, A
13. 1, C; 2, A; 3, C; 4, B
14. 1, C; 2, A; 3, B; 4, D
15. 1, A; 2, D; 3, C; 4, A

GLOSSARY

Ablution The act of washing or cleansing. Early hydrotherapists used ablutions in the form of sponge baths or towel baths, mainly to bring down fevers.

Activated charcoal A substance made by heating or burning wood or other organic matter in the absence of air. Charcoal is used for its absorbent ability: it can absorb many times its weight in liquids or gases.

Acute Sudden in onset and not prolonged.

Adhesive capsulitis Extreme stiffness caused by adhesions between a bone and its joint capsule, often painful.

Adrenalin A hormone produced by the adrenal glands that increases the heart rate, among other effects.

Affusion The act of pouring water on the body or any of its parts for therapeutic purposes. Often refers to the hosing or pouring of water on a patient who is sitting or standing in an empty bathtub.

Aneurysm A weak spot in a blood vessel that can balloon out and then burst.

Aqueduct An artificial channel, usually raised on pillars or arches, that conveys water from one place to another.

Aquifer Underground rock, sand, clay, or gravel formation that stores significant amounts of water.

Arrhythmia Irregular heartbeat.

Arteriosclerosis Hardening of the arteries.

Arthritis Inflammation of joints, usually accompanied by joint pain. The two most common types are rheumatoid arthritis, an immune system disorder, and osteoarthritis, which is more directly related to overuse of joints.

Ascites An accumulation of serous fluid (serum, the fluid portion of the blood) in the peritoneal cavity, caused most often by cirrhosis of the liver or cancer.

Atrium The upper chamber of each side of the heart.

Autoclave A closed boiler that produces steam to kill fungus, bacteria, viruses, and other microorganisms. Used to sterilize surgical instruments, glassware, and other objects.

Banya Russian sauna, similar to a Scandinavian sauna; a heated room with water poured on the stove to make steam.

Baroreceptors Sensory nerve endings, found in the walls of the heart, vena cava, aortic arch, and carotid sinuses. These nerve endings are very sensitive to stretching of the vessel walls due to increased blood flow, and they are responsible for monitoring blood pressure. They report this information to the central nervous system.

Basal metabolic rate The energy required to perform all the functions that keep a resting body alive, such as keeping body temperature at its optimum (98.6°F), repairing injured tissues, digesting and assimilating food, providing energy for muscles to move, and removing waste products. This variable is sometimes expressed as the rate at which an animal consumes oxygen or produces heat.

Bladder stones Stones in the bladder, usually made of crystallized uric acid, caused by problems such as urinary tract infections or prostatic hypertrophy.

Buerger's disease (thromboangiitis obliterans) Inflammation of the entire wall and connective tissue surrounding medium-sized arteries and veins, especially of the legs of young and middle-aged men; associated with thrombotic occlusion and commonly resulting in gangrene.

Buoyancy The upthrust that is equal to the weight of the fluid displaced when a body is partially or wholly immersed in water.

Bursa Closed sac filled with synovial fluid, found over exposed or prominent body parts or where a tendon passes over a bone.

Bursitis Inflammation of a bursa.

Caldarium Steam room in a Roman bath.

Carpal tunnel syndrome Chronic entrapment of the median nerve at the wrist, accompanied by pain and numbness in the distribution of the nerve in the hand.

Cholera A bacterial infection that causes severe vomiting and diarrhea, often leading to death. The most common way cholera is transmitted from one person to another is through contaminated water.

Cholesterol A fatlike substance made by the body, with many important functions.

Chronic Lasting longer than 3 months and showing virtually no change.

Claudication From the Latin verb *claudico*, to limp. Ischemia of the calf muscles, causing lameness and pain when the patient tries to walk, because the blood supply to the calf muscles is insufficient for increased blood demand during exercise. Generally the pain caused by this ischemia stops as soon as the patient stops walking and starts again after the patient resumes walking, leading to the term *intermittent claudication*.

Cold mitten friction A whole-body friction performed with a terry cloth mitt or washcloth that is dipped in cold water.

Cold wet sheet wrap   A body wrap in which the client is wrapped in a cold wet sheet and two blankets. It is initially cold and gradually becomes warm and then hot.

Compress   A folded cloth dipped in water, with or without additives such as essential oils or mineral salts, which is applied to the body.

Concussion   An injury to a soft structure caused by a blow or violent shaking.

Condensation   The process by which a gas or vapor changes to a liquid.

Conduction   The transfer of heat by direct contact of one heated or cooled substance with another.

Constipation   Reduced or difficult bowel movements.

Constitutional hydrotherapy   A treatment consisting of a series of hot and cold towels applied first to the chest and abdomen and then to the back, combined with application of sine waves; constitutional hydrotherapy treatments are designed to strengthen the immune system, stimulate the circulation, improve the function of the digestive organs, and promote detoxification.

Continuous bath   A bath in which the patient is placed on a hammock suspended in a bathtub. The tub with the patient in it is covered with a canvas sheet that has a hole for the bather's head; then warm or neutral water is run continuously, often for extended periods.

Contracture   Myofascial shortening due to tonic spasm or paralysis of antagonist muscles, leading to fibrosis and a permanent loss of motion in related joints.

Contralateral reflex effect   The phenomenon of heat applied to one limb causing vasodilation in the other limb as well.

Contrast compress treatment   A treatment consisting of hot compresses alternated with cold ones.

Contrast treatment   A series of alternating hot and cold applications, with the hot application generally being longer than the cold.

Convection   The giving off of heat by moving currents of liquid or gas.

Coronary artery disease   A condition in which the coronary arteries are partially clogged, usually by deposits of cholesterol, cellular waste products, calcium, and fibrin on the artery's inner lining.

Coronary artery   An artery that supplies blood to the heart muscle itself.

Counterirritant   A substance that stimulates nerve endings on the skin and distracts the central nervous system from deeper-seated pain.

Depletion   Decrease in blood flow to one area, created by decreasing the size of local blood vessels.

Derivation   From the Latin words *derivo*, draw off, and *rivus*, stream; the decreased flow of blood and lymph to one particular part of the body caused by increasing the flow of blood and lymph to another part. When local blood flow is decreased, local blood pressure also falls; then excess tissue fluid will be drawn into the local blood vessels by osmosis, and this will relieve congestion.

Derivative   Refers to treatments that decrease flow of blood and lymph to one particular part of the body by increasing the flow of blood and lymph to another part.

Detoxification   Removal of toxic materials from the body.

Diabetes   A disease characterized by glucose intolerance, excess discharge of urine containing glucose, and disturbances in the metabolism of fat, protein, and carbohydrates.

Diastole   Rest period after each heartbeat, during which time the heart fills with blood.

Douche   A spray of water directed against some portion of the body. Douches may be of various temperatures, various directions (horizontal or vertical), and applied locally or to the whole body.

Dry brushing   A friction technique using a dry brush applied to the skin surface.

Dry sheet wrap   A body wrap consisting of two blankets and one sheet, with external warming devices placed on the client's wrapped body.

Dysmenorrhea   Significant pain before or during the menstrual period.

Embolism   The plugging of a blood vessel by an embolus that has broken loose and traveled through the bloodstream. The embolus cuts off the flow of blood to the part of the body supplied by the blood vessel.

Embolus   A blood clot formed inside a vein.

Emetic   An agent that causes vomiting.

Encephalitis   Inflammation of the brain, usually caused by a viral infection.

Endothelium   The inner lining of blood vessels.

Enema   A rectal injection for administering fluids, medication, or nutrients, or for clearing out the bowel. Enema ingredients may vary widely, depending upon the purpose of the enema.

Erythrocyte   Red blood cell, a disclike cell without a nucleus that contains hemoglobin, which carries oxygen from the lungs to body tissues.

Evaporation   The process of changing water, a liquid, into water vapor, a gas.

Eyestrain   A feeling of discomfort and pain in and around the eyes, without any eye disease or pathology.

Fibrin   A protein made up of long, sticky fibers.

Fibromyalgia   A musculoskeletal pain and fatigue disorder, with these symptoms: chronic pain in muscles and the soft tissue surrounding joints, tenderness to pressure at specific sites in the body, stiffness after rest, low pain tolerance, sensitivity to cold, nonrestful sleep, and chronic fatigue.

Fomentation   Any warm, moist application that delivers heat to the body for healing. This book refers to fomentations as the large pads made for moist heat applications that are made of many layers of thick laundry flannel or toweling.

Fracture   A break in a bone.

Frigidarium   Cold pool in a Roman bath, sometimes used to describe the room in which the cold pool was located.

Frostbite   A cold injury caused by the freezing of body tissues and occurring most often in the hands and feet. When a person's body temperature decreases due to cold exposure, constriction of the blood vessels of the arms and legs keeps warm blood in the body core and if necessary sacrifices the extremities to maintain the internal organs and brain.

Glomerulonephritis   Kidney disease caused by inflammation of the glomeruli.

Glucose   A sugar that is carried to the cells and serves as their main energy source.

Gout   A disease of the joints, primarily of the toes, ankles, and knees, triggered when sodium urate crystals collect in the fluid around the joints. This causes inflammation, irritability, and attacks of excruciating pain. Gout is primarily an inherited disorder, but small, regular doses of lead can induce it in susceptible people.

Heart attack   See myocardial infarction.

Heatstroke   A condition produced by exposure to excessively high temperatures, especially when the person is exercising vigorously. Symptoms include a rise in body temperature, hot dry skin, headache, confusion, and vertigo; in extreme cases, when the person's body temperature rises very high, there can be vascular collapse, coma, and death.

Hematoma   A localized mass of blood that has leaked out of broken blood vessels, usually clotted or partially clotted.

Hubbard tank   A very large whirlpool for therapeutic exercise, designed in 1928 by engineer Carl Hubbard for therapeutic exercise.

Hydropathy   The treatment of any disease by the internal and external application of water. Formerly known as the water cure.

Hydrostatic (derivative)   Causing blood to migrate either toward or away from an area of the body.

Hydrostatic pressure   The force that water exerts on a submerged body, which is equal on the entire surface.

Hydrotherapy   The therapeutic application of water for the treatment of musculoskeletal disorders and promotion of general wellness.

Hypothalamus   A small part of the brain in the lower front brain that is considered the central controller of the autonomic nervous system. It monitors many visceral functions, such as skin temperature, blood temperature, and the amount of water in the blood.

Ice massage   A method of cooling tissues by applying an ice cube or ice cup over an area with a rotating motion.

Ice stroking   Stroking the length of a muscle with ice to induce temporary release of muscle tension and suppress pain.

Iced compress   A wet towel that has been placed in a resealable plastic bag and then frozen; when removed from the freezer and placed on the client's body, it remains cold for as long as 20 minutes.

Intermittent claudication   See claudication.

Kidney stone   A small mass caused when certain natural chemicals such as uric acid crystallize in the kidney. Kidney stones may have a variety of causes.

Laconium   Hot dry room or sauna in a Roman bath.

Late-pregnancy toxemia   See preeclampsia.

Lateral epicondylitis   Inflammation of the wrist flexor tendons at their insertion on the lateral epicondyle of the humerus.

Lower leg compartment syndrome   Increased pressure inside the anterior compartment of the lower leg, leading to pain, compression of blood vessels and nerves, and possibly nerve damage. Usually caused by excessive muscle swelling or compression from a too-tight bandage or cast.

Lumen   The space in the interior of a tubular structure such as an artery, vein, or lymphatic vessel.

Lymph   From the Latin *lympha*, clear spring water. Lymphatic fluid is clear (a slight yellow tinge comes from the presence of a few red blood cells) and consists of white blood cells, mostly leukocytes, and a few red blood cells. It is carried in the lymphatics, the veinlike vessels of the lymphatic system.

Lymphedema   The accumulation of lymph in subcutaneous tissue resulting from the obstruction of certain lymphatic vessels or nodes. People with this condition have chronic swelling in at least one arm or leg. The most common cause of lymphedema is mastectomy surgery for breast cancer, when the surgeon removes not only the breast but also numerous surrounding lymph nodes. Less commonly, lymphedema can be caused by trauma, radiation therapy, mechanical constraint (such as a tightly fitting cast), and some types of tumors.

Macrophage   Phagocytic white blood cell, found throughout the body.

Mechanical treatments   Friction treatments, such as salt glows, and percussion treatments, such as sprays or jets of water.

Medial epicondylitis   Inflammation of the wrist flexor tendons at their insertion on the medical epicondyle of the humerus.

Migraine headache   A severely painful headache, usually limited to one side of the head and often accompanied by vertigo, nausea, hypersensitivity to light, a perception of flashing lights, or other visual disorders. Migraine headaches begin with an extreme vasoconstriction of the blood vessels of the brain on the affected side of the head.

Moist blanket wrap   A body wrap in which the client is wrapped in a cotton blanket wrung out in 110°F water and two additional blankets. External warming devices are applied on the outside of the wrap.

Multiple sclerosis   A progressive autoimmune disease that causes the body to attack the myelin in the brain and spinal cord, resulting in a variety of symptoms including fatigue, muscle weakness, spasticity, bladder abnormalities, visual loss, and mood alterations. Some people with multiple sclerosis have all these symptoms; others, just a few of them.

Muscle cramp   Strong, painful, short-lived involuntary contraction of skeletal muscle.

Muscle spasm   Low-grade, long-lasting involuntary contraction of skeletal muscle.

Myocardial infarction   An episode of diminished blood supply to the heart muscle; without oxygen, parts of the heart muscle begin to die.

Nerves   Bundles of individual neurons—single-cell fibers that transmit electrical impulses, each wrapped in its own fascial sheath together with its own tiny blood vessel—wrapped together with connective tissue. They carry sensory information or motor commands.

Nociceptors   Nerve receptors on the skin or in deeper structures that can carry pain signals to the brain.

PCB (polychlorinated biphenyl)   Industrial compound produced by chlorination of biphenyls, which when accumulated in tissue can have pathogenic effects, including abnormal prenatal development.

Percussion douche   A very strong spray of water, generally applied to either the entire front or the entire back of the body.

Peripheral neuropathy   A condition of damage to peripheral nerves, caused by poor circulation, chemical imbalance, or trauma. Symptoms may include burning, itching, numbness, and excessive sweating of the hands and feet. Burning or tingling pain will eventually be replaced by numbness. Most cases of peripheral neuropathy are caused by diabetes, when high blood sugar levels damage the capillary circulation in the hands and feet.

Pewter   An alloy (mixture of metals) composed mainly of tin and copper along with lead and other minerals.

Phlebitis   Inflammation of a vein.

Physiatrist   A physician specializing in rehabilitation.

Plantar fasciitis   An inflammation of the plantar fascia that causes pain on the underside of the foot, most often in the heels or arches.

Plaster   Pastelike mixture made of ground herbs mixed with water, spread upon a cloth and applied to the body.

Polio (poliomyelitis)   An acute infectious viral disease affecting the central nervous system. It can cause paralysis and muscle wasting. Compensatory movement patterns—overuse of some parts of the body to compensate for paralyzed or weak muscles—can cause severe musculoskeletal pain, discomfort, and deformity.

Precordium   Area on the anterior chest overlying the heart.

Preeclampsia   In a pregnant woman, hypertension occurring along with protein in the urine, edema, or both. This condition usually develops after the twentieth week of pregnancy and occurs in only 4% of pregnant women. Blood pressure often rises dangerously high. Preeclampsia is associated with retarded fetal growth and dramatically increases the risk of death for both the pregnant woman and her baby.

Prolotherapy   The injection of natural substances at the exact site of a ligament injury. It stimulates the person's immune system to repair damaged ligaments and can significantly increase ligament mass, thickness, and strength.

Pyrotherapy   The treatment of disease by inducing an artificial fever in the patient.

Radiation   Giving off heat, such as when a part of the body that is not insulated is exposed to very cold air.

Raynaud's syndrome   A condition involving spasm of the arterioles in the extremities. Episodes of vasospasm can be triggered by exposure to cold or emotional stress. Tissues, especially in the hands and feet, can be damaged from lack of oxygen.

Reflex   An involuntary reaction to a stimulus, generally a body action or movement that happens rapidly and automatically in response to possible danger.

Repetitive strain injury   An injury to muscles, tendons, or nerves caused by repeated, unvarying movement of a part of the body

Revulsive   From the Latin *revulsum*, plucked or pulled away. The drawing away of blood and lymph from one particular part of the body by increasing the flow of blood and lymph to another part.

Rheumatism   A poorly defined term that has been applied in the past to various chronic conditions of pain in the soft tissues and/or swelling of the joints.

Rheumatoid arthritis   An autoimmune disease that primarily affects connective tissue and causes inflammation of the synovial membranes, leading to pain and stiffness in many joints, especially those of the hands and feet.

Rhinovirus   The virus that causes the common cold. *Rhino* refers to the nose.

Russian steam bath   A steam bath given in a tiled room with a circular hole in one wall so that the client can lie on a bench inside the room while the head protrudes out of the hole. Sometimes applied to any head-out steam bath.

Salt glow   A friction treatment performed on the bare skin by rubbing it with moistened salt.

Sauna   A heated room used for sweating. Dry saunas can be changed into wet saunas by pouring water on the wood stove, electric heater, or sometimes on rocks atop the stove.

Scar tissue   Tissue made of collagen fibers, which replaces tissue that is damaged or killed by an injury or a disease.

Scotch hose or spray douche   A small high-pressure hose designed to blast areas of pain and tension with a strong stream of water. The spray is applied to the client from a distance of 6 feet or more.

Sebum   The secretion of the sebaceous (oil) glands of the dermis.

Shin splints   A catchall term for a variety of lower leg problems that are characterized by aching pain along the medial border of the tibia.

Shower   A stream or streams of water from a showerhead directed upon one or more parts of the body.

Silica gel hot pack   A pack made from canvas material, filled with a silica gel, and heated in water in a special metal container with electrical heating elements inside.

Sinus headache   A headache caused by sinus inflammation or congestion.

Sitz bath   A bath that immerses the pelvic region, covering about the same area of the body as a pair of shorts.

Solvent   A liquid that can dissolve a substance.

Spasm   A sudden, involuntary contraction of a muscle.

Specific heat   The amount of heat required to raise the temperature of 1 g of a substance by 1° Celsius.

Spinal cord injury   Damage to some or all of the fibers that make up the spinal cord resulting from the fibers being torn, bruised, or severed by mechanical force.

Sprain   A tear of a ligament, ranging from a slight tear of a few fibers to the entire ligament being torn away from the bone.

Spray   A stream of water from a showerhead that is applied to the client by the therapist.

Steam cabinet   A cabinet in which a person may sit and receive a steam bath, with a hole for the head and a port through which steam can enter.

Steam canopy   A body-length canopy made of sturdy water-resistant fabric placed over a supine client. The canopy is filled with steam made in a slow cooker at the foot of the massage table.

Steam room   An enclosed room with a port through which steam can enter.

Stress fracture   A bone fracture caused by a repeated stress, such as the repeated pounding of the leg bones by long-distance runners. Also known as a fatigue fracture.

Stroke   Death of brain cells caused by cut-off of blood supply to a part of the brain.

Subacute   Less than completely acute but not chronic.

Sweat lodge   Native American version of a steam bath. A low dome-shaped structure, constructed of willow branches covered by animal skins and heated by pouring water over hot rocks inside it to produce steam.

Swiss shower   A shower with multiple (9 to 12) showerheads at different levels and varying pressures that spray the whole body.

Tendonitis   Inflammation of a tendon.

Tepidarium   Warm dry room in a Roman bath.

Thalamus   A part of the brain that receives sensory information, sorts out the information, and then projects it to the sensory area of the cortex that is specific for that type of information. For example, information about touch is relayed to the brain's touch center, the somatosensory cortex.

Thalassotherapy   Bathing for health in sea water.

Thrombosis   Occlusion of a blood vessel by a thrombus, which is formed inside it.

Thrombus   A blood clot.

Toxin   Any substance that can cause illness or poor general health if absorbed by the body.

Turkish baths   Buildings that house hot rooms and hot pools, developed directly from Roman bath and bathing culture. They consist of a series of dry hot air baths, given in three separate rooms, each of which is hotter than the one before. The first room is at 130° to 140°F, the second room at 160° to 180°F, and the third room at 180° to 220°F. In Turkish baths, unlike in Roman baths, exercise is not connected to the bath experience at all, there is no cold pool, bathing is done in individual basins, and massage, which takes place in the main hot bathing hall, is done with soapsuds lather rather than with oil.

Typhoid   A severe bacterial infection spread by infected water, food, or fecal material. It causes malaise, headache, high fever, and often diarrhea. Patients can die of dehydration.

Urea   A water-soluble compound that is the main end product of nitrogen metabolism in animals, usually formed in the liver and excreted in the urine.

Vasoconstriction   Narrowing of a blood vessel through muscle contraction.

Vasodilation   Widening of a blood vessel through muscle contraction.

Venules   Minute veins that connect capillaries to larger systemic veins.

Vichy shower   A horizontal shower given with the person lying on a table. Water showers down from a swinging arm, which contains about seven jets and is positioned at a height of about 4 feet.

Water cycle (hydrologic cycle)   The life cycle of water. In this process, surface water evaporates from the sun's heat and becomes water vapor in the atmosphere. After condensation, it falls back to earth as rain or snow and begins the cycle again.

Watsu   A water massage therapy invented by massage therapist Harold Dull that is based upon traditional shiatsu techniques but is performed in a swimming pool filled with warm water.

Whiplash   An injury to the muscles, bones, ligaments, nerves, or other soft tissues of the head, neck, or spine caused by rapid hyperflexion and hyperextension of the unsupported neck, most often in a motor vehicle accident.

INDEX

Note: Page numbers followed by f, t, and b refer to figures, tables, and boxed material, respectively.